P9-CEC-608

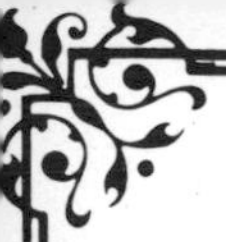
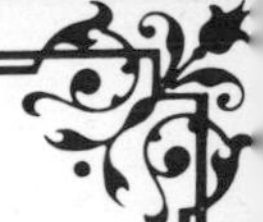

A VETERINARY GUIDE for ANIMAL OWNERS

Cattle • Goats • Sheep • Horses
Pigs • Poultry • Rabbits • Dogs • Cats

by C. E. Spaulding D.V.M.

Illustrations by D. Erick Ingraham

Rodale Press, Inc.
Emmaus, PA 18049

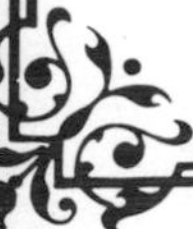
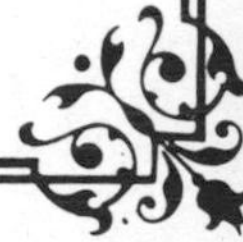

16 18 20 19 17 15 hardcover

Printed in the United States of America on recycled paper

Library of Congress Cataloging in Publication Data

Spaulding, C.E.
A veterinary guide for animal owners.

Includes index.
1. Veterinary medicine. I. Title.
SF745.S63 636.089 76-10641
ISBN 0-87857-118-3 hardcover

CONTENTS

INTRODUCTION

The back-to-the-land movement, which picked up momentum in the late sixties and early seventies, brought a lot of city discontents to the country for the first time. These people didn't come necessarily to become farmers, but only to slow down and really live a little, and to attain a degree of self-sufficiency. A garden certainly, but also a few chickens, a pig, maybe a small herd of goats or a family cow, a beef steer, and a horse have often become parts of this new life-style.

What these new animal owners find out soon enough is that when they acquire livestock they take on full responsibility for the animals under their care. Things can go wrong, and they often do, even for the best of us. Animals are going to get sick sometimes and have occasional trouble breeding, giving birth, and such.

Many of these people (and maybe you're one of them) have had little or no contact with farm animals before. Even if they have, there are so many old wives' tales and untruths about preventive measures and cures that it is often confusing and difficult to decide on the best methods of caring for livestock, in both sickness and health.

As a practicing veterinarian, veterinary columnist, and homesteader, I'm often asked by animal owners, "How do I know if my animals are sick, and if they are, what do I do?"

In *A Veterinary Guide for Animal Owners* I try to answer just such questions. I see my book as a bridge between animal owner and veterinarian, and animal owner and veterinary books (of which a comprehensive library weighs several hundred pounds and costs a few thousand dollars). With this for reference, plus some common sense and a little barnyard experience, I feel sure that new homesteaders and even seasoned animal owners will be better equipped to prevent many livestock problems, spot others early enough to control and rectify difficulties, and know what to do in a crisis situation.

CLIENT-VETERINARIAN RELATIONSHIP

If you have moved into an area where there are several veterinarians it is usually easier to find one that you believe in. Veterinarians, after all, are people, and like people in any profession, some are better at it than others. When trying to pick a veterinarian for your stock, try not to let personality or "bedside manner" (stallside manner?) affect your choice. A good veterinarian doesn't necessarily have to kiss your ass (donkey) or hug your goat to be able to do a good job doctoring them. On the other hand, you wouldn't trust someone who kicks your dog or swats your steer with a 2 by 4, vet or not.

It's a good idea to pick a veterinarian just as you do a family doctor: by results and attitude rather than by superfluous details. A $300,000 clinic can house a poor veterinarian. Those impressive stainless steel operating lights, table, X-ray units, and scary-looking instruments are no good if they are used more to impress clients than to help sick animals. On the other hand, you can't have much luck with a veterinarian who uses only a stethoscope and a bottle of Combiotic.

Look for a veterinarian who seems interested in your problems and will, when you ask, explain the trouble and explain what he's doing. Remember that many veterinarians will not explain things without being asked, for the simple reason that a lot of people won't bother to listen. More than a few times I've been trying to explain what I was doing, only to have the client butt in with how little rain he's had on his corn, etc. I've actually stopped talking midsentence and the client never noticed. So you can't always really blame a vet for working in silence.

Watch out for a veterinarian that tries too hard to be superprofessional. His every word sounds like a tape-recorded medical dictionary; his clinic and office help are an exact copy of an M.D.'s setup; everything is perfect. Fine—he may well be a supervet, but his fees may be super too.

Better this type, though, than a veterinarian who is a slob. Dirty needles, crusty syringes, and filthy instruments are used by very, very few veterinarians, but occasionally you may be unfortunate enough to find one. Don't make the mistake of judging a veterinarian by the inside of his car or truck, however. Eighty percent of the busy large animal practitioners' cars look pretty cruddy at times, mine included. Rough, dusty roads, rutty fields and driveways can somehow shake loose those neatly packed bags and boxes, dump drawers upside down, and spill used throwaway syringes, empty vials, bags, or boxes all over the place. An hour's ride can dust-cover the outside of bags that were previously shining.

In brief, you should look for an interested, honest, up-to-date veterinarian that works on your animal as if it were his own. By honest I mean a person who, if he doesn't know the answer, will say so and try to find out and not snow you with medical jargon. As veterinarians, we are called to treat such a wide variety of animals that it is impossible to be totally informed on all species. One day it may be cattle and sheep, another day a canary, deer, and boa constrictor; and still another day, a goat, monkey, and turtle. *No* veterinarian knows *all* animals equally well. He may be an authority on sheep and cattle but be in the dark on horses. But he can brush up if he knows he is going to have a client with horses.

Okay, we'll say you've found a veterinarian you can trust. Now when you have a problem with one of your animals and you make arrangements for the vet to come out, have the animal in the barn or tied up, and be there yourself. It is frustrating for a veterinarian, late on rounds, to have to wait while a cow is herded in from a 200-acre pasture by a neighbor who does not know anything about the signs of illness the animal has shown.

Next, let your veterinarian diagnose, choose the method of restraint, and treat the animal. This is why you called him. Offer help, such as describing symptoms and temperature or giving help in restraint. Ask any questions you have and *listen* to the answers. Most veterinarians are overjoyed to go to a place where the owners are truly interested in learning and will do as they are told to the letter. After all, good nursing sometimes is as important as drugs or surgery. It's always a pleasure for me to go through a rough operation or serious illness with an animal and return the next day, seeing everything just the way I have told the owners to have it, and seeing the animal munching on its feed, on its way to a good recovery.

It's always a good idea to have your veterinarian refer you to another veterinarian you can call in case he is out of town or ill. This eases the panic you feel when your pet goat is down with milk fever—you dial Dr. Smith, and his secretary says he'll be back next Tuesday. Okay, you say, fine, but I live in the boonies and the nearest veterinarian is 60 miles away. In this case, it is best to take a drive and visit that veterinarian. Explain your problem and ask if you may call for over-the-phone advice. It is not as good as having a veterinarian out, but it may save an animal you might have lost without help. In cases where surgery is needed, you can haul goats, sheep, pigs, or calves, to him. Many vets in farming areas have facilities for cattle and horses, so with the aid of a borrowed or rented trailer most animals can be hauled to the veterinarian if necessary. (A hint: when calling long distance, call person-to-person, as most large animal practitioners are in and out all day, and you may save a couple of dollars by doing this.)

THE IMPORTANCE OF PREVENTIVE MEDICINE

The importance of preventive medicine cannot be strongly enough stressed. If more people practiced preventive medicine, there would be a lot less work for me (and other vets), and a lot more healthy animals and happy owners.

Every animal should be checked daily. Danger signs, such as lack of appetite, listlessness, unthriftiness, weight loss, diarrhea, constipation, or noises of pain (grunting, whining, etc.) should bring prompt thorough examination *at once.* Tomorrow may be too late.

The most important "drug" you can give your animals is good husbandry. This means having a warm, dry, well-ventilated, draft-free shelter in the winter; cool, shady, rain-proof shelter in the summer; and room for exercise in the sunshine. It also means having different-sized animals separated to prevent injuries and giving all of them the correct amount of the right food.

A good health program is essential, too. Routine fecal examinations by your veterinarian, and worming if necessary, will increase your profits as well as the health of your animals. Even with a house dog, you will save money if your dollar buys dog food, not food to support worms.

Talk to your veterinarian to find out what routine vaccinations are a good idea in your area. Don't be afraid he will try to sell you a bunch of expensive, unnecessary vaccinations. He doesn't want to treat a hopeless animal that could have been saved with a 30-cent vaccination, any more than you'd want to have it.

Have your animals tested for any diseases prevalent in your area. Cattle and goats should receive a yearly TB and brucellosis test. Swine and dogs should be tested for brucellosis and leptospirosis, horses for infectious equine anemia, and so on. Any new animals, especially, should be tested before they are added to your herd or flock.

Any sick or new animals (even your own animals that have been to shows) should be isolated from the others. This simple precaution will not only ease your mind, but may prevent spread of a disease like shipping fever.

Remember to check things like teeth, ears, eyes, and feet. Cleaning or floating teeth can prevent a lot of dental problems later. Cleaning dirt and wax from the ear canals can prevent ear mites or a bacterial or fungal infection from getting a start. Any white spots in the eye, discharges, or foreign bodies spotted right away may save the sight of that eye. And it is a lot easier to trim a toenail or hoof regularly than to try to teach that animal to walk again after it has been crippled badly by a toenail or hoof that grew too long.

CATTLE

General Care and Management

HOUSING

Cattle are more likely to become sick due to too much shelter, rather than too little. Therefore, I recommend open housing where it is possible. This consists of a barn or loafing shed, with an opening to the south (unless the prevailing winds come from this direction) where the cows can wander in and out at will. Even in the North, the south side of the barn stays warm in the sunlight and the cows love to lie out in the sun and chew their cuds.

Inside the shed, it is best to have individual bedded stalls. (This is for dairy cows. Beef cattle do not need the stalls, as they don't have to be kept quite as clean as do the dairy animals.) This only leaves the aisle to clean manure from and really saves labor and bedding, while at the same time keeping the cows clean. Cattle have the nasty habit of plastering each other with manure when walking over each other. These stalls should be raised six inches from the aisle by placing a 2 x 6 across the back of the stalls and filling with sawdust and/or sand. This will also save cleanup time.

Sizes of stalls differ greatly with the breed of cattle you are housing. For instance, a 600-pound jersey needs a far shorter stall than a 1400-pound holstein. The stalls should be just long enough for your cattle to lie in comfortably, with the platform dropping off just behind the tail. Remember, the cows are free to come and go as they need. A hay rack outside encourages them to exercise, as does a salt and mineral lick. After all, the exercise is one of the most important reasons for having loose housing. Open housing works as well for a person who has only one cow as for a person who has a hundred.

There are a couple of things you have to watch with open housing in the North in the winter months. Make sure each cow's teats and bag are dry after milking before you turn her back out. This will help prevent cracked and chapped teats. Also, try not to have your cows freshen during the coldest part of the winter, as the full, tight bag, along with the cold, can cause frozen teats.

Cattle that have to be confined are better off in comfort stalls rather than stanchions. With comfort stalls, the cows are kept on chains, thus giving them more freedom of movement. This is nice for the cows, but not for the veterinarian! Be sure to have at least one sturdy stanchion or a chute as a place to treat the animals. A chute should not be over 28 inches wide, and some stockmen prefer 26 inches. This measurement holds true for all breeds of cattle, even large beef animals. If it is built any wider, they *can* turn around, exploding chute planks in all directions.

The temperature in the barn should not get much above 50°F. in the winter. When it gets too warm, the humidity goes up due to urine, body moisture, breath, and manure, and the animals are much more prone to pneumonia than they would be in a subzero dry barn. True, it's nice and comfy to work in a toasty barn. But I'm trying to save you vet bills. If necessary, invest in one or more ventilating fans to keep fresh air circulating through the barn.

When cattle are on cement platforms with gutters behind, check to make sure the manure is going in the gutter and that all of the cow is lying on the platform. If your barn was built for jerseys and you have holsteins, the platforms will be too short

Parts of a Cow

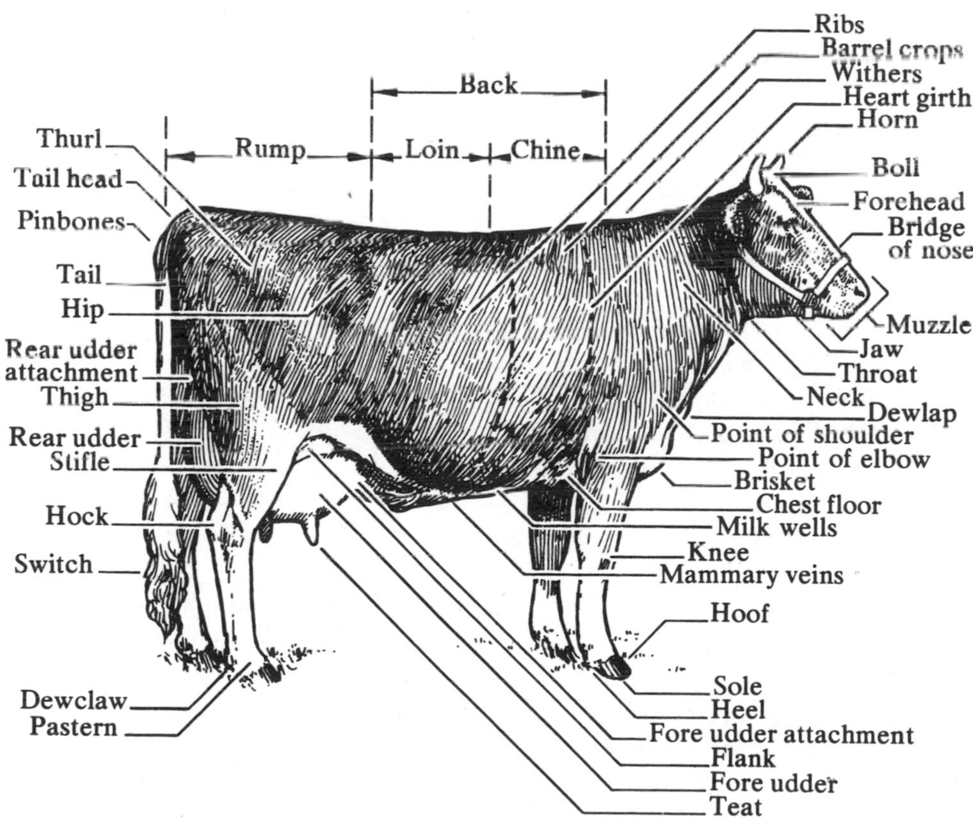

and your cows will have to lie in the gutter, which causes swollen hock joints. If the barn was built for holsteins and you have jerseys, the platforms will be too long and you will have a bunch of dirty cows.

Be sure to place plenty of bedding under the cows when they have to be confined in the stalls for some time, otherwise you may end up with arthritic, lame cows. There is no use in trying to save money by skimping on the bedding and shortening the useful productive life of your cows.

Calves should be kept separate from each other until past weaning age. This prevents them sucking on each other's ears and udders. There is no use keeping a nice heifer calf and having her freshen with only three quarters, or freshen with mastitis because her stall mate sucked her udder. Another reason for keeping calves separated is to reduce disease problems. Calves from birth to three weeks of age are prone to scours, and after that age, to pneumonia. If they are kept separate, they will not be so apt to pass bacteria back and forth.

Keep your chickens away from your cattle. Aside from the little leavings the chickens present you with in the manger, they can bring more ominous trouble. Birds can carry avian T.B. This type of T.B. isn't transmittable to humans, but when your cattle are tested for T.B. they may have picked up avian T.B. through the chickens and will react to the test. Until the animal is slaughtered, there is no way to differentiate avian T.B. from bovine T.B.

When I was testing for the state of Michigan, I found a herd of cattle that had several reactors to the T.B. test. They were shipped for slaughter, at some monetary loss and worry to the owner, and found to have "no visible lesions." I found out later that the farmer who owned this herd had a habit of throwing his dead chickens out on the manure pile, where the cattle had access. Evidently the cows picked up avian T.B. This is one of those lessons that is better learned from someone else's mistake.

FEEDING

As for feeds, during the summer dairy cattle should have access to all the lush pasture grass they can consume. A word of caution here, though. Don't just turn cattle that have been wintered on dry feeds onto lush green pastures, or you may have a bunch of bloated cattle. Feed hay as usual in the morning, water, then turn them out. Plan to spend that day home. Let the cattle graze for an hour or so, then drive them back to the barn. This may be easier said than done, though. A small fenced off area and several people help some, but cattle don't like to leave such goodies to go back to the barn. After a week of extending their stay in the pasture by an hour each day, it is usually safe to let them go. Here again, it is a lot of bother, and some neighbors will probably tell you just to let them go the first day, but I've treated several herds bloated by too much grass. (What do you do with twelve cows down and bloated, twenty more like balloons with legs, one farmer to help, and only two stomach tubes and a trochar?)

In the winter, a good, clean (no dust or mold) legume hay is best for cattle. This can be fed free choice. As for grains and grain rations for cattle, I'm going to pass the buck to your county extension agent (usually located at your county seat) for the reason that there's a wide geographic variation in grains available, protein supplements, etc. Call for an appointment. He can give you several pamphlets describing feeds for your area and help you decide what will be best and most economical for you to use.

One thing to be extremely careful of in formulating a ration is the use of urea as a protein supplement. Personally, I would not use it at all, but if you do, be very careful. Sometimes an elevator operator makes a mistake and dumps too much urea in a mix: result, dead cows. Or someone may use urea in the silage, and then unknowingly buys dairy mix with urea in it also. Then there's the person (feed store or farmer) who thinks that if he adds more urea to the mix the cows will surely milk better. Urea can cause a variety of problems such as sterility, muscle incoordination, or diarrhea, when fed at a slightly toxic level. Uremic poisoning is tough to treat successfully.

Be sure to have trace minerals and iodized salt available at all times for your cattle. There are areas throughout the country that are deficient in certain minerals, and it's a lot easier and cheaper to prevent a mineral deficiency than to treat it. A vitamin A and D supplement in the winter is a good idea, because of the instability of the vitamin A in the hay in the winter, and the lack of vitamin D during the less sunny winter months.

Feeds And Feeding by Morrison is a must to read, for it is the stockman's bible of feeding. This book covers practically every feed available in the world and lets you know just *what* you are feeding. It covers feeds for all livestock and poultry, and it is available at most libraries.

RESTRAINT

Here we get into perhaps the most important part of cattle raising. For without knowing and understanding the effective methods of restraining a bovine, you can become a bruised and bloody pulp trying to do some simple thing like pulling a sliver out of Bessie's hide. There are two ends to every cow. The butting, trample-you-in-the-manure end, and the kick, smash-you-into-the-wall and swat-your-face-with-the-tail end. First we'll restrain the front part.

A beef animal is most easily restrained by driving it into a funnel-shaped pen which leads to a narrow (26 to 28 inches) hardwood chute. Cattle can smash pine 2 x 4s like matches if they get upset enough. Have your hardwood planks, preferably bolted, on the inside of the posts, which should be set three feet into the ground. A few poles slid in close behind—and a sturdy stanchion to catch the head in—wrap it up nicely. In this chute you can snare legs to treat foot rot, dehorn, deliver a calf, vaccinate, sew up wounds, etc., in safety. (Well, almost. I've been knocked down by a kick through a six-inch opening in the planks.)

To restrain a dairy cow, drive her into a stanchion. Get a strong, moderate length rope, or better yet, a nose lead. This is a handy, inexpensive tool that is worth investing in, whether you have one cow or fifty. The blunt, rounded ends are

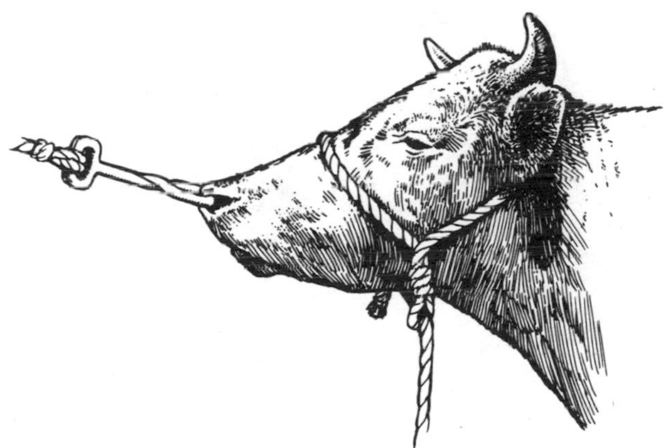

A nose clamp is applied to nose for restraint of cattle.

clamped in a cow's nose. Her head is then pulled as far through the stanchion as possible and to one side, and tied there. Make sure she isn't fooling you and is *tight* against the stanchion with her shoulders, or she can still jump around a lot. If you don't have a nose lead (also called bull lead or nose clamp in different locales), make a halter and pull her head around as with the nose lead. Tie the rope with a knot that can be jerked loose in an emergency. This goes when tying any animal, anywhere!

Don't wear gloves when working with ropes and livestock—especially thick, fuzzy gloves which can get tangled in ropes. Many fingers have been lost that way. Also, don't get between the rope and the post when tying an animal. It's a good way to get killed.

To restrain a cow's hindquarters, the most readily available method is to grab her tail close to the base (yes, I know it's usually slimy with green stuff) and raise it straight up above

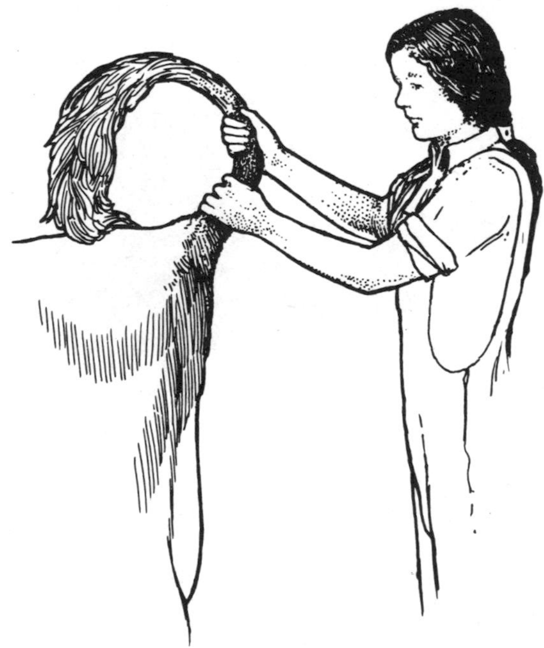

Restraint of cow to prevent it from kicking during medication, exam, or treatment. Grasp base of tail and raise firmly over the back of the cow.

her back. Really push. This nearly eliminates getting kicked, as it puts pressure on the nerves, making it hard for her to quickly raise her feet. When working with a sore teat, sometimes it is necessary to place a figure 8 around the hocks with a light rope. Don't tie this rope, but have an assistant keep tension on the rope to prevent the cow from stepping around.

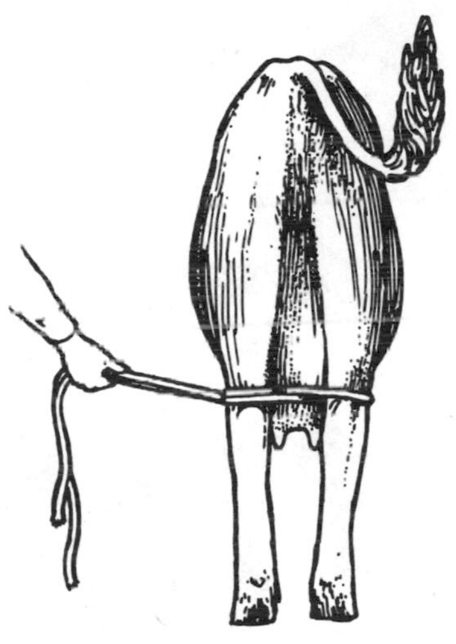

Figure 8 around hocks, the rope is held just tight enough to prevent kicking or stepping around. Do not tie the rope, as the cow may fall on you.

Restraining to Give Medication To restrain a calf to give it a pill, or to drench it, the easiest "one person method" is to straddle the calf's neck facing the same way as the calf, grasp the mouth, raise the head, and dose. To give a pill or bolus (pronounced "bowl-us"), coat it lightly with shortening. This makes it slide down easier. Did you ever try to swallow an aspirin without water? Invest in a balling gun. This only costs a couple of dollars and saves your hands from getting all skinned up on those sharp teeth, and also makes dosing easier. Shove the balling gun way in, past the hump in the tongue. Then pop the pill down junior.

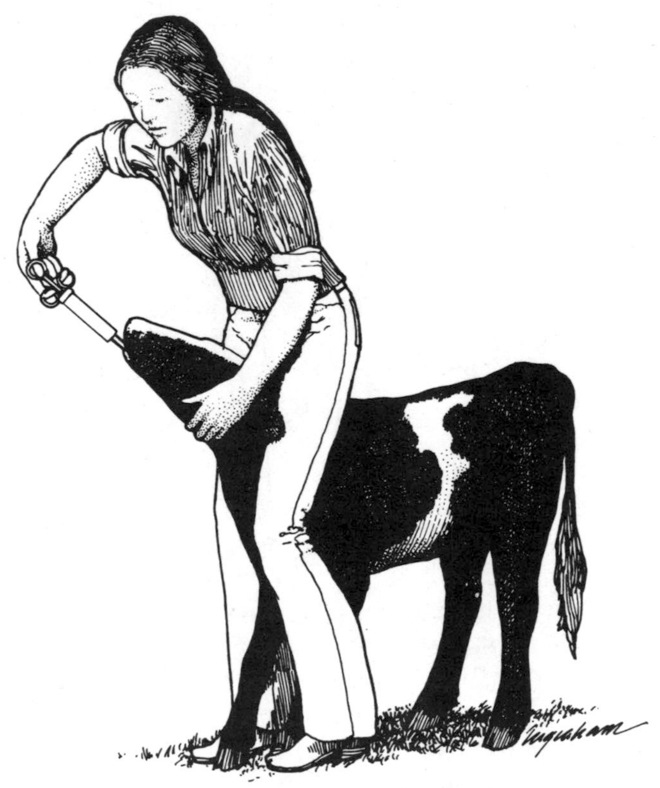

To give a liquid, use one of those plastic squeeze-type soap bottles that shampoo or dishwashing soap comes in. There is no danger of broken glass, and you can better gauge the size of the stream you are putting into the calf. You don't want to give it so fast that you choke the animal.

A larger calf can be held by tying the head and pushing a knee under the flank, forcing the calf up against a wall. With a large, active calf, it is best to have two people work with it, one to restrain and one to dose.

When trying to restrain a bovine, don't let your temper show. Screaming and hollering doesn't help. It only riles up the animal, making it even more wild or stubborn. And there's only one thing more stubborn than a stubborn cow, and that's two of them. Take your time; go slow and do a little at a time. You'll avoid high blood pressure. Sometimes a little grain at the right time will help, or driving several cows in to get one stubborn one. Remember that cows are herd animals. It's awfully hard to only bring one cow in out of a herd.

If you're going to have the veterinarian or inseminator out for an animal, leave it in the barn in the morning. You probably won't be able to get it back in the middle of the afternoon. Cattle are creatures of habit. If they're used to coming in at six to be fed and milked, no amount of persuasion will make those cattle think that they should go in at 2:30.

BREEDING

When A heifer should not be bred before she reaches 18 months of age or nearly all of her mature size, in order to make the best cow. If she is bred earlier than this, she may have trouble calving or may never reach the potential she would have if not bred too early. For the first calf it is wise to breed her to either a bull of her own breed known for small-sized calves at birth, or a breed known for small calves. These breeds are jersey, Angus, Hereford, and shorthorn. Jersey and Angus calves are the smallest, but if you are after a calf to sell, choose Angus, as Angus calves bring higher beef prices. Don't breed a small cow or a first calf heifer to a Charolais or holstein unless that's what the heifer is, or to any other breed known for large birth-weight calves. To do this is asking for trouble. Most of the really hard deliveries that I have to assist with are such cases. This is not to say that a jersey heifer cannot have a Charolais calf, but chances for trouble are greatly increased.

A heifer can begin coming into heat while she is still sucking on her mother, or as young as five months. Therefore, it is best if you do not run the bull with a bunch of young heifers even if they seem too young to be bred. I have delivered calves from 15-month heifers, and it is usually a rough job.

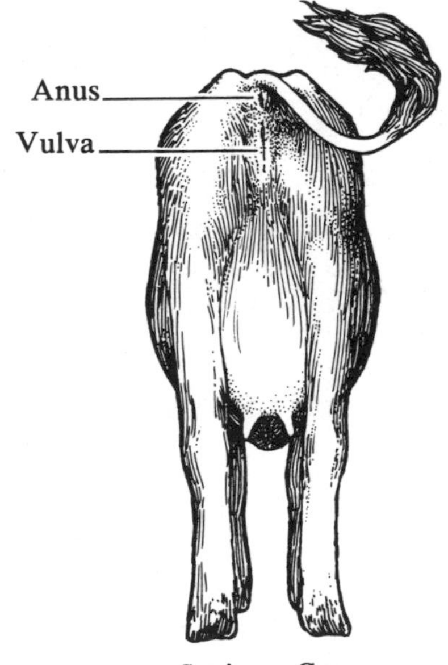

Sexing a Cow

The Bull When a heifer is of the age and size to breed, there are two alternatives. One is to turn her in with a bull. This is the general practice with beef animals. If you only have one or two head to breed, keeping your own bull is not practical. He costs too much to buy and feed for the use you will get out of him. There is quite a bit of risk involved with one, especially if you have a dairy bull. No matter how tame a bull seems, you always have to remember that he *is* a bull. Most people are not hurt by a mean bull because these bulls are watched constantly. It is the tame, friendly bull that is dangerous. He may not mean to hurt you, but a 1000–pound–plus playmate can get unintentionally rough in his play, and smash you through the barn wall.

A ring in his nose is no good unless you have a bull staff and use it. I'll bet over 90 percent of all the farm bull owners do not have a staff, or if they do, don't know where it is. The staff is a pole with a snap in the end that clips to the bull ring. Leading a bull with a staff gives you a lot more handling power, as the bull can't get any closer to you than the length of the staff. Leading him by a chain in the ring lets him run over you at will. And never really trust the ring, as I have seen bulls rip a ring out when they got angry enough.

Never rub a bull's head or wrestle with his horns. This teaches him to use his head, and when he finds his strength, he is very dangerous. I've seen a bull lift the front end of a tractor like a tinker toy, and another push out the whole end of a barn, beams and all. I've seen one who walked through a five-strand barbed wire fence as if it were string, and another get a man down, kneel on him, and ignore pitchforks stuck into him in an effort to get him off. These are not scare stories but facts to consider before bringing that bull home.

In most areas, there are two alternatives to owning a bull. One is to use a nearby neighbor's bull and let someone else deal with management responsibilities.

Artificial Insemination The other is to use artificial breeding or insemination. In most cases this is the best choice.

Here you have many choices as to bull, several breeds to choose from, and complete information on them. You can see what he looks like, what he's produced, and his ancestors. If you plan to keep calves, this gives you a great chance to upgrade your herd at a really economical price. If you plan to sell your calves, it gives you a chance to make a few dollars more by having the most saleable calf possible.

In order to have the best supply of milk, your family cow will have to be bred each year, so keep breeding in mind when buying that milk cow. Two of the best ways to find out about AI (artificial insemination) or a nearby good bull are to ask your farm neighbors, or ask your county agent or veterinarian to recommend someone.

The Heat Cycle Most cows come into heat every 21 to 27 days all year around. If you have only one cow, you can tell she's in heat by several signs. She may bawl much more than usual—really roar. She may suddenly decide to wander off (looking for a nice bull). She will usually show strings of clear mucus on her tail or hindquarters. She may try to ride you. If you are not too sure whether your cow is in heat, jot down the date on your calendar, wait 21 to 27 days and see if she repeats the same behavior. If so, chances are you were right. Most cows are in heat for one full day, some longer. The best time to breed is near the end of the heat cycle, or with some cows, just after they quit showing signs of heat, since some cows ovulate later.

After the cow is bred, just let her return to normal and keep track of the date she would be due to come into heat in case she didn't conceive. Usually, the average cow (if there is one!) settles with one or two services.

Pregnancy Exams If there is much doubt as to whether or not the cow is really bred, you can call a veterinarian to do a pregnancy exam for you. He can examine her uterus rectally and give you a good guess as to whether or not she is bred. I say a good guess, for at an early date it often is only that, an educated guess, as the fetus gains size only during the last four months of pregnancy. (The gestation period for a cow is nine months.) The size of the fetus at two months is about the size of a walnut. The vet will, however, be able to tell whether the cow has a uterine infection or if she definitely is not bred.

When there is no veterinarian around, you just have to be patient and watch your cow carefully for signs of heat. At five or six months along in her pregnancy, you will with some practice be able to "bump" the calf. That is to say, make a fist and gently but firmly bump into her right side in the flank region. If successful, you will feel a hard, abnormal lump bump you back. This is the calf.

Drying Up The Cow If you are milking the cow, it is best to dry her up six to eight weeks before she is due to calve. This gives her a rest and gives her time to build a good strong calf. There are many arguments as to how to dry up a cow. These range from just stopping milking to only milking once daily, or only milking when she looks uncomfortable. I firmly believe in just stopping milking and not touching her bag until she starts to dry up. She will look miserable for a couple of days but will then quickly dry up, usually uneventfully. Any milking just stimulates her to produce more milk, and this slows down the time it takes her to dry up. If her bag gets too hard, a brief rub with a warm bay balm will help, but if you spend too much time rubbing, this will also stimulate her milk production.

Several days after you stop milking her, you will notice quite a change in her udder. Where before you saw a nice round, full udder, there will only be flabby skin. It's sort of like letting most of the air out of a balloon. Don't worry, that nice udder will return in a few weeks. Most cows start to spring bag (begin to round out that udder) about a month before calving. This slowly fills out and soon starts to look beautiful again. Some cows don't bag up until they calve, so don't panic if Daisy looks like she's going to give very little milk. Wait until after she calves, then panic. Even then, a veterinarian can give her a shot of oxytocin, a hormone, that is an aid in forcing her to let the milk down. That is, unless of course there is no milk to let down. This, fortunately, is rare.

Getting Ready for Calving It is normal for a cow heavy with calf to throw off strings of clear mucus, usually after she stands up. Many times people have thought this was the beginning of calving. It is not; I think it's a false alarm she gives just to see if you are watching her! When she's through kidding around, she'll pass a cloudy mucus, followed by a pinkish or bloody discharge. She may or may not lie down to have her calf. Some cows just strain a few times in between mouthfuls of hay and out plops the calf. More usually, though, the cow will lie down and strain for a half hour to an hour before calving.

It is best, if at all possible, for you to have a maternity stall ready and put her in it a few days before she is due to freshen. This should be a box stall about 12 x 12 feet unless you have really huge holsteins or other large breeds. Then it should be about 14 x 14 feet. If there is a cement floor, haul in eight inches of sand, or four of sand and four of sawdust. Don't cheat.

I advise this stall for several reasons. Most of the really hard calvings and the delivery of dead calves could have been prevented if someone had seen that the cow was having trouble and helped her, or called the veterinarian if it was too much to handle. In the maternity stall you can check on the cow several times a day and at night, if necessary, whereas if she is in the pasture, sometimes it's hard to locate her, especially after dark.

And when cows know they're about to calve, quite often they instinctively go off somewhere secluded to have the calf. They can really hide! So it's best to have them where you can find them.

If she should have trouble calving, it's a lot easier to help her when the rain or snow isn't blowing, or it isn't so dark that you can't see what is happening. In case she should throw her uterus out after calving (not many cows do this, but it is something to remember), she will be a lot easier to work on if she is in the barn.

If she should be a little weak in the hindquarters after calving, she won't slip and slide around if she's in a maternity stall, and thus won't be so apt to tear ligaments and get into really serious trouble. I'd say that 70 percent of the "downer" cows after calving (cows that are unable to stand) happen because of injuries to ligaments, muscle, and bone, caused by sliding around and ending up spread-eagled on the cement.

NORMAL DELIVERIES

Front Presentation Most cows deliver their calves front end first, so after your cow has strained good and hard several times, the first part of the calf that you will see is the tip of a hoof, usually followed closely by the other hoof. These tiny hooves are whitish and soft and have flaky, spongy bottoms. This is normal, so don't worry. They are this way to protect the mother from injury at birth. They will soon become hard.

The calf is born in the position of a diver, or front legs stretched out with its head in between. The legs will protrude about a foot, and then you will begin to see the head. Quite often the tongue will be out and appear swollen. There will be a momentary pause, then the cow will bear down hard and the whole head will come into the world. This is soon followed by the shoulders, and the calf slides out onto the straw. Usually the afterbirth comes along too but if it doesn't, don't worry. Most cows lose the afterbirth within a few hours after calving.

After calving, let the cow clean off her calf, and let her relax.

Rear Presentation Less frequent, but still considered normal, is the rear presentation. The first hint of this kind of birth is that the hooves will appear upside down. Instead of seeing the toes, you will see the underside and sole of the hooves. As the cow strains, the tail will become visible. A backward delivery in many ways is easier for the cow, as there is no bulk at the shoulders to block up.

There are two things you may have problems with in this type of birth. Sometimes the umbilical cord breaks while the calf's head is still in the birth passage. When the cord breaks, it is natural for the calf to start to breathe. But unfortunately, in this position, its head is still covered by afterbirth and mucus. As soon as it gets halfway out, you should take hold of its legs and quickly get it the rest of the way out. Be careful that its head doesn't drop to the ground, especially if the floor is cement. I've seen several calves with severe concussions because of this, if the cow is standing.

As soon as the calf slides free, quickly clean out any mucus from its throat and nose. If it isn't breathing or isn't breathing strongly, whack it HARD on the side with the flat of your hand. Remember, the doctor whacked you when you were born. And the calf weighs a heck of a lot more than you did. Sometimes, poking your finger up its nose or poking it in the eye will make it gasp and start it breathing. Again, let the mother clean off her baby, and let them rest.

ABNORMAL DELIVERIES

There are three groups of abnormal deliveries. First, there are the deliveries that can be assisted by the owner, with a little knowledge and common sense. Second are the births that need to be helped along by a veterinarian. Third, and most uncommon, are births which require caesarean section.

Helping with the Delivery When an abnormal delivery is suspected, the best thing to do is to scrub up (if you have long fingernails, trim them), use some ordinary liquid dish detergent as a lubricant, and go in and reconnoiter. If you find the head and one front leg, loop a binder twine or thin rope around the head through the mouth. An obstetrical chain works better, but a one-cow homesteader can't afford to purchase a veterinary O.B. kit merely for one cow who might have trouble some day.

Keep tension on the rope so you don't loosen the head, and push the head and leg back far enough to be able to work the retained leg—usually doubled back, butting up against the pelvis—out through the cervix. While you are bringing the stubborn leg up into position, try to keep a hand over the hoof so it doesn't poke a hole in the wall of the uterus. Once the leg is into position, she should pop the calf out with no more trouble.

If you find two front legs and no head, you're in for a little more work. Try to push the legs back. This in itself is quite a chore, as a cow can really bear down, just about crushing your arm at times. However, if the legs can be shoved back enough to make a little room to feel around, it will make finding the head easier. The easiest way (if there is one) is to follow a leg up from the chest with a hand, around the bulge of the neck and up to the nose. Sometimes you may be able to force the head around into the correct position by just pulling on the nose.

Other times you have to grasp the eye sockets with your thumb and finger in order to have enough traction to pop the head around right. This will not injure the calf's eyes. Once the head is through the cervix, you can easily place it between the legs and the delivery can proceed.

If you find the head but no legs, place the rope through the mouth and behind the ears. Keep this tight enough that the head doesn't drop out of reach in the uterus. Shove back on the

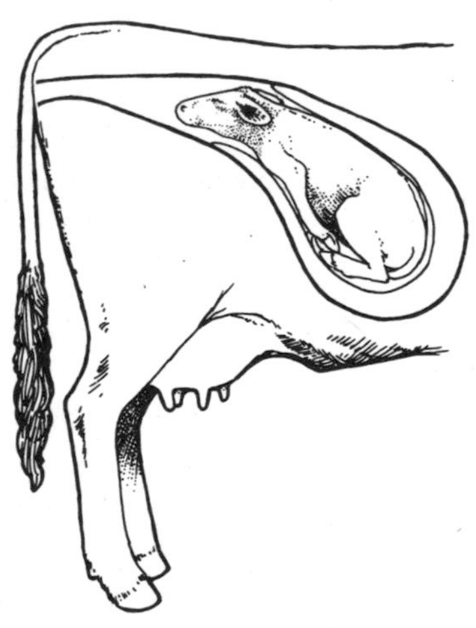

Calf in abnormal position. Front limbs have caught the brim of the pelvis and doubled under.

head. You will have to force it back far enough to be able to bring up both front legs. Here again, this is a tiring job but it can be done. Keep a hand between the hooves and the wall of the uterus to guard against tears.

If the head and front legs are in position but the calf is large or the birth canal is narrow, you can help by fastening ropes to the legs. Here again, obstetrical chains are better as they do not shut off circulation. Be sure they are above the first joint of the foot (the fetlock joint) because if they aren't sometimes the leg will break there.

As the cow strains, pull down on the ropes. Don't jerk, but keep a steady pull as the cow strains, and hold the calf where she pushes it. Sometimes a pole or a pitchfork can be used as a lever. Brace the end or tines against the floor and put the handle through the ropes and pull down. I'll never forget asking for a pitchfork at a farm and having the owner reply, "Four or five tine, Doc?" Or the farmer who gasps, "You're not going to run *that* into her, are you?" Don't use a fence stretcher or tractor, as these pull the cow around and pull at the wrong angle, only jamming the calf worse.

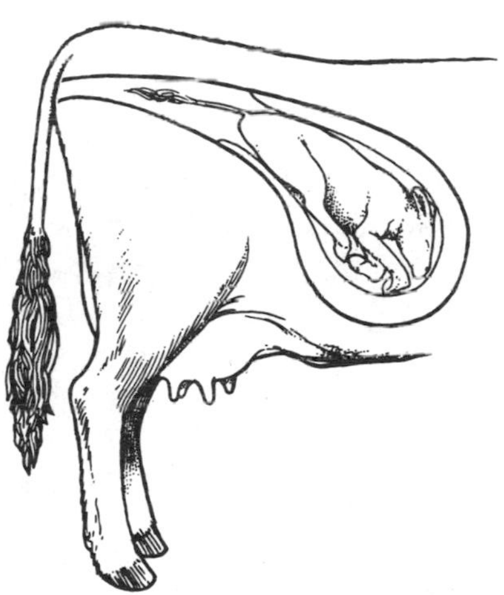

Calf in abnormal position. Buttocks first, legs doubled up.

If the calf should be coming backward but only the tail is showing (no legs), you will have to shove the hindquarters in as far as possible. Then you will be able to bend the legs into the correct position, doing each leg separately.

Calling the Vet There are some instances when you should call a veterinarian in on a difficult calving. If you have tried any of the above methods and still cannot get the cow to expel the calf, don't work on her until she is exhausted. Call. The veterinarian has special obstetrical equipment that can greatly speed up the delivery of a difficult calf, sometimes saving the calf and the cow. He also has the experience and knowledge of the "inside" of a cow, giving him access to "tricks of the trade," so to speak. Just when to pull, which way to push, how hard to pull—all these come with practice.

If the cow quits straining on the calf and just lies there, call the vet. He can give her an injection that will start uterine contractions. Even with a calf jack to help him, the veterinarian can have a hard time pulling if the cow doesn't help.

If you check the cow and find a foot, or two feet, tightly encircled by something that feels like a tough bag twisted shut, call. It may be a torsion of the uterus. Here the uterus twists on itself, thus preventing the birth of the calf. The vet can use a torsion rod inserted between the legs to rotate the calf, something like a barbecue spit. It's quite tricky, and can be a real job.

If the calf is dead and the cow can't deliver, call the vet. He may have to cut it apart with an embryotomy knife, as dead calves tend to absorb fluid and swell up. The embryotomy

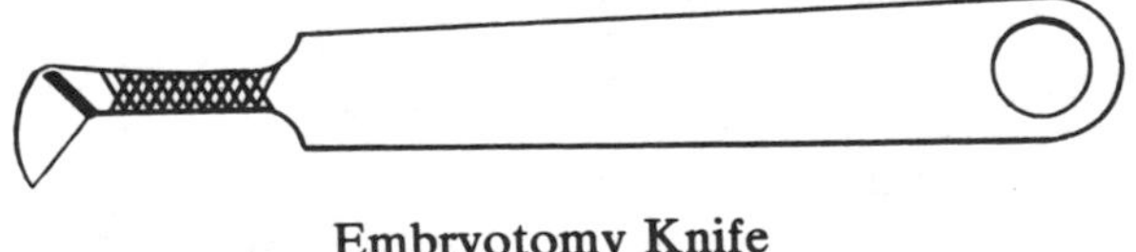

Embryotomy Knife

knife is a special curved knife with a small blade, made to cut the skin of a dead fetus and still protect the wall of the uterus.

Caesarean Section Once in a while, there is a need to do a caesarean section in order to deliver a calf. The usual cause for this is a too-young heifer having been bred. No matter how hard you push and pull, you can't get a 29-inch sofa through a 24-inch door. The same applies to cattle.

Many times a caesarean is a poor risk, as quite often the veterinarian is called as a last resort and the cow (or heifer) is just too tired to be a decent surgical risk. Any major operation performed on a sick animal, as a cow with a foul, dead fetus in her or an exhausted cow, is risky to say the least. If, however, the need for a caesarean is discovered soon enough and the veterinarian alerted, the chances for a successful operation are greatly increased.

For other problems related to calving, see "Ketosis," "Milk Fever," "Retained Placenta," and "Eversion of the Uterus" in the section, **Diseases and Other Problems** later in this chapter.

CASTRATION

Clamping or "Pinching" This is the method that I recommend as best by far. There is no blood, very little shock or setback, no chance of infection or tetanus, and it is very easy to do, even on large bulls. The only disadvantage is the cost of the clamps. The only types of emasculatome or clamp that are consistently good or worth using, in my opinion, are those made by Burdizzo. There are many imitations, but if you look closely at the place where the jaws meet to crush the cord, you will see a tiny crack of daylight in other brands. This is what causes so-called "slips," or animals that were thought to have been castrated and found to have one or both testicles still in operation.

If you have only an occasional bull to clamp, it is usually very inexpensive to have your vet do it when he is doing something else at your farm. The cost here will usually be less than a lunch uptown.

The purpose of clamping is to crush the cord, thus causing the testicles to atrophy and shrink up. They do not drop off. When preparing to clamp a bull, the first thing is to have the animal restrained as well as possible, making the job quicker and safer for the operator. With a calf up to, say, 600 pounds, the best way to restrain him is to have the head tied or in a stanchion and have a helper crowd alongside, grasping the tail at the base. The tail is forced straight up over the back, making it nearly impossible for the calf to kick. The helper's knee should be pressed under the belly, just in front of the hind leg. This prevents the calf from dancing around or sitting down. The same method is used to secure a larger bull, but a couple more helpers are always appreciated.

In applying the clamps, locate the cord leading to the testicle. With the cord positioned between the jaws of the clamps, slide them to a point above the testicle at a sufficient distance above to avoid mashing the testicle. With the cord safely between the jaws, press the handles together all the way. While the jaws of the clamps are still together, check to see that the cord did not slip out of the way when the jaws were being closed. Release the handles and move on to the next testicle. Do one cord at a time. DO NOT CLAMP ACROSS THE CENTER SECTION OF THE SCROTUM: There is a septum separating the two testicles, and if this is crushed you can have serious trouble.

Surgical Castration This is the surest method but a little trickier. As I tell many cattle raisers, when you see the testicles lying on the ground, you can be sure there were no slips. This procedure requires the use of an emasculator (an instrument that crushes and cuts the cord and blood vessels at the same time), as this greatly minimizes bleeding. You also need a sharp knife or scalpel.

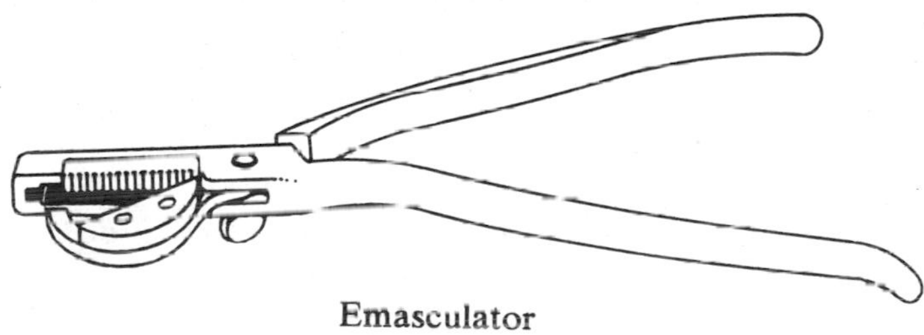

Emasculator

Using the same method of restraint described above, with the operator standing behind the animal, the scrotum is grasped by one hand and the lateral surface of the scrotum is turned back toward the operator. An incision is made along the side to the bottom of the scrotum. The incision should be long enough to easily expose adequate drainage. There is a layer of tough tissue covering the testicle. This should be removed with the testicle. The cord should be cut as high as possible. Cutting high, along with removal of the tunic (the covering of the testicle), prevents the animal ending up with a scirrhous cord which must be peeled out by hand—and is one finger-cramping condition to correct!

When the cord and testicle are exposed, the emasculator is applied. Be sure the crushing part of the emasculator is towards the animal, or it won't do any good. The second testicle is then grasped; proceed in the same manner on the opposite side of the scrotum. A mild antiseptic is applied to the area after both testicles have been removed. A fly repellent may be used if the flies are bad.

DEHORNING

The best time to dehorn cattle is when they are calves. It is easier on all concerned, does not require a veterinarian, and heals quickly.

Caustic Ointment This is applied when the calf is several days old. The hair is clipped around the tiny horn bud. Vaseline is rubbed in a wide ring around the eyes to prevent burning them in case the ointment should run. Don't use caustic if:

- It is raining—it'll run, burning the face where it goes.
- Several calves run together. They'll burn each other.
- The calf and mother (or nurse cow) are together, even just at meals. The calf may burn the cow while nursing.

The caustic ointment is applied in a ring around the base and on the button, which kills the horn cells so that no horn grows. Be sure you follow the directions on the product you use, as all are a little different.

Electric (or Dehorning Iron) This also burns, killing the horn cells, but is safer all around. There is no caustic material on the head after a few seconds, thus no danger of face burns or burns to other animals. The one problem many people have is that of not leaving the iron on long enough. Thus a deformed horn or "scur" forms. This may turn into the head, pressing right into the skull. Of course, the dehorning iron costs more than the caustic paste, so if there is only one calf involved, the paste would be more economical.

Be sure to follow the directions with your dehorning iron, and leave it on the full time, even though the calf bawls bloody murder. Better to dehorn once for the proper length of time than to have to repeat the process later.

Gougers These are simple instruments with two round wooden handles with a sharp blade which fits down over a horn button. The handles are pulled quickly apart and the horn button is snipped out. This is the method I prefer for calves up to five or six months of age. Gougers are easy to operate and quite sure. When the horn button pops out, there are very few scurs to grow back—unless the button was cut *off* not gouged *out.*

As soon as both buttons are out, sprinkle blood-stopping powder on the wounds. The bleeding will usually stop in five minutes. It may spray in a fine squirt for a minute. Don't be alarmed. It will stop shortly. If not, place a clean cotton pad on each side and wrap gauze snugly around the head to put pressure on the wounds. This is seldom necessary to do, but it will stop the excessive bleeding.

Keep freshly dehorned calves indoors for a few days so the flies can be controlled. Either use a face wipe or fly repellent antiseptic such as scarlet oil on the wounds.

Elastrator (Rubber Band Method) I must confess that I'm not really in favor of this method of dehorning, so if I sound prejudiced—I am! First, the base of the horn is clipped. The elastrator is slipped tight against the head, placing the rubber band between the head and base of the horn. The band is released, shutting off circulation to the horn. Basically, gangrene develops and eventually the horn falls off.

Painless? I really doubt it. I don't think I'd like an arm amputated this way.

Improper use results in scurs or one horn on–one horn off, as does a broken or lost band. There is no blood or fly problem, but once in a while an infection develops when the horn is part way off.

Dehorning Adult Cattle This may be done by a layman but usually is best handled by your veterinarian. The animal is restrained in a chute. A stanchion may be used, but you may not have totally good results if the head is not immobilized. The nerve around the base of the horn is usually injected with an anesthetic if the horns are to be manually sawed off. If an electric dehorning saw or large manual cutting dehorner is used, most veterinarians do not use an anesthetic—as it is over with so fast, there is little more than afterpain. The dehorner is pushed up close to the head and quickly closed. If done close enough, the arteries are near the surface and can be picked up and clamped off with a heavy forceps.

If the horns are left an inch or so long, a piece of binder twine can be drawn tight around the base of both horns, then tied together over the top, further tightening it. Once the arteries are clamped off or the twine is tied, dust some coagulant powder on the wounds. There will then be very little bleeding. When the horn is cut, there can be a stream the size of a small pencil spraying for a second!

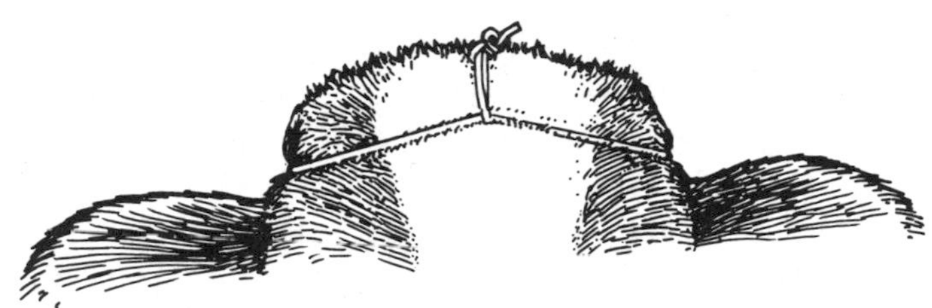

Twine is tied around horn stumps to prevent bleeding after dehorning.

A large-based horn must either be taken off with an electric dehorning saw or a manual saw, as blade dehorners can crack the horn or the skull at times. These horns are most often seen on bulls and older beef cows.

FOOT TRIMMING

Due to the lack of exercise most cattle receive and the type of ground they walk on (usually grass—not rock and sand), their feet are prone to quick growth. If left untrimmed the toes often either cross or curl up like elf shoes. This puts a strain on the tendons and can make a cow lame. Any harassment of this sort soon lowers milk production of dairy cows and growth of beef cattle.

There are special hoof trimmers for cattle, which are used while the cow is standing, all four feet on the ground; lifting the feet is not necessary. One side is braced between the toes and the other on the outside of the hoof. A few snips and those long toes are sound again. If you see pink while working, stop, as the next cut may bring blood. If you should hit blood, it can be stopped with a dehorning powder or hot iron used as a cautery.

If not taken back to the quick, hoof trimming is like toenail trimming on people—no pain or blood.

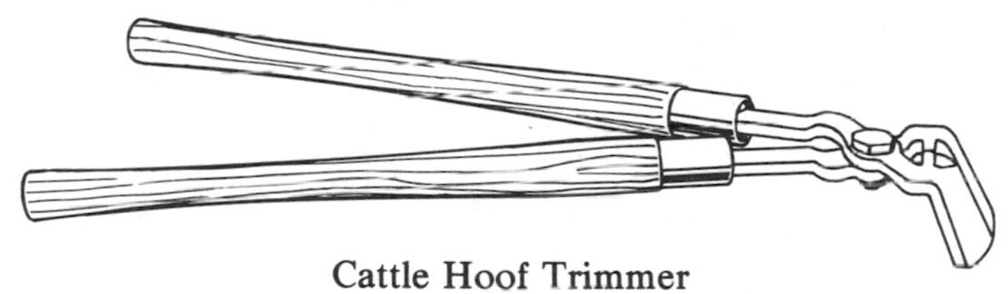

Cattle Hoof Trimmer

Diseases and Other Problems

BLACKLEG

In many parts of the country blackleg is a disease that causes severe losses in cattle from three months to two years of age. It is caused by one of the clostridia, *Clostridium chauvoei,* which is related to the organism that causes tetanus.

Blackleg organisms live in the soil for years, which explains why some farms can be bothered by blackleg year after year until the young stock are vaccinated. Blackleg organisms enter the body through the digestive tract or through small puncture wounds. They don't grow when exposed to the air, but when they enter the body, in the absence of oxygen the organisms grow and produce a toxin which when strong enough kills the animal. Blackleg is a sudden-appearing disease: the animal may be okay at night or just a little lame on one leg, and when morning comes, it's dead.

Blackleg is usually quite easy to diagnose. On skinning out the legs, one usually appears purple, as if it were bruised badly. If the legs are all normal, the neck is sometimes involved. If you find yourself in an area where blackleg is a problem—ask your veterinarian and your neighbors—arrange to have your young animals vaccinated. It costs only a few cents a head and takes only a little while to do a whole herd. It is certainly worth the preventive steps, because there is no sure treatment after an animal contracts the disease.

BLOAT

The usual cause of bloat in cattle is overeating. Pasture, especially lush clover and legume pasture, is a common culprit. Overeating of this type pasture produces what is called frothy or foamy bloat. There is an abnormal amount of gas formed in numerous small bubbles which the animal is not able to belch up. Thus the gas continues to form and the animal becomes bloated. If not treated, the animal will become staggery, have respiratory trouble, pant, and finally collapse in a heap. Unless immediate treatment is given, death is usually not far away.

In nearly all cases, the animal will recover promptly if a defoaming agent is given. Some very effective defoaming agents are corn oil, peanut oil, soybean oil, and safflower oil. Cream and mineral oil have also been used with quite good results. Four to eight ounces are usually sufficient for a calf, and a pint is about right for adult animals. A trochar should be in every barn that has cattle, for in an emergency (where the animal is weak and staggering) it may be necessary to use one. A trochar is a pointed instrument like an awl that has a small,

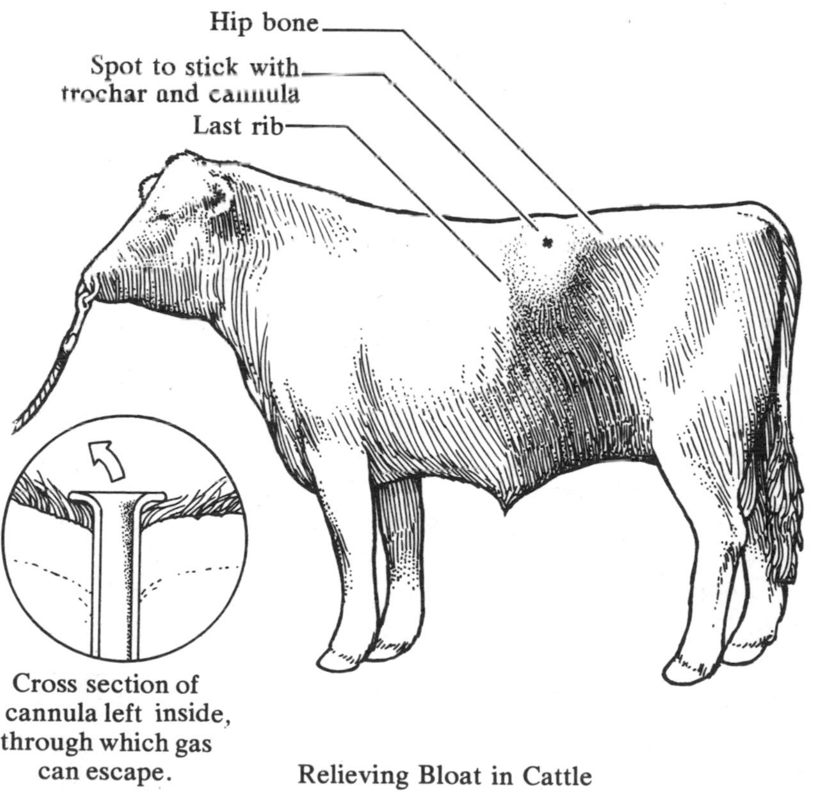

Relieving Bloat in Cattle

pipe-shaped accompanying piece, the cannula, which is left in the animal after inserting the trochar to let gas escape without contaminating the peritoneal cavity with debris from the stomach. If needed, stick the bloated cow at the highest point of the bloat, on its left side just in front of the hip.

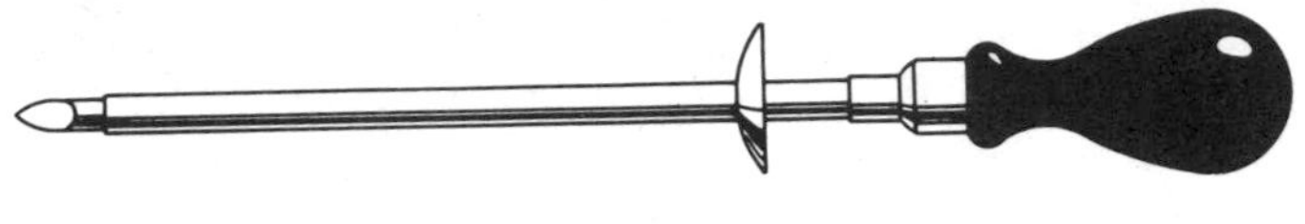

Cattle Trochar

If a trochar and cannula are used, sometimes it becomes necessary to make a small incision through the hide with a sharp knife. I'll never forget the first bloat I treated, just after completing vet school. The cow was really sick, so I got out the trochar. I hauled off to stick it, but the trochar just bounded off the tight hide, nearly knocking me on my whatchamacallit. To say the least, I was embarrassed!

Sometimes a cow will overload on dry feed, usually ground grains, and bloat. In cases such as this, the gas is usually in larger pockets, as compared to frothy bloat's tiny bubbles. Here the quickest way to relieve the bloat is to pass a stomach tube and manipulate it to relieve each pocket, one at a time. Caution: use only a stomach tube, not a garden hose, milk hose, or the like. These can tear. I know a lot of farmers who use them, but I also know of several cases where they've caused the death of a cow. You can get a stomach tube from any veterinarian, and the cost is minimal. If you have a large number of cattle, it is a good idea to buy one, plus a mouth speculum to prevent a cow biting the tube, especially if your nearest veterinarian is a long distance away.

After the gas is released, a bloat medicine can be given to prevent the further buildup of gas until the animal has had a chance to digest the grain.

BREAKS

Most broken bones occur in cattle in the legs and pelvis. This excludes the broken tails given to them by people twisting them, trying to get a cow to go somewhere it doesn't want to go. We have one cow that came to us with *four* breaks in its tail!

Broken Legs A sudden, severe lameness in a leg, especially if the leg appears floppy or dangling, is a prime suspect for a break. Do not move the animal unless it is in a really bad place (swamp, willow scrub, etc.). If it must be moved, do it a few steps at a time. Keep it quiet and call the veterinarian. If the bone has not come through the skin, there is a good chance the animal can be saved without it costing you a fortune. That old idea of "shoot a cow or horse with a broken leg" is okay for movies but can be rather costly and foolish in reality.

A plaster cast or a cast-brace combined works quite well in many cattle. The weight an animal carries and its disposition have a lot to do with the success, as does the aftercare it receives. Some animals are quite clumsy with a cast on and need to be helped up after lying down. The cast must not stand in wet bedding or barnyard muck as the plaster will soften, making the cast worthless. An inner tube slipped over the bottom helps, but must be changed often due to wear.

The healing time varies, but a calf's broken leg is usually healed in a month, and a cow's in twice that long. With a severe break on an adult cow or a break where the bone tears out through the skin, it is sometimes necessary to have the leg amputated. I have done this on a large holstein cow and later she calved normally and went on to milk 80 pounds of milk a day. It is surprising how well an animal amputee can get around, and how unnoticeable the missing leg is to it.

Culverts with holes in them, bridges with holes or rotten planks, woods with many down trees, and swamps all rate high in causing breaks and are best repaired or fenced off.

Fractured Pelvises Most fractured pelvises in cattle occur with a difficult birth or a bad fall on the cement in the barn. With a hard calving, call your vet. Many times the calf is dead and can be cut apart with a special embryotomy knife, allowing it to be delivered with little risk to the cow. Forcing too big a calf out by using a tractor, a fence stretcher, or chain fall, can easily fracture a pelvis. Slipping on the cement in the barn, either when the cow is weak as in milk fever or just clumsy and on slippery footing, can result in a spread-eagle fall that can fracture the pelvis. The usual result in either case is a cow that cannot get to its feet for several weeks.

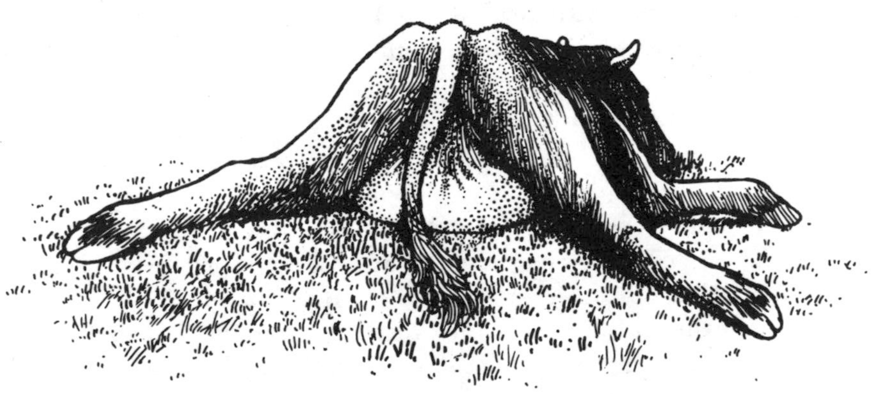

The "spread eagle" position of a "downer" cow.

Here again, we have a "shoot her she's no good" situation. And again you'll have to give the animal time and some effort. Many of these "downer" cows will lay for a month or more before rising. As long as they are eating and appear bright and alert they have a chance of getting to their feet. There are cow lifters which fit over the hips and are used to lift down cows, but a cow with a broken pelvis should *not* be hauled up. This will only aggravate the problem and make the healing take longer.

Down cows must be kept bedded and kept on their brisket, not lying flat out. Bales of hay or straw can be used to prop them up if they tend to lie flat. They should be turned twice a day, so as to keep up circulation in their legs and prevent "bed sores." A sun shade is a must if they are outdoors. Plenty of fresh water and fresh feed are appreciated. A happy cow will get better quicker than a miserable one, and won't quit as easily.

BVD

Bovine virus diarrhea, or infectious bovine diarrhea, is a viral disease that is quite common in cattle. It is not always a severe disease, and is more of a chronic infection.

Affected animals will show a rise in temperature for several days, lose their appetites and have diarrhea. There are sometimes sores around the mouth, eyes and nose. Drooling or foaming at the mouth is often a sign of the disease.

Treatment is often difficult. Vaccines are available to protect against the disease before it strikes.

CAKED BAG

Udder edema, or caked bag, is a condition usually found in cattle just prior to or soon after freshening. The bag becomes swollen and feels doughy to the touch. If you press your fingers into the bag, fingerprints or dents will remain when you take your hand away.

In udder edema there is increased circulation to the bag, the bag swells, and the blood is being carried into the udder faster than it can be carried away. Some of the fluid settles into the tissue, causing the edema. Diuretics cause the animal to urinate more often, drawing fluid from the body and from the congested udder.

I have had very good luck in reducing udder edema by using an injection of diuretic, followed by oral diuretics given until the bag becomes normal. Hot compresses and warm udder ointment or udder liniment can help to increase circulation and carry away the edema.

If a caked bag is let go, it can cause a breakdown in udder attachments and result in a pendulous udder, which in turn leads to other udder problems. It can also lead to gangrene mastitis, if the blood supply becomes completely shut off.

CUTS

Most cuts do *not* need to be sutured. Believe it or not, 75 percent of the cuts I am called on to suture do not really need it, and I end up not doing it. It is purely a waste of time and money to try suturing up a number of wounds, either because of the area in which the wound occurred or the type of wound it was. Consult your vet to be sure, then believe him. There are some cuts that heal better if sewn up, but many times Mother Nature plus your good nursing will heal up a cut better than will stitches.

A three-cornered tear, with skin hanging, should either be sewn up or the flap should be snipped off. The hole left where the flap was snipped off will fill in, leaving little or no scarring. It is best not to sew up a gash in areas that are heavily muscled or in "stretch areas." Stitches will just tear out in a few days.

Most important is cleanliness, followed by fly control. Clip all the hair away from the edges of the wound, as hair is irritating to a wound and will double the healing time if left in the wound. Keeping a cut clean and dry, by use of good old soap and water (not Lysol) plus an antiseptic that is also a fly repellent, such as scarlet oil, will greatly cut down on the healing time. A six-inch gash can be completely healed in three weeks with good nursing.

Flies must be kept out of a wound as they deposit their eggs there, and in a day the wound can be crawling with maggots. Maggots, in moderation, are not a bad thing as they eat necrotic tissue, cleaning up a wound nicely, but when they run out of the dead tissue, they go on further and can literally eat up an animal alive. So it's best to keep them away.

EVERSION OF THE UTERUS

Not to be confused with a retained placenta, the eversion of the uterus is an emergency and requires immediate attention. Where the placenta is stringy and thin, the uterus is heavy and bulky and the buttons or caruncles stand out plainly. The uterus may be out from the size of a basketball to the size of a bushel basket.

There is much shock to the cow when this problem occurs, so call your vet immediately. Tell him your cow has thrown her uterus out. I've had farmers that were too embarrassed to say this; they just said their cow needed me. It helps the vet if he knows exactly what the problem is.

Keep warm wet towels on the uterus, and do not let it swing and flop around or get in the manure. If at all possible, get the cow's hind end up a foot or two higher than her front. An old door or sheet of plywood propped up on hay will work nicely. The extra trouble you take may save her life. Don't let her get near barbed wire or brush. If she snags or tears the uterus, she will quite often die. Don't run her or excite her, as she is in shock and her heart cannot stand exertion.

When your vet gets there, have a couple of pails of warm water and several towels handy. If there are a couple of helpers, it will greatly speed up things and may also help save the cow. I have seen cows die with a uterus out only fifteen minutes, but then again, I had a shorthorn cow whose owner thought she had a retained placenta and only needed cleaning. This poor cow had her uterus out for *three days*! She lived too, but she was an exceptional case.

A bale or two behind the cow, draped with a sheet or towels to rest the uterus on, may be needed as your vet returns the uterus to its proper place. A spinal anesthetic is given to cut down the straining both during and after the veterinarian returns the uterus. Even with an anesthetic, this is at best a rough, tiring job. It's like picking up 60 pounds of liver and stuffing it carefully through a crack, while someone on the other side is shoving it back at you!

Once back into place, it is usually necessary to lace the lips of the vulva to help keep the cow from throwing it back out, although *nothing* will absolutely prevent it from coming out again if she strains hard. Thus, a spinal may be given a few hours after replacing the uterus to hold her until it shrinks down and the swelling leaves.

After the uterus is replaced, it is a good idea to build up the back of the stall with hay or to keep the door under her so that when she lies down, the weight to her bowels will not be pressing against the uterus, shoving it towards the vulva.

FLIES

The most common trouble flies cause is plain irritation, both to animals and people. Cows bothered severely by common flies will drop off in milk production and even lose weight, just from worrying and swishing their tails at the pests. It has often been said that the most expensive fly swatter in the barn is a cow's tail.

Keeping the barn spotless, both inside and out, will aid in keeping flies down. So will completely eliminating a manure accumulation outside the barn, either in a manure pile or in a messy barnyard the cows can get into at other than milking time. Fly traps and those horrible (but useful) sticky spiral fly catchers help keep flies down in some areas, but are not practical in others. Spraying the barn in the morning and at night when the barn is empty can be used as a last resort, as can spraying the cows. Many of the sprays on the market, however, can do more harm than good because of the dangerous chemicals they contain, so check all the warnings on the label before buying a can of spray.

Biting insects, such as horseflies, horn flies, deer flies, and mosquitoes, often can be more than just irritating. These flies not only bite hard, bothering the cattle, but can drive them into a run, through fences and fields. There are sprays and wipes that may be used on dairy animals to cut down these pests' attacks. Here again, be sure to thoroughly read the label before purchasing one of them.

FOOT ROT

The first sign of foot rot is usually a sudden lameness, often in just one foot. On checking the foot, you may find it swollen and possibly with pus oozing from between the toes. If left untreated, the swelling will increase and as the animal is in pain, the milk production will drop, the cow will lose weight and "dump around."

In winter months, foot rot (caused by a fungus) may result from cattle stepping on the mud that was cut up by cattle tracks and then frozen, making very bad walking conditions. The flesh between the toes chaps, splits, and is irritated further by walking daily on the rough ground of the barnyard. The fungus gains entrance through these broken areas in the skin and suddenly—foot rot. During the summer, the cattle congregate in the swampy areas, and the alternate wet and dry condition chaps the feet, and cracks form.

The fungus that causes foot rot is in the soil, and thus some farms are plagued with it while others never are bothered. Keeping the cattle away from muddy places in the summer and rough places in the winter will help keep down foot rot. Also, feeding an iodine preparation in the feed or salt will help a lot in some herds. Making dairy cows walk through a foot bath containing a fungicide as they come into and leave the barn at milking time will slow down foot rot, but not stop it.

Treatment consists of using a broad-spectrum antibiotic or sometimes an intravenous sulfa. The foot must be kept clean and dry. Any walking in mud or manure should be avoided. A drying powder containing an antibiotic will help, as will a drying liquid such as Kopertox.

When the foot rot has progressed too far, sometimes it becomes necessary to remove the infected portion. Many times a hay rope can be drawn through the crack between the toes several times, the friction burning the necrotic tissue away. Don't be gentle, as you won't accomplish anything. If this is not successful, one claw can be surgically removed. It is much better, of course, to notice the lameness and begin systemic treatment at once.

Foot rot should not be confused with a condition sometimes occurring in cattle known as "corns." This quite often occurs in heavy cattle and is not a swollen, pussy foot but an extra chunk of tissue that extends further than normal between the toes. Check the other three feet to see the difference. These corns can be very painful and are often best taken care of by surgical removal.

GRUBS

Like screwworms, grubs are also parasitic fly larvae, but they are not usually so dangerous. The botflies lay eggs on the legs and lower belly of cattle. On hatching, the maggots burrow directly into the flesh. They migrate and end up just under the skin in the back. Each grub makes a breathing hole and remains there, until they drop out of the holes to the ground, to start the cycle over again. There are many sprays, pour-ons, and powders on the market for grubs, but extreme care must be used, as many are not safe for milking animals. In mildly affected animals, it is usually best to just leave the grubs alone; it is when they show on the back that most people want to get rid of them. Pinching or squashing them in the back can cause an anaphylactic shock.

HARDWARE DISEASE

Hardware disease, as the name implies, is caused by swallowing hardware (nails, wire, bottle caps, tin cans, and whatever). These metal objects stay in the reticulum. As feed is churned by the stomach, the sharp metal penetrates the wall of the reticulum and often travels into the thoracic cavity and the pericardium. A nail or wire may migrate to other organs such as liver, spleen, and so forth. I once did an autopsy on a cow I had diagnosed as hardware disease. There was a black hole clear through the heart where a wire had passed through, and there was no finding the wire. Where it went or whatever happened to it was anybody's guess!

Hardware disease can produce a wide variety of symptoms, depending on where the wire is in the body. The animal may go off feed, go down on milk production, stand with the left elbow cocked out, move slowly, grunt on expiration, have an above normal temperature. All can indicate hardware disease, but an animal may have swallowed hardware and never show any of the above.

When suspecting hardware, call your vet in to thoroughly check the cow over. In early cases, a magnet can be fed to the cow. It's shaped like a bolus so that it can be easily swallowed by the animal. This gathers the loose objects in the reticulum and keeps them from traveling about, causing harm. Antibiotics given after a wire has pierced the reticulum, causing peritonitis, will often calm the infection. Sometimes a rumenotomy can save a valuable cow that would have to be shipped (sold for meat) without the operation.

Prevention consists of keeping the cattle away from junk, places where buildings have been torn down, old wire fences, and nails. Do not chop the wire on hay bales with an axe to open them. Little pieces of wire break off and are swallowed with the hay. One farmer I knew swept out his cement manger with a steel broom. What he didn't realize was that the broom shed bristles in the manger and these were eaten by his cows.

JOHNE'S DISEASE

Johne's disease is caused by the bacteria *Mycobacterium paratuberculosis.* Affected animals show a recurrent diarrhea with a foul odor. Johne's disease is most often seen in cattle, but has been found in goats and sheep.

An animal with Johne's disease will lose weight until weak, then die. There is no treatment.

It is most often seen in females between two to seven years of age. Any new animals brought to the farm in an area where Johne's disease has shown up should be tested, as should any animals with a chronic diarrhea.

KETOSIS

Ketosis, or acetonemia, occurs mainly in high-producing milking cows after calving. It most often happens while the cattle are being fed hay and dry feed while being kept in the barn.

There is primary ketosis, which happens by itself, and secondary ketosis, which happens along with or because of something else, such as mastitis, a displaced abomasum, etc. The cow will usually go off feed, drop in milk, and act generally depressed. These symptoms in themselves could be caused by any number of ailments, but if the cow is in the barn, has just recently freshened, and is a fairly good producer, it would pay to check her for ketosis. There is a powder that can be used very easily to check her milk. The only hitch with the powder is that the colostrum milk does not combine with the powder to give an accurate reading. In such cases you may have to take a urine test, and stand around (nearly forever!) with your little jar ready, waiting for her to urinate. Then, just try to catch a tiny jarful without getting drowned. If a urine test is too inconvenient, have a blood test taken.

If the test indicates a positive for ketosis, there are several treatments that are effective. Some cows respond to one but not any of the others, so if possible, get your veterinarian out to look at your cow and make the choice of treatment. For instance, some cows respond to drenching with one or two pints of molasses. If you're using this treatment, mix the molasses with the same amount of warm water, or else it could be quite a mess getting it in the cow. Sometimes a heavy concentration of molasses in the grain ration before and for a few weeks after calving will prevent ketosis, and it surely won't hurt anything. Sometimes cortisone injections are given, on the theory that adrenal cortex becomes exhausted and quits producing enough glucocorticoids. Drenching the cow with propylene glycol, or giving an intravenous injection of 500 to 1000 cc. of 40 percent dextrose daily, will work in many cases.

Cattle can also exhibit a craziness with ketosis. They may run with their head up against the barn wall, or circle to one side or try to attack a person. In cases like this, try to work the animal into a stall or a chute where it can't do much damage to itself or hurt someone, as it has no idea what it is doing.

LICE

Lice can appear on any cattle at any time of the year, but are most often seen during the winter months. They do not like sunlight and exposure, so they wait until long hair and dark days come along. Unless you are specifically looking for lice, the first sign that your cattle are lousy is the rubbing that suddenly begins. The affected animals, usually all of them, will begin to rub and scratch their necks on fences, the stanchion, the brush, or anything handy—you for instance!

Pretty soon the hair will be worn away, especially on the neck, making them look moth-eaten. They may look as if they have dandruff. On parting the hair and peering around on the skin, you will see little gray bugs, smaller than a small grain of rice. They are oval shaped with a head at one end that often appears to be red. Suddenly you feel crawly. Don't worry, they prefer cows to people and very seldom stay on a human to dine.

Lice may be small, but if there are sufficient numbers on a cow, the animal can become anemic and literally be bled to death by them. So plan to get rid of the pests as soon as possible. There are many louse powders on the market, carried by your vet, the drug store, or feed store. Caution: Be sure you use a dairy powder for dairy cattle, as some powders can get into the milk and cause problems for you.

MANGE

There are several types of mange that can occur in cattle. All true mange is caused by tiny mites that burrow into the skin. These cause itching, moth-eaten appearing spots, scales, crusty spots, pustules, or thickened skin.

The most common mange found in cattle, chorioptic mange, is treated effectively by use of lime-sulfur dips or lindane—which is, unfortunately, on the "no-no" list for many classes of livestock. Check with your vet, at any rate, when you suspect mange. Many cases of suspected mange turn out to be something different. A mange remedy will not help an allergy, vitamin deficiency, etc. Complete isolation of a mangy animal is a must, as it is hard enough to treat one animal with it without having to treat ten or twenty.

MASTITIS

Mastitis means the inflammation of the mammary gland. There are many bacteria that can cause mastitis, including streptococci, staphylococci, Pseudomonas, *Corynebacterium pyogenes, Escherichia coli,* etc. There may or may not be lumpy or abnormal milk, but in most cases there is some change in the milk. The most economical test for mastitis that is easy to use is the California Mastitis Test, or CMT. This can be purchased at most rural community drug stores, or your vet can pick up a kit for you. This kit is best used routinely, say monthly, and in between times should you suspect mastitis. With regular testing the mastitis can be picked up in its early stages and treatment can be started before it becomes worse and harder to treat.

Acute Mastitis There are several types of mastitis, but here we'll try to explain three—acute, chronic, and gangrene. Acute mastitis has a rapid onset. The cow may be all right one night and sick the next day. When first noticed, there is usually a marked reduction in milk production. There may be flecks in the milk, or gummy strings, or sometimes a watery fluid that in no way resembles milk. The bag is quite often hot and swollen on one or more quarters. The sick cow very often runs a temperature of 103°F. or higher. Quite often she will also go partly or completely off feed. She looks and acts sick.

If possible, milk samples should be taken and sent by your vet to a laboratory for culture and sensitivity tests. If such a test is not possible, the next best thing is to treat the animal systemically with a broad-spectrum antibiotic or to use a sulfonamide, either orally or injected for a period of at least three days, even if the animal seems to recover. Be careful in your choice of injectable antibiotics, as the milk from affected animals must be withheld from market for several days (check the label) after treatment with an injectable antibiotic. I do not use intermammary injection very much any more, as systemic treatment seems to clear up the mastitis quickly in most cases. I believe in many cases the mastitis is actually prolonged by using mastitis tubes, due to the unintentional injection of unwanted bacteria along with the tube tip. No matter how careful a person is in washing the teats and disinfecting the tube tip, there are still bacteria there just waiting to catch a ride on the tube into the teat canal. It is nearly impossible to disinfect skin. Merely rubbing alcohol on doesn't immediately kill off all bacteria.

Acute mastitis is quite often brought about by stress, such as a bump, beesting, or cold, which enables the bacteria to multiply and become dangerous. Along with drugs to treat the animal, massage with warm cloths, a warming udder ointment, and milking the animal out several times a day will all help to bring about quick relief in most cases. Milking the cow out every two hours or so is like draining an abscess. It helps carry out the bacteria, thinning their numbers, making the drugs work faster.

Never milk a mastitis cow with the milker you use on your other cows. You can't disinfect it thoroughly enough in between cows, or even in between milkings, to risk spreading the mastitis to others. Milk by hand, then scrub your hands. If you milk by hand normally, milk the mastitis cow last when milking your cows. Always scrub your hands after milking her until she is well cleared up.

I believe that misuse of the milking machine is one of the main causes of mastitis in cows. I have been in barns where one man working alone had three milking machines going at one time. This is not physically possible, that is, if the milking is done right. A milker should not be left on a cow for over three minutes. When left on longer, there is more chance of doing damage to the udder. Figuring the time it takes to do a good job washing and drying the bag, belting the cow, dumping the milk, and dipping teats after milking, plus walking back and forth, NOBODY can use more than two milkers at once without help.

I was in a feed store once buying grain, when a client who had had a lot of mastitis troubles came in. This was about noon, so I figured he'd been done milking for about six hours, as he milked early. On seeing me, his face paled, and he gasped, "My God, I forgot to take the milker off that last cow this morning!" and tore out to his pickup. I could just picture a big holstein trying to claw her way out of a milker that had her all sucked in but the horns.

Chronic Mastitis With chronic mastitis, the same cow or cows will show repeated periodic flare-ups of mastitis. She is not usually as sick as the acute mastitis cow, or may not appear sick at all. The udder may swell, but usually the first sign of trouble is when her milk will not go through the strainer. The four quarters should each be separately stripped into a strip cup BEFORE each milking, but not many farmers do this, because they feel it's too much trouble. It's a lot easier to strip check than to explain to the dairy why you've got mastitis milk in today's shipment!

I believe that once a cow has a problem with chronic mastitis, it is seldom completely knocked out, but lies hidden in scarred, walled off, areas of the mammary gland, and any stress lets it break out again. The chronic mastitis cow should be the last cow milked in the herd and should, if possible, be milked with a separate milker. When culling time comes, it might be best to choose her, rather than a cow that doesn't give quite as much milk, perhaps, but is mastitis-free. As long as a chronic mastitis cow is in the herd, she is a potential source of infection for all the others.

Gangrene Mastitis This type of mastitis can follow acute mastitis or appear suddenly by itself. When the bag feels hard and cold, worry. Once the bag or part of the bag becomes cold and has a "dead" feeling, help must be gotten soon or there is a good chance the cow will die. Many times gangrene mastitis is caused when the swelling shuts off the circulation in one or more quarters. That part with no blood supply actually dies, and will literally rot off if the animal doesn't die first. If the animal receives no treatment, she quickly becomes toxic and then is a poor risk for successful treatment.

Some cows' bags will swell a bit and feel harder than normal to the touch a few days or weeks after freshening. If the milk checks normal with a California Mastitis Test and her temperature is normal, don't worry. In a few days the bag will go back to normal.

Some cows will pass a few "plugs" or "strings" in their milk while drying, or when first fresh. This also can be normal. A cow can and does sometimes freshen with mastitis, but unless her milk stays stringy for a day or so, or she shows signs of sickness, don't worry. There are physiological changes in the milk during freshening, drying up, and even some heat periods, which cause abnormal or bad-tasting milk.

MILK FEVER

To begin with an animal with milk fever has no fever. In fact it usually has a subnormal temperature! Milk fever occurs in high milk-producing cows, with a greater incidence in jerseys. A cow that only produces 20 pounds of milk a day will very seldom come down with it. I have only treated one beef cow with milk fever, and she was part holstein. It doesn't occur very often in heifers, but usually in cows that have had two or more calves.

Milk fever is caused by low blood calcium. So far, there is nothing that will prevent it, only treatment after an animal has it. A cow can come down with it several weeks before calving, but it usually happens a day or several days after calving.

Milk fever causes an ascending paralysis, beginning with the hind legs and progressing up the body. I would be very suspicious of any newly fresh cow that was staggery in the hind limbs, or staggered when trying to rise. If it's milk fever, the condition will get progressively worse until the cow is unable to rise. The next thing you will notice in most cases is the characteristic bend or kink to the neck. The cow will twist her head to one side and be unable to hold it straight. Not all cows will exhibit this, but in my experience many have.

Milk fever is classified as an emergency, for if the cow doesn't get prompt treatment she may well die. It is also one thing that should, if possible, be treated by a veterinarian. There are several reasons for this. First of all, the calcium-phosphorus solution that is given for milk fever must be given intravenously for the quickest results. It can be given intraperitoneally, but that way it is absorbed more slowly. This may be all right in a mild case or one that is caught early, but many times the cow is quite sick when the problem is discovered. I treated a little jersey recently that wasn't breathing regularly and had dry, open eyes (like paper). She lived, but I wouldn't have had a chance if I had administered the calcium intraperitoneally. Calcium is also a stimulant to the heart and can be hard on the heart. Some cows with milk fever show abnormal heartbeats before the calcium is given. Sometimes an amphetamine injection can be given to regulate this, as calcium given to a cow with heart abnormalities can kill her.

Some stubborn cases need more than one bottle (500 cc.) of calcium. But this decision should be made by a veterinarian if possible, as he has had the experience to make the right decision. There is no need to give two bottles if the cow is simply tired from her efforts to get up. Too much calcium or calcium given too fast can kill a cow. Even the vet can be wrong, as nothing is ever sure in medicinc, but his chances for a correct decision will be better than an inexperienced layperson.

If you do not live fairly near a veterinarian (30 miles or so) and you have one or more high milk-producing cows, it would be a good idea to obtain an intravenous outfit and two bottles of calcium to keep on hand. See if you can get your vet to show you how to use them in an emergency. And I would advise home treatment of milk fever *only in an emergency situation.* If it becomes necessary to treat it yourself, work carefully. Take your time and do it right, as you will be more apt to save the cow than if you rush around making mistakes. When starting the intravenous injection start slowly. Bubbles should rise in the bottle one or two at a time, not in a continuous stream. Calcium given too fast can kill.

Make sure the needle is threaded well into the vein, as calcium is sometimes irritating to the skin, and if some leaks out under the skin, it can make a section of the neck slough off. I have been called to treat cattle with this problem, and there isn't a whole lot that can be done. And it looks pretty ugly for quite a while. (See "Intravenous Injection" in final chapter.)

After you have given the whole 500-cc. bottle, your cow should begin to shake, look brighter, and manure as the paralysis wears off. Don't be in a big rush to get her to her feet as many cows are hurt trying to get up when they are still too wobbly. Make sure she has plenty of footing and that her head isn't in a corner or up against a wall, as cattle have to throw their head and neck out to balance themselves when getting up. Don't let her slip and slide around on cement. Throw a bushel or two of sand down under her. If she is in a stanchion, release her head. When it is time for her to get up, she will have a better chance of making it.

If she still can't get up after several hours, you may have to give her the second bottle. Also, some cattle relapse into milk fever after getting to their feet, so be sure to watch a cow that has been treated for several hours, and check in on her regularly for a couple of days.

I don't like to treat a cow for milk fever until she goes down, because it is dangerous and sometimes the cow is just a little wobbly from calving and really doesn't have milk fever at all. It is, however, a good idea to call your vet and let him know you have a cow you think is coming down with milk fever, as he will try to stay within phone reach in case you do need him.

Don't milk out a cow that has freshened for three days. Take just enough of her milk, from all four quarters, to feed her calf. Also cut down on her grain for a few days. These steps will not prevent milk fever, but if not followed, they may help cause it.

Once a cow has had milk fever, she is quite apt to have it each year after (or before) she calves for several years, as may her daughters, since she is probably a good producer and will pass this problem on to them. If you have no problem in getting prompt veterinary help, I wouldn't necessarily advise selling a milk fever cow, as they are good producers, but it does mean watching them like a hawk around calving time. I have two such cows in my own herd. Both give over 60 pounds of milk a day, and I feel their good production justifies the extra bother they cause. Of course there is more risk in having cattle such as these as it is possible for them to die either from the milk fever if undiscovered in time, or the treatment. But I find I gamble on animals a lot.

PINKEYE

Pinkeye, or infectious keratitis, is usually seen during the summer months. It is spread by flies. The first sign of trouble is a watering or tearing eye. Soon the eye will begin to squint and appear bloodshot. If left untreated, a cloudy film will appear in the eye, spread, and cover the eye, which in turn will become bluish white. The cow will lose sight in that eye, or if both eyes are affected she will go totally blind. Sometimes pinkeye will clear up untreated, but not all that often. Since the flies walk on the tears of the infected eye, then on to other animals, the disease is quickly spread.

There are several eye powders on the market that usually stop the pinkeye before it gets past the tearing stage. These powders contain antibiotics plus sometimes a local anesthetic to cut down the pain and itching. Some contain a dye, so if you have many cattle you can easily tell which animals have been treated.

In cases where the eye has clouded over, I have had very good luck using foreign protein injections. Antibiotic injections don't usually work very well as the eye has a natural protective barrier to matter foreign to the body, which also keeps out much of the antibiotic. The foreign protein stimulates the body to produce nonspecific antibodies which are natural to the body, and thus can get through this barrier into the eye and attack the infection. These injections are given daily or every two days until improvement is noted. I've found that 90 percent or better of these white-eye cattle clear up entirely with treatment.

Fly control during the summer will help prevent pinkeye, but there's nothing that will completely stop it.

PNEUMONIA

This is another disease brought about by stress, such as a change in the weather, shipping, changes in the feed, or confinement in damp quarters. I have found that the latter seems to cause many problems in the winter months, and the problem is not one confined to old, rickety, overcrowded, dirty barns. I have treated pneumonia in damp barns that were designed by agricultural engineers. But they were too warm (I don't like a barn warmer than 50°F. in the winter) and "sweat" dripped constantly from the ceiling. That is too damp. Animals are much more comfortable in a cold but dry barn than a warm, damp one, even though it is comfy for you to be in while milking. Remember, you leave after a little while but the animals stay and become chilled.

Dry, clean bedding and adequate ventilation do much to help a barn stay dry. So does not packing the animals in too closely. You would be better off to let the young stock run in and out of an old shed that is cold but dry and draft-free, than to put them in the barn in a pen which might crowd the cattle you already have inside. Here again I recommend free housing, where at all possible. When cattle are free to come and go, they can go outside and stand in the sun, come in out of the wind, or move about if chilled, where as a confined animal has to take whatever conditions you and the barn provide.

Pneumonia has been caused by several bacteria, quite often a *Pasteurella,* and also viruses. Usually the animal or animals are stricken suddenly, with no warning. The first signs are unusually quick breathing, a drop in milk production, and perhaps a few dry, unproductive coughs. Next the cow begins to pant, quite often running a temperature of 104°F. to 106°F., and goes off feed. If let go longer, the animal begins to show signs of difficulty in breathing. The neck is extended, the nostrils flare, and the cow will grunt heavily on each breath. The animal usually dies shortly after beginning to grunt and foam at the mouth from lack of oxygen.

At the first signs of rough breathing or panting, it is best to isolate the animal as well as possible in a comfortable, draft-free stall. Take the cow's temperature. If the temperature is above 102°F., or the breathing doesn't improve overnight or during an afternoon, call your vet. A pneumonia suspect must receive prompt attention if the animal will ever amount to anything. I've treated animals in advanced stages of pneumonia (neck stretched out, grunting and down) and had them live. But when there is too much damage done to the lungs, nothing can be done to repair them and you will end up with an animal that acts like a person with emphysema. A beef animal will remain thin, using every bit of energy to breathe, not to eat and gain weight. A dairy animal will not milk as she should. A young animal won't grow like one that breathes normally, and will not milk well. It is possible to successfully treat an advanced pneumonia case, but the chances for complete recovery are much better if the animal is diagnosed and treated in the very early stages of the disease.

If a veterinarian is not available to make a positive diagnosis, or a probable one, you will have to do a little guesswork and treat the sick animal for pneumonia. Let me stress not to go ahead and treat a pneumonia cow if you do have a vet handy, since he can sometimes advise other ways to help save the animal. For example, he knows from past experience about steaming (or not steaming), use of cortisone, use of injectable expectorants to help clear congested lungs, or feeding the cow special "goodies." He will advise whether to take the animal outside or not, to force exercise or not, and so on.

A wide-spectrum antibiotic, such as penicillin-streptomycin or oxytetracycline, seems to work best. Antibiotic treatment should continue for at least four days, or until the animal seems well (no temperature, eating again, breathing better) for 24 hours. If the antibiotic treatment is stopped, or worse yet, only one shot given, an animal may develop resistant organisms to that antibiotic and suffer a relapse. This is much harder to treat than the original pneumonia.

Sulfonamides, oral or injectable, also usually work well in pneumonias. Remember, there are MANY sulfa drugs, and MANY more combinations. Make sure the sulfa you use is for pneumonia! I have had very good luck with triple sulfas, such as sulfadiazine, sulfamerazine, and sulfathiazole combined. When using any sulfa drugs, make sure that the cow or calf is drinking plenty of water, as sulfas can be hard on the kidneys if inadequate water is consumed.

PUNCTURE

A puncture wound in many ways is more dangerous to cattle than a wide open gash. A typical puncture happens when Bessy steps on a nail out in the field and comes hobbling home. Most times the nail has come out, leaving a tiny black hole which does not bleed, or if it does, only a few drops. The nail carries in bacteria, which are sealed in a nice, moist, warm incubator by the swelling, perfect for growth and multiplication. In addition to blackleg and tetanus organisms, many other bacteria can cause a severe infection, making the treatment of a puncture wound important.

As soon as the wound is noticed, the cow should be tied in a clean place where you can work on it. It should be a place where you can clean out the puncture as well as possible and keep it clean. The wound should be scrubbed well with hot, soapy water and irrigated with an antiseptic, such as iodine. An old syringe may be used, or any number of improvised things. Scrounge around the house—a doll bottle with a stiff plastic nipple or an ear syringe usually work fine. The important thing is not what you use but to get the antiseptic clear down to the bottom of the wound.

After treating the wound, it is a good idea to give a three-day systemic treatment with a broad-spectrum antibiotic, as an added precaution. A tetanus antitoxin injection is also a good idea. Cows do not get tetanus as often as horses do, but often enough to respect its presence.

RETAINED PLACENTA

A cow usually expels her afterbirth within a few hours after calving. If she has not expelled it 48 to 72 hours after calving, she is said to have a retained placenta and should then be checked by your vet.

Sometimes the placenta comes away by manual removal quite easily. The afterbirth is attached to the uterus by caruncles or "buttons." These buttons are the size of a potato and have a surface like a sponge, into which fits the placenta.

When the placenta is manually removed, the hand gently peels each "button," freeing the afterbirth. There are quite a few buttons, so it takes quite awhile to clean each one.

Sometimes the caruncles are swollen or there is an infection, making a thorough cleaning impossible. Many farmers insist on "having the cow cleaned" and pull and yank on the placenta until it comes away. This could be dangerous, as some of the caruncles can easily be pulled off too, and the cow may not carry another calf, not to mention the chance of severe bleeding.

In cases where the cow cannot be cleaned, your vet can give the cow an injection which will help the uterus cast off the placenta and place uterine boluses or powder to prevent infection and help dissolve the afterbirth. It is important to keep as much of the placenta hanging through the cervix as possible, keeping it open, since if it closes before all the shreds have passed out there is more chance of infection.

RINGWORM

Ringworm is not a worm nor is it caused by a worm or worms. It is a fungus-caused dermatosis, most often caused by *Trichophyton verrucosum.* It appears as rough, scaly, round patches of baldness, most often on the face and neck. It is most often found during the winter, since, like lice, the fungus is a lover of dark days and long hair. Although in small patches it is not dangerous, it can, if not treated, spread over quite a bit of the body, making the skin nonfunctioning, and is in this way harmful.

Treatment consists of removal of the thick, scaly dandruff by soaking with warm, soapy water and applying any one of the antifungal drugs. Tincture of iodine is one of the best and most easily obtainable drugs. The antifungal drug should be scrubbed into the lesion, working from the outside to the inside. Don't scrub from the inside out, as this can spread the lesion.

SCOURS

In Calves Scours is a term used for diarrhea in farm animals. Calves in the three-day to three-week age group are the usual victims of this problem. In the ideal situation, a newborn calf is allowed to nurse from its mother three times daily. If, after three days of colostrum milk, you need the cow's milk, the calf can be switched to goat's milk or allowed to suck its mother after she has been milked (this strips her milk and saves you from doing it). Colostrum is the first milk secreted after birth by the cow; it is necessary to provide antibodies for the calf but is generally discarded for human use.

The calf should not in my opinion be switched to powdered calf milk replacer. I do not believe in medicated feed, especially for very young calves. There is not enough antibiotic in a pound of feed to prevent scours or other diseases, and the antibiotic fed daily can damage enough of the natural and necessary bacteria in the gut to cause scours. Also, many of the powdered calf milk replacers on the market are quite insoluble and settle to the bottom in a layer of silt to be eaten by the calf, causing digestive upsets.

Unmedicated calf pellets are very good to start a calf on, along with a minimal amount of milk from its dam, a goat, or a nurse cow. Be careful here too, for nearly all *are* medicated. In fact, I only know of one in my part of the country that isn't—Carnation's Calf Manna.

When the calf consumes a full pound of pellets, along with a fair amount of good hay or pasture, it can be weaned. When feeding goat's milk to the calf and sometimes its dam's milk, it is necessary to use a calf bottle. If fed from a pail, the calf has a tendency to gulp great mouthfuls of milk, which can form large curds in the stomach while being digested. These large curds can easily upset the delicate digestion of a young calf. A nipple pail is better, as the calf sucks and gets less at once than drinking directly from a pail. The nipple pail does have disadvantages, though. They are hard to clean thoroughly. Also, dust, manure, hay, etc. can be flung by an overzealous calf into the open pail and can thus be swallowed along with the milk. With a bottle, the nipple pops off easily (for people, not the calf) and the bottle can easily be cleaned out and rinsed for next time.

Sometimes, even with the best of care, a calf will come down with scours. The usual causes are overeating—especially milk—and stress. Stress is *any* drastic change, and may result from changes in the weather, moving, emotional upset, changes in feeding routine, a switch from timothy hay to legume hay, and so forth.

A loose stool in a calf in the scour age bracket (3 to 21 days) warrants immediate attention. A normal calf stool is yellowish and like gooey putty. It should be formed. You know a calf has trouble when you see puddles in the bedding instead of manure, or a slime of manure stuck to its tail.

At the first sign of loose stools, discontinue all feeding, or if they are not too loose, cut the feedings in half. If the stool is quite loose, or you think you may have trouble getting to town tomorrow, try to get some oral electrolyte solution at your vet's or at the drug store. While you are there it may be a good idea to get some scour medicine, just in case you need it later. I have had good results with a kaolin-pectin-bismuth solution containing antibiotics. The kaolin solution soothes the gut and the antibiotic works on the destructive bacteria present.

I do not recommend giving scour medicine every time a loose stool is passed, as many times just laying off feeding milk for a day will effect a prompt return to normal. The electrolyte solution will provide fluid intake and restore the electrolyte balance in the body. (For discussion of this balance see "Electrolytes in the Body" in the final chapter.) If an electrolyte solution is impossible to get, feeding barley water will often help. This is made by simmering half a pound of barley in a gallon of water until the barley is tender. Drain off the gruel for the calf and save the barley to eat yourself! Feed the barley water, a pint at a time, every two hours for the day.

Keep a close watch on a calf that has shown an abnormal stool. If, as you are treating it with oral electrolytes or barley water, the stool progressively becomes worse, start it on scour medicine. Please read the directions on the label and follow them exactly. Scours is nothing to play around with. If the cure doesn't come quickly, the calf will die. It may not seem that a 100-pound calf full of bucks and kicks can die in a couple of days just from diarrhea, but it's true.

If you have any trouble in clearing up the scours in two days, call your vet. Sometimes an intravenous electrolyte injection over a 24-hour period is necessary, and a blood transfusion sometimes works miracles. I knew one Angus calf that was so sick it was laid out flat for two days, unable to raise even its head. We had it in the office with an intravenous drip for 36 hours and a heat lamp on. The only way we knew the calf was still alive was by its breathing. Then at night, we heard a bawl from the office. We went in and it had its head up and the eyes were open and bright. Two hours later it took some oral electrolytes from a bottle. The calf had stopped scouring and steadily improved. Two days later it nursed by itself from our old nurse cow. Today it weighs 800 pounds and its owner is glad he gave it a chance and gambled on such a poor risk. We are too, as it's things like this that makes being a veterinarian worthwhile.

Buying young calves at the stockyard is the surest way to buy calves that will get scours. There the calf is subjected to more stresses than possibly anywhere else. First is the emotional trauma of being separated from its mother, stallmates, or the company of other cattle it knows. Then comes the strange ride to the yards, in a trailer, truck, or worse, jammed into a trunk, sack, or crowded in a truck with a bunch of other animals. Next, the calf is unloaded and pushed into a strange pen with a bunch of calves, where they trade germs. Maybe one or two sick calves are in the bunch, to make matters worse. You buy the calf and take it home, changing the diet, schedule, and again changing its surroundings.

If you do buy a young calf at the stockyard, be prepared for scours and start medication as soon as the first loose stool hits the ground. Also be very stingy with the first three days' meals. If you can, give only a quart but feed every three hours; this is better than giving two quarts twice a day.

After the calf is older than three weeks, give or take a few days, it is usually past the calf scour stage, so you can relax a little.

In Adults During the summer months when cattle are on pasture, their stool becomes quite loose and is sometimes mistaken for scours. If in doubt, bring the animal into the barn or a dry barn lot and feed it hay for a day or two. If the looseness was simply due to eating lush green grass, the hay will return the stool to normal. If not, it is best to take the animal's temperature. Some diseases, such as shipping fever, have diarrhea as a symptom. (And, with shipping fever, the animal does NOT have to have been recently shipped anywhere.)

If the temperature is normal, take a stool sample into your veterinarian. By stool sample, I mean just a sample. A teaspoonful—not, as one farmer brought in, a whole bushelful. The vet can examine the sample under his microscope and tell if the animal has trouble with worms or other intestinal parasites, one of the commonest causes of diarrhea in cattle. You will not necessarily see worms in the manure when the animal has parasites, as some dangerous ones are microscopic. If the sample is negative for worm eggs, there is no reason to worm unless another test reveals the presence of them. Once in a while a test (almost any kind of test) results in a false negative, but with one examination negative for worm eggs, you can be fairly certain that they are not causing the scouring. It can kill an animal just to worm it if it acts sick. You assume the trouble must be worms, but it isn't.

Ask your veterinarian to give you some astringent antidiarrheal medicine. This comes in various forms: bolus, powder, or liquid. Give it according to directions. If this doesn't help in a short time—a day or two—ask your vet if he'd come out to thoroughly check the animal. There are many things that can cause scours in cattle, but it is usually something easily remedied. An allergy to a certain plant, slightly poisonous plants in the pasture, a moldy chunk of hay, too much feed, etc. can all cause scouring.

There are some more serious problems that can show scouring as a symptom. Johne's disease, BVD, hardware disease, poisons, and other ailments must pass through a veterinarian's mind as he examines a case of stubborn diarrhea.

During the winter months, especially with cattle that are confined in a barn, they become susceptible to what is called "winter scours" or "winter dysentery." This comes on suddenly, with several animals in a herd or perhaps just one or two developing a terrific diarrhea. If there are many animals in the herd, it usually will spread quickly until all or nearly all of the animals are affected. In milking animals there will be a sharp drop in milk production. One farmer whose entire dairy herd came down with it said, "I didn't get any milk this morning. Just manure!" He was sloshing around in two feet of sloppy manure in what had previously been a spotless barn.

The affected cattle can pass mucus and quite large quantities of blood. If the problem is noticed quickly and treatment is started (with an astringent antidiarrheal such as one percent copper sulfate solution 75 to 150 ml. daily for no more than three days, or catechu along with ferrous sulfate and copper sulfate several times daily), it will usually hold the animals until the "bug" (believed to be a virus) dies out.

SCREWWORMS

The screwworm used to be a very severe pest in the warm southern and southwestern United States. But now they have been found in nearly every state because animals have carried them to every part of the country. The USDA began an eradication program in the late 1950s in which they raised male flies which were sterilized by gamma radiation, and then they released them to breed with females. Since the female only mates once, if she mates with one of those USDA flies she would never be able to reproduce. The USDA program has been successful in cutting down markedly on the screwworm population in many parts of the country.

Blowflies must have a wound to deposit their eggs in. On hatching, these larvae become screwworms, crawl to the wound, and begin feeding. In approximately one week they drop to the ground, leaving an oozing, larger wound which attracts other flies, which in turn lay eggs, and so on.

In areas where screwworm is a very bad problem, routine spraying of the cattle is recommended. The cattle must be watched for wounds, and if one is found, an effective treatment is Smear 62. This is a lasting fly repellent which kills maggots, enabling the wound to heal.

SHIPPING FEVER

Shipping fever is a pneumonia enteritis complex, also known as hemorrhagic septicemia. It is most often brought on by stress, and shipping *is* a stress. But an animal does not have to be shipped or moved to come down with the disease.

Shipping fever can be quite contagious. The temperature is often high, sometimes reaching 105°F. There is rapid breathing with a rasping cough. There may be a heavy nasal discharge. The animal will often have diarrhea.

Death can be caused by lung consolidation or dehydration. Sulfas, tetracycline dihydrostreptomycin, and antiserum have been used to treat the disease. The use of antiserum is argued by researchers; some say it works well, others say it is worthless.

Antidiarrheals, good nursing, and expectorants will be of use. Adding one percent cobalt chloride to the water (one oz. per animal) will aid in stimulating the appetite.

TEAT AND UDDER INJURIES

Cows, due to their weight and clumsy ways, and also intentionally inbred "deformities" like huge bags and long teats, are more prone to udder and teat injuries than any other domestic animal. Two of the most common accidents which befall cows' udders and teats are stepping on and snagging those parts. If a cow doesn't manage to step on her own teat, some kind neighbor seems willing to do it for her. Sometimes nothing more serious than a bruise results, but many times there is a cut, tear, or mashed teat to contend with. If caught while the cut is still new or "fresh" (not dried up and scabbed over), the chances are good that if your veterinarian comes out and sews it up, healing will be rapid. To suture a cut that is a day or so old means putting in stitches that will probably not hold well, and may also mean sewing in bacteria that will cause an infection. With an old cut, it's best to let your vet decide what to do with it.

A cow objects to being milked when she has an injured teat, so the easiest course of action is to use a milk tube inserted in the udder to let the milk run out as needed. Some milk tubes have caps on their ends that can be unscrewed to let the milk out at certain times of the day. Tubes like these are good, as it is a bit unsanitary to have a cow leaking milk out all over the barn floor, especially in the summer. The flies might like it, but people don't.

It's not uncommon for cows with large, low-hanging bags to snag their udders on almost anything handy and rip them. Barbed wire fences and old dead brush seem to rank high on the list of causes of cow snags. Many bloody rips can be successfully sewn up, leaving little or no scar, so don't be talked into shooting your cow by some nice neighbor (they always seem to be so experienced with problems such as this, and so free with advice). An udder rip can be quite ugly. Many times they gape widely, bleed profusely, and leak milk. Of course, after such an injury the affected quarter or quarters may not give as much milk as before, but generally it pays to have them taken care of.

To stop excessive bleeding, pack clean cloths against the injury quite hard until the blood stops flowing. This may take several minutes. Leave a cloth on the wound, as the blood will clot between the cloth and the injury; when you pull the cloth off, it will quite often start to bleed again. Don't put anything on the wound before the veterinarian arrives. It is sometimes hard to suture a wound—and see what you're doing—if it is gobbed up with powder or gooey salve. The important thing is to call the vet as soon as you see the rip, and to keep the area as clean as possible. No barn surgery is sterile, but it won't help an animal to lie down in six inches of manure and dirt with a gaping wound.

Milk Vein Injuries While we're on this part of the cow, let's move just a little forward to an injury that is fairly common in larger cows. On each side of a cow, viewed from underneath, runs a very large blood vessel known as the milk vein. On a large, high milk-producing cow, this vein is as big as three inches across, making it a prime target for injury. Cows sometimes catch this vein on a nail, step on it while rising, hook it with a sharp dewclaw on a front leg, etc. When this vein is nicked or cut, it bleeds profusely, to put it mildly, and if cut badly the cow can bleed to death.

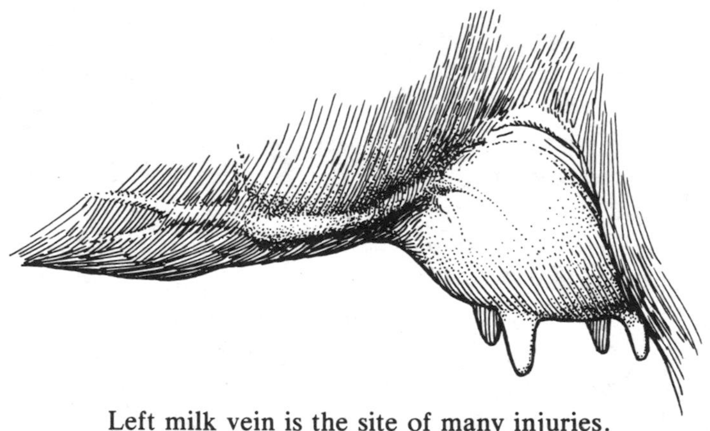

Left milk vein is the site of many injuries.

If a cow should get this sort of injury, check to see how badly it is bleeding. Remember, a little blood sometimes looks like a lot. If it is dripping, leave it alone (unless you should have some blood-stopping powder for use when dehorning; this will sometimes stop it) and call your vet. If it is running out in a stream as big as your little finger, sometimes a pressure pack will stop it or at least slow it down to almost a standstill. Keep the pack on and have someone else call the vet. Make sure you tell him you think she cut a milk vein. He'll know it's an emergency call and get there as soon as possible.

When a milk vein is cut badly enough that the blood is pouring out in a heavy stream, get a rope ten to twelve feet long, or several binder twines fastened together, and tightly pull it around the cow's body to form a tourniquet while someone else RUNS to call the vet. The rope will usually slow down the blood to a slow drip, but will not stop the bleeding permanently. The wound must be sewn.

Once the wound has been taken care of, you will have to keep the cow in and keep her very well bedded so that she doesn't catch the stitches and rip them loose, starting the whole thing over again. It is sometimes necessary to wrap a sheet around her belly to keep straw from poking the injury for a few days, to be sure the healing is quick and complete. There are usually no bad aftereffects.

TETANUS

Tetanus is caused by *Clostridium tetani.* Although it is more often a problem of horses, it does occur quite often in cattle. Tetanus organisms grow only in the absence of oxygen, so are only a hazard in a puncture or otherwise sealed-off wound.

I have seen several cases of tetanus in bull calves that have been castrated with elastrators (the rubber band method) and have seen it following dehorning and surgical castration. When tetanus follows castration, it is almost always due to the operator making too small an opening. After the castration this tiny incision closes off, making a dandy incubator for tetanus organisms.

A cow or calf with tetanus will usually be reluctant to move, stand with its neck stretched out, possibly drool, and be unable to eat or drink. The membrane in the corner of the eye typically covers nearly half of the eye. The stiffness progresses until death follows. There is no sure treatment although massive doses of tetanus antitoxin or penicillin have worked.

Cattle are usually not vaccinated for tetanus but there certainly is no reason why they should not be or cannot be, especially where a case has been diagnosed. Tetanus can be prevented by giving *antitoxin* when there has been an injury. This immediately builds up immunity, and thus gives quick protection. But this protection, though quick, does not last long. Tetanus *toxoid* is given routinely to protect against an unknown injury causing tetanus. But it still is a good idea to give the antitoxin if an injury is known to have happened, as *NO* vaccine is 100 percent sure.

TICKS

Ticks are the same type of creature as lice, but larger. They are flat and differ in size; they may be the size of a small pea or nearly that of a fat nickel when full of blood. Empty, they are usually a darkish color—brown or black. When full of blood and attached to an animal, they become grayish. In some geographic areas cattle are not particularly bothered and only pick up an occasional tick which may be picked off at milking time. In other areas it becomes necessary to dip, spray, or powder cattle periodically. Check with your vet or county agent on this.

Other than sucking blood and looking ugly, ticks can spread disease. Who hasn't heard of Texas tick fever from all those Westerns on TV? There are still areas of the country where ticks can spread disease, so it's best to find out what is happening in your area.

Where lice are most prevalent in the winter, ticks prefer the summer months and seem to have a "season" when they are the worst.

WORMS—INTERNAL PARASITES

Volumes can—and have been—written about internal parasites of cattle. There are many families and many individual worms involved. A few are the common stomach worm, medium stomach worm, small stomach worm, hookworm, tapeworm, threadworm, lungworm, and large-mouth bowel worm.

When suspecting worms in your cattle (weight loss, potbelly, bad hair coat, weakness, and coughing are all possible symptoms), take a small fecal sample to your vet for examination. It is not enough that you don't find any sign of worms in the manure, as many are invisible to the naked eye. He can check this sample under the microscope for the presence of worm eggs or larvae. When you know the type of worm your cattle have, you can use the right medicine to rid them of the parasites. But if they do not have worms, you could kill them by using a toxic wormer. It has often happened this way. Cattle, weak from pneumonia or lice, have been killed by a well-meaning farmer who figured the trouble must be worms ("So I gave 'er a little more than the label said, just to make sure I got rid of all of 'em."). Cattle should be checked for worms more frequently than they are, as many cattle, both beef and dairy, would do better if they didn't have to feed all those worms.

Liver fluke is a serious problem especially in swampy or lowland areas, because liver flukes are carried by snails. The snail passes encysted larvae which adhere to grasses and leaves. When they are eaten by a grazing cow, the cyst breaks and the new liver fluke penetrates the intestine and migrates to the liver. Here, along with fellow flukes, it rambles about, destroying liver tissue.

An affected cow or heifer may keep its weight and just suddenly die. On autopsy, you'd wonder how it possibly seemed well for as long as it did. The cow may also begin to act dumpy and progressively get worse, no matter what is done to help it. If you know you are in a liver fluke area, it is best to fence off any lowlands you have on the farm, if possible.

Intramuscular injections of carbon tetrachloride and hexachloroethane have been recommended, but to use these on dairy cows in production or cattle that have liver damage and are acting sick could do as much damage as the flukes at times.

If you suspect you have flukes, have your vet do an autopsy to be sure. He may be able to steer you onto something that is working for him, as there are new discoveries every day in veterinary medicine.

GOATS

Goats are fast becoming the dairy animal for the "little people"—people with only a few acres or a need for only a small amount of milk and dairy products. (Dairy goats have been

Parts of a Goat

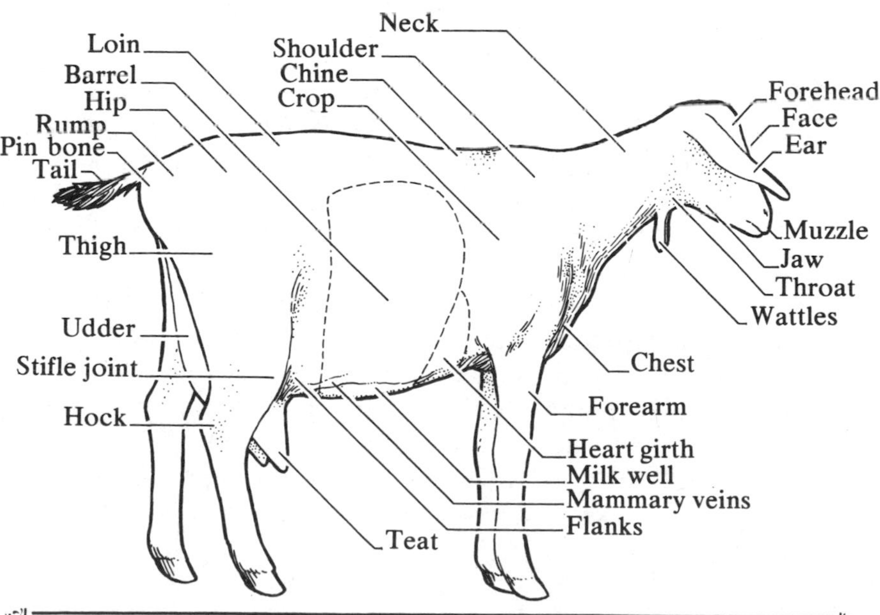

bred up in milking ability so that a doe that milks a gallon daily isn't rare.) They are such a clean and pleasant animal with a nice, intelligent personality, it is no wonder they are becoming popular.

People are being educated away from the "goats smell and eat tin cans and butt people" image that cartoons instilled in their minds as "facts." It is only the buck that carries that musky odor, mainly in the fall breeding season. And since they can be descented by a minor operation, few have any odor at all.

Although many people think of goats as replacements for cows, goats are not just small cows—they belong to an individual species and have their own particular problems, along with several ailments shared by many domestic creatures.

General Care and Management

HOUSING

Dry and milking does do best if allowed free housing where they may wander in and out at will. The only exception to this would be if the kids are allowed to nurse their mother. Eager kids that are nursing will sneak a suck or two (or the whole bagful if permitted) from several does, not just their mother, if the does are around. This can cause digestive upsets and is a waste of milk. It can also cause injury to the kids, as angry does kick and butt the thief. Does that are kept tied short or are kept in stanchions are more prone to arthritis, lameness, and leg swellings. Large, draft-free, well-bedded loafing pens, with an outside paddock for exercise and sun, keep does healthy and happy.

Don't forget the buck when allowing room for pens. All too many bucks are shut away from the herd in a small, filthy, dark pen, and no attention is paid to them other than at breeding season. He needs exercise and sunshine as much as the does. After all, he *is* half your herd. Another buck can often be kept with him or a wether—castrated buck—or a doe that is not being milked. A buck needs companionship and will not do as well without it. Nervous habits such as chewing on wood, beating the wire with his head or horns, or masturbating can many times be prevented with a companion and outside run.

Goats are not basically grazers as are sheep and cattle, but browsers, preferring tender willow tips and other brush. This is the most important reason for having a goat-proof fence to contain them. Apple and other fruit trees rank high on a goat's goodie list, as do flowers and ornamental shrubbery. As a rule, goats are hard to contain. Barbed wire won't do anything, and plain woven wire stock fence does little. Many goats can be successfully kept in with a two-strand electric fence, but I've found some determined caprines that grit their teeth and dash through or under the fence, in spite of the shock they receive.

When planning to use electric fences for goats, you must train them, that is, teach them that flimsy-looking wire jolts when touched, making them fear to even get near the wire. This is accomplished by putting the goat in the fence and setting a pan of grain just outside. Then walk away so the goat doesn't think *you* did the dirty trick to it!

I've found on my farm that a combination electric fence and woven wire will contain anything placed inside. This is more formidable than just the electric wire and yet the electric wire is there to keep animals away from the woven wire. (It seems that one of the goats always has to graze on the other side of the fence, smashing the wire down if it's there by itself.)

If you have only one or two goats, they may be kept staked out, but there are many problems with staking. A dog can

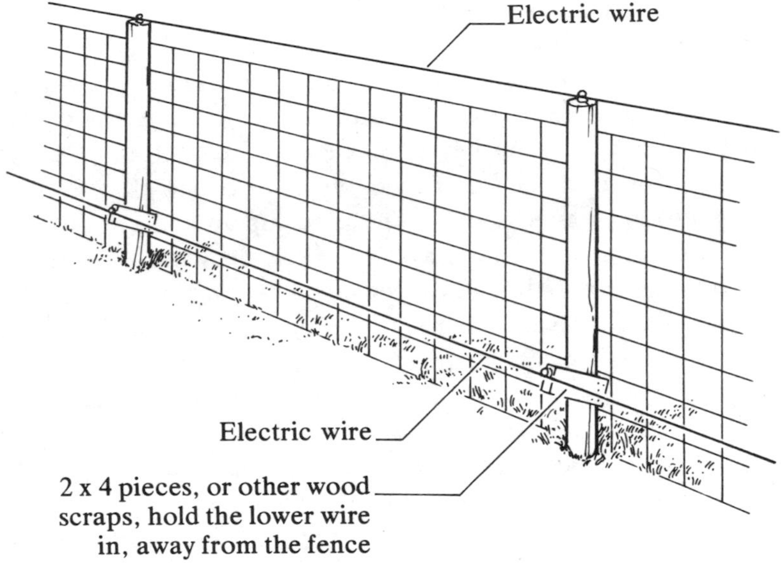

Goat-Proof Fence

worry and even kill a goat, as goats haven't much defense when tied. Sunstroke is also a problem. The amount of shade during the day must be taken into account when staking a goat. Where there is shade in the morning, there may be none for the hot afternoon. If it goes unnoticed, there may be a dead goat in the evening. It is hard to provide water for a staked-out animal. It seems they *always* tip the pail over ten minutes after being watered. A goat doesn't get much exercise if tied short, and gets tangled up if on a long rope. Goats have been known to break legs after wrapping them up in a chain or rope, then panicking and thrashing about.

A goat hates getting wet. A few drops of rain will send a herd stampeding for shelter, screaming as if they were being eaten alive by wolves, so be sure your goat pasture has access to shelter.

I believe that many of the problems encountered by goat people stem from either overcrowding or too much warmth in the winter months. Many goats may be run together in the loafing-barn/free-access-paddock system, but not where the goats are penned inside. In any group of goats there is a "pecking order," with the toughest goat being boss, and on down the line. The strongest or bossiest goats will hog the hay rack, grain trough, and even sometimes the water pail and salt block. When one of the meeker ones tries to eat or drink, the bossier ones butt it away, keeping it in its place. Sometimes severe injuries and even death can result. The boss goat does not necessarily have horns either. A small group of goats may be kept in a large stall, but hay should be on hand at all times in a long manger to reduce the fighting, and the goats should be separated when receiving their grain.

A doe that is due to kid should be separated from the others. She should not be tied, but put in a roomy pen near the other goats, but kept apart so the others will not bother her while kidding or be hurt themselves by an overprotective mother.

A heated barn for goats is not necessary, even in the coldest climates, and really does more harm than good. As with cows, it's more comfortable to milk and do chores in a nice warm barn, but a warm barn is quite often a damp one, and with the dampness comes trouble with pneumonia. If you must have a cozy place to milk, build a small milking parlor in one corner of the barn and heat that. The goats won't be in it long enough to have trouble from it, and you won't have cold hands.

FEEDING

Goats, like dairy cattle, must have good food to produce a decent amount of milk and maintain their own weight. Speaking of weight, a dairy goat to many people looks thin. It is perfectly normal for a milking doe to have a "bony topside." So many new goat people are shocked at the "underfed" appearance of their new goat and swear the previous owner starved her. They immediately begin to fatten her up. In six months the previously healthy goat looks like a fat beef steer and is having breeding or kidding problems. A high milk-producing doe many times puts her all into the milk pail and loses much fat. She is not skinny but trim, like a race horse on the track.

A naturally chubby goat quite often does not milk well. This is not to say that a skinny goat is in good shape. A goat with backbone sticking up and no flesh on at all certainly needs weight and cannot produce milk if she is emaciated. If unsure of the proper weight for your goat, ask an experienced goat breeder in your area or a veterinarian who is used to goats.

In the ideal situation, dairy goats should have access to a pasture, preferably seeded with a legume-grass mixture. There may be small brush to browse, but once in a while goats may eat brush which may give off-flavors to the milk. There should be a rack of hay in their shelter to munch on while inside for shade or rain protection, as well as wintertime. This hay should be changed daily, as some hays become dusty or moldy and can become a health hazard, causing bloat and bowel upsets. There should be a constant supply of trace mineral iodized salt available. Many areas of the country are lacking in one or more minerals, which if not provided in the form of salt or feed supplements may cause a variety of problems.

If a water supply is not available all the time, goats must be watered at least twice daily, being allowed to drink as much as they need. The watering should be done *before* giving grain, since if given after the grain, they may bloat. In the summer the water should be cool, and the winter water should have the chill taken off. During the summer, if a pail of water is left for the goats, make sure they are drinking. Goats will very seldom drink unclean water. Manure, a dead mouse, or other unsavory material falling in the water will usually keep the goats away. And drinking less water will mean a cutback on the amount of milk produced. Goats *can* get by on the snow they eat in the winter instead of regular water, but don't expect much production from them in the way of milk or kids. They can sometimes produce both, but it is a risky way to farm because of the chances of dehydration.

A dry doe most of the time requires little if any grain. Good legume hay or lush pasture will usually keep the dry doe in good flesh but not overly fat. It is the fat, sluggish doe that quite often has kidding problems. As the doe becomes heavy with kids, it is usually wise to increase her grain, as it is during the last month or so that the kids begin to grow large enough to become a drain on her. It is wise to cut back on the amount of grain given just before she is due, as sometimes this will prevent milk fever in a high milk-producer. After freshening, you may gradually increase the amount of grain fed, bringing the doe to full production. There is no hard and fast rule about the amount of grain needed by goats, as each animal is an individual and must be fed as such. Also there is a great variety of feeds available. However, you won't go too wrong feeding the following (assuming you are using a good mixed grain ration):

Kids, birth to four or five months: free choice.
Older kids to dry yearlings: one pound daily.
Bred does, dry: one to two pounds daily or less, depending on other feed available, such as lush pasture or good legume hay.
Does heavy with kid: two pounds daily.
Milking does: ½ to one pound for each two pounds of milk given daily.
Bucks with heavy service: two to three pounds daily.

These are not hard and fast rules, and the amounts may be

increased or decreased as the animal's condition and production indicate.

DO NOT FEED UREA OR FEED CONTAINING UREA TO GOATS. Much mixed dairy ration today contains urea, a cheaper protein supplement. Read the label on the bag, ask the feed store owner, but make sure. Goats are easily poisoned by feeding urea; feed meant for cattle often contains urea, but goats can't handle it without disaster.

Goats are naturally friendly animals that like plenty of attention and handling, if raised from the start without mistreatment or fear. They love to have their necks scratched, shoulders rubbed, and sides petted. They *hate* to have their ears pulled. I have Nubians, and it seems that visitors simply must pull their ears, so be on the alert with your company. And pulling or wrestling with a goat's horns is a sure way to invite trouble. The most mild-mannered goat can become nasty with its horns, if taught to do so by its owners. We know of a little horned buck that was teased this way, that is until he finally put his owner in the hospital with 18 stitches in his leg.

RESTRAINT

The goat, being smaller than a cow, is easier to restrain. Usually the only restraint needed is a stanchion—the milking stanchion works well because it is raised, giving them less area to dance back and forth on—or a secure place to tie it with a halter or collar. Goats, distracted by a measure of grain, easily learn that hoof trimming or routine clipping of the hair does not hurt and soon ignore it.

Working on an injured teat or breaking a young doe to milk calls for patience on your part. You have to use your arm, pressed against her leg to guard against kicks and to hold her from dancing around so much. It usually does no good to hold one of your legs up, especially when breaking a doe to milk, as you can't milk her the rest of her life with one of your legs off the ground. Sometimes when it's necessary to work on a bad injury to a teat, it becomes necessary to slip a figure 8 around the hocks. The end of the rope or twine is held by a helper. Do not tie it, because if she should fall or get panic-stricken, she could break a leg.

Pressing your head firmly into her flank, holding her against a solid wall with her head tied, is a good way to hold a jumpy goat with little danger to either of you. Don't quit or give up if she does jump around a bit. She may just be trying you to see if she can make you quit, and not succeeding, she will often quit herself.

To catch a goat running around in a pen, especially one which is not used to people and does not have a collar or halter on, get as close as possible to it, reach out quickly, and grab the beard, or with a beardless goat, put a hand under the chin. Tip the head up and push it against the side of the pen. This will keep it off-balance and easy to hold.

To drench the goat or give a bolus, straddle the neck, facing the head. Tip the chin up and dose. When giving a drench, pour slowly enough that the animal doesn't choke or get any of the fluid in the lungs. This will cause aspiration pneumonia and quite often kill the goat. A bolus can be greased or coated with Vaseline before being given, which will make it slide down easily. If you must give a very large bolus, it is usually best to break it in half or thirds, to prevent choking. Many boluses are made with cattle in mind and are a little too big for a goat to swallow with ease.

When taking a goat's temperature, it is usually easiest to crowd the animal against a solid wall with your knee. Goats do not like their tail pulled, so it is easier to get them to stand still to have the temperature taken if the tail is not handled.

To restrain a small kid, you may hold it between your knees while seated, or have an assistant hold it while drenching, giving pills, treating cuts, etc. When more restraint is needed, a kid box or bag can be used. The box can be of heavy cardboard with a head hole in it, with the cover tied with heavy twine. The box should be just big enough for the kid to fit into, but not roomy enough to squirm around in. The bag should serve the same function. It is made of heavy canvas with either an enforced hole for the head or a drawstring, making the bag snug around the neck to prevent the front feet from coming through. Such a bag or box is used for dehorning, descenting bucklings, or treating facial lacerations, and can be modified by cutting a small hole to give intravenous injections in the leg vein, which is sometimes easier than hitting the jugular vein on a kid.

BREEDING

The Heat Cycle The doe normally comes into heat every 21 days, more or less, mainly in the fall and early winter. Many continue coming into heat until spring or early summer, provided they have not been bred, so it is not impossible to have does kid every month of the year. The doe will be in heat from one to three days. Bear in mind that each doe is an individual. She may differ from the "normal" and still be normal.

When there are several does with a buck running with them, signs of heat are very easily detected. The most obvious is the extreme interest of the buck in one or two does. He will paw at the doe, sticking his tongue out, or nibble along her body, making guttural grunts. She will respond by wagging her tail, urinating, squatting, and bleating.

If the buck is not running with the does, the doe in heat may suddenly start hanging around as near to the buck pen as possible. She may bleat, run back and forth, wag her tail, ride other does, or be ridden by them. Her vulva may be red and swollen. She may have strings of mucus on her tail or sides. When stroked across the back, she may wag her tail. When she is taken to the buck, he will show extreme interest in her. (There are some bucks that show extreme interest in any doe, regardless of whether or not she is in heat, so know the buck.) If the doe is in heat, she will allow the buck to mount her. The hard part comes when there is no buck, and there are no other does to help indicate heat in a single doe. There are many cases where a doe is sold as sterile, simply because she didn't make it to the buck while in heat.

Many times there is a drop in milk production when a doe comes into heat. Be alert for changes in personality. She may get bossy, nervous, or act strange when in heat. When stroked across the back, she may wag her tail and bleat. If possible, it is best to take her to the buck you plan on using (make reservations first, in advance of the heat) and leave her for a month. If he breeds her the first day you take her there, fine. But it is possible to be just a tiny bit late or early, and to make sure, it is wisest to leave her there until she is a few days late with her next scheduled heat period. It may cost a few dollars for boarding fees, but you will save in the long run by not having to feed a doe you thought was bred, missing out on all that milk in the spring.

The Pregnancy After your doe is bred, let her come home and settle back to routine life. Do not try to get her fat by graining her to death. Just continue feeding on the basis of how much milk she gives and her general condition. Be sure she gets daily exercise, especially during the winter when many goats are kept confined. A doe that gets little exercise will be in poor muscle tone when kidding time arrives; she will have a harder time kidding and will have weaker kids. The exercise should not be violent, such as climbing and jumping, but gentle, such as walking about for hay, salt, and water.

Approximately five months from the date of service, the doe will kid. Four months from the time of service, the doe will have begun to increase tremendously in girth and begin to "build bag," or to fill out in the udder.

KIDDING, NORMAL

There are two positions for birth which are normal. The most common is the front presentation. The doe just prior to kidding may or may not lose interest in feed, paw, appear restless, grunt, or lie down and get up repeatedly. When she passes strings of bloody mucus, you'll know she's beginning labor in earnest.

Front Presentation With the front presentation, the first thing usually to appear is a dark round bulge (the water bag). This is closely followed by two feet and a nose. The average doe (if there is one!) usually works 15 to 45 minutes to deliver the first kid. If all appears well, leave her alone. Too much "help" can upset her and cause trouble.

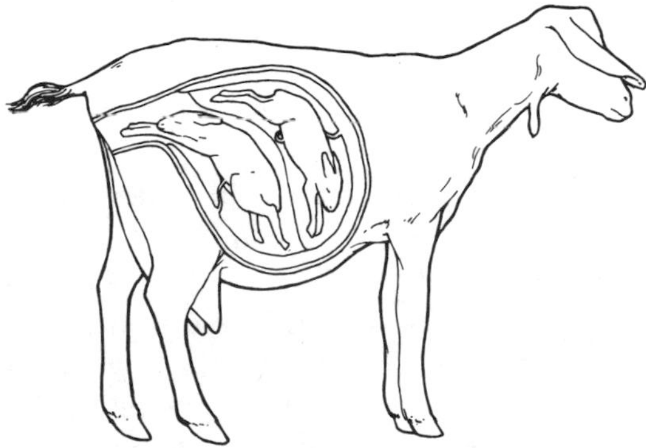

Normal Presentation of Twins

The kid is born in three stages. First the head and front feet, then shoulders, and finally, the hips and back legs. The nose and mouth should be cleaned of afterbirth and mucus to prevent suffocation or inhalation of fluids. If the kids are born in very cold weather, and it is below freezing in the barn, dry them immediately and provide a heat lamp. Ears and feet freeze very easily, and frozen parts will become gangrenous and fall off.

Posterior Presentation The other normal birth position is the posterior presentation. Here the water bag is followed by two feet but no head. The toes will point up instead of down, as seen in the front presentation. It is easier generally for the doe to give birth to a kid when it is in this position, as there is not the bulge of the head and shoulders so abruptly.

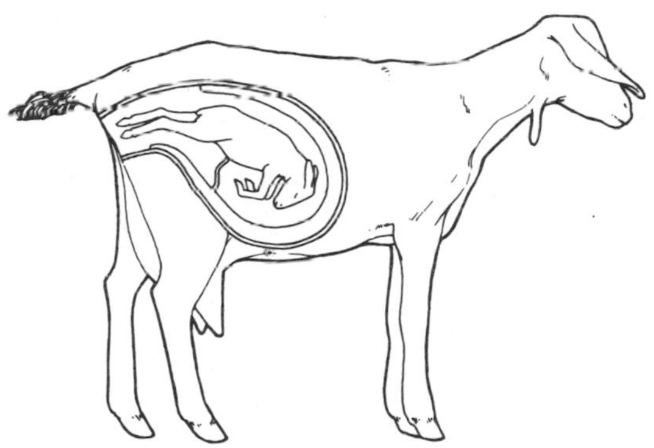

Normal Birth—Rear Presentation

The only problem encountered with the rear presentation is that as soon as the umbilical cord breaks, the kid begins to breathe. If the head is in the birth canal, the kid can suffocate or inhale fluids, causing death. For this reason, it is best to help the doe having a backward kid as soon as the kid is out up to the shoulders. Don't yank, but apply firm pressure downward as she pushes. Clean out the mouth and nose well. If the kid is not breathing well, hold it upside down by the hind legs and smack its side with the flat of your hand, quite hard. This will generally force any mucus and fluid out and begin normal breathing. This is what doctors do with human babies. The shock of that slap causes the kid to draw a deep breath, and holding it up by the feet drains the fluid out.

After the kid is breathing well and is dried off, apply an antiseptic such as iodine to the navel. This will help prevent navel infection, scours (diarrhea), and crippling joint infections later on. A wide-mouthed jar is good. Just hold it tight to the belly and slosh well, completely drenching the whole umbilical cord. Daubing a little on isn't enough for thorough coverage.

There are more possible abnormal positions in goats than other animals due to the multiple births and legginess of the fetuses. This is not to say there are more problems with goats, but a wider variety of *possible* problems.

KIDDING, ABNORMAL

Front presentation—head back When the doe has been in labor for some time, producing only two front legs and no head, you can strongly suspect that the head has deflected off the brim of the pelvis and is turned back. DO NOT PULL ON THE LEGS. It will only make matters much worse.

Scrub up with a mild dish soap and lubricate your hand and arm with it. Carefully slip in and check. Work down one front leg to the chest. Make sure both legs belong to the same kid (keep twins in mind). Then follow up the neck and locate the head. Usually the head can be cupped in your hand while being drawn back into position. A grip can also be had in the eye sockets (this will not hurt the kid) or in the lower jaw. You may have to push the forelegs back in order to gain room enough to slip the head into the birth canal. Once the head is in between the legs, gentle, firm traction will aid the doe in moving it on its way into the world.

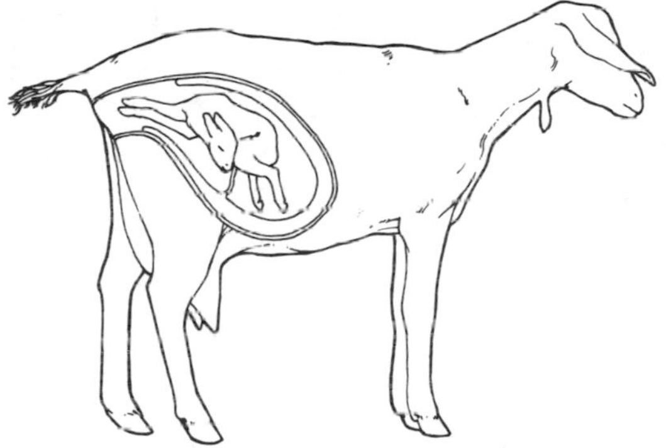

Abnormal Birth—Head Turned Back

Front presentation–one or both legs back If the doe labors a while and produces nothing but the water bag or perhaps just the tip of the nose, suspect the front legs are folded back, stopping the birth. (If only one is back, you will see one hoof and perhaps the nose.)

Again, scrub up and lubricate your hand and arm. Follow the neck down to the chest, then to one leg. Be *sure* it belongs to the kid whose head is in the birth canal. It can be easy to grab its twin's leg. Two can't be born at once! You may have to shove the head back to get space to slip the legs up. Shield the uterus from the hoof by cupping your hand over it. Slip the leg over the brim of the pelvis and through the cervix. Repeat this procedure if the other leg is back.

When everything is in position, a little traction (remember, pull down!) applied will help the doe, as she may be tired.

Breech presentation—both legs back The doe will strain for some time, but may not work as hard as usual. Nothing but the water bag is produced. When you examine, you will run into a round ball—the buttocks. Work your hand down to find the stifle, then the hock. Gently shove forward, just above the hock, and at the same time, try to slip the leg back over the brim of the pelvis. Keep the hoof covered as soon as you can grab it, as a torn uterus can mean a dead doe. Work carefully. Once one leg is up, you can grasp it, shoving the kid back. This makes the other leg easier to bring up. Once in proper position, treat as a normal rear presentation. Be sure to clean out the nose and throat.

Mixed delivery—tangled twins Here, there can be a wide variety of possibilities: a leg of one twin, head and leg of another, rear leg of one and front leg and head of another, three legs and one head, and so on. If a doe labors over half an hour without giving birth, it is advisable to go in and see what's happening. Be *sure* of what you are feeling. Don't just assume that things are as they appear. If all seems okay, withdraw and give her a bit longer. Some does are just slow, or may only require a bit of gentle traction.

If there are tangled twins, all you have to do is untangle them (ha!). Take your time and work carefully and slowly enough that you know what you're doing. It may take some doing, but once the twins are untangled, delivery should proceed fairly easily. One twin, usually the one without the head in the birth canal, is shoved back, allowing the other twin to move ahead. Traction may be needed to slide the first kid far enough that the second kid will not interfere with the first birth.

Abnormal births that require veterinary help Any doe that is in hard labor for over 45 minutes without producing a kid should be examined. If it is just an abnormal position, most kids can be delivered by the owner using common sense plus a little knowledge. Sometimes, though, a really difficult birth needs added experience. If you work with the doe for longer than 15 minutes without results, it is best to call your veterinarian.

I'd say a general rule to follow in a complicated delivery is to examine the doe. If you feel competent to make the necessary correction, work for no longer than 15 minutes. If you haven't been successful by then, call your vet. An exhausted doe is a poor risk. Also, too much trauma is a huge stress which can easily put a doe into shock. Such a doe is also bad to work on. No vet likes to work on a half-dead doe, and will usually charge accordingly.

Too Large a Kid If the kid is just too large to pass through the birth canal, a caesarean may be done, generally with very good results provided the doe is not exhausted when the surgery is performed.

A Dead Fetus Sometimes a kid dies before birth. When this happens, the fetus may absorb fluids and swell up. If it becomes too large, it sometimes is necessary for a veterinarian to remove a leg and shoulder in order to gain room for the rest of the fetus to pass. This is done by a special hooked knife called an embryotomy knife. This has a small blade that can be shielded by the hand to protect the uterus from accidental cuts.

Torsion of the Uterus Occasionally a doe experiences a torsion of the uterus. This most often happens in older does with twins or triplets heavy in the uterus. The uterus gets twisted, making delivery impossible until the torsion

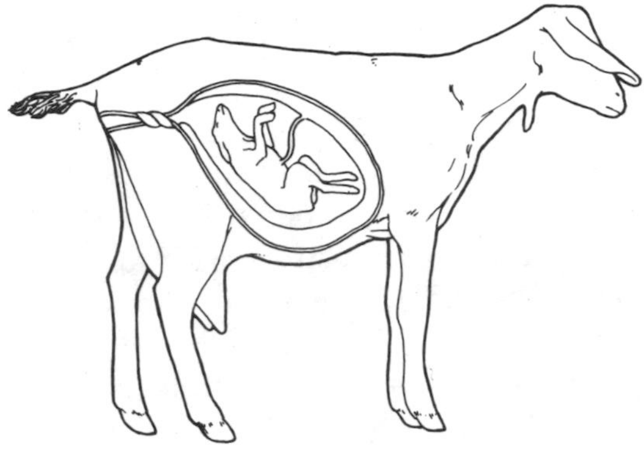

Abnormal Birth—Torsion of the Uterus

is corrected. This can be quite a job, as it is hard to figure out which way it has turned. A torsion rod is often a great help. This is fastened to the kid's legs, making turning the uterus easier. The only problem is space. If the uterus was twisted tight before any part of the kid entered the birth canal, there is no way to get hold of the legs or work the rod in. In cases like this, rolling the doe over will often flop the uterus over into proper position. This is tricky, even with experience, because if you roll her the wrong way, there is a chance of making the uterus twist tighter instead of going into proper position. Sometimes a caesarean is the only course of action.

For other problems related to pregnancy and kidding, see "Milk Fever," "Retained Placenta," "Eversion of the Uterus," "Freezing" (especially of kids), "Ketosis," and "Infertility" in the section, **Diseases and Other Problems**, later in this chapter.

CASTRATION

Only the best of bucklings should be left bucks. Selling a buck born from an inferior doe or an accidental breeding to be used as a buck will only injure the reputation of dairy goats in general. And keeping such a buck "because he's pretty" or some such reason will only degrade your own stock. Surplus bucklings should be castrated. Wethers then can either be used for meat or sold as pets. (It takes a real goat lover to have a *buck* for a pet!)

There are three main methods of castrating, only two of which we'll talk about. The other is the use of an elastrator or "rubber band" method. I do not advise use of this method at all. I've treated too many "mistakes" because of it. It is painful—for an extended period, not just a few minutes. Tetanus and infections can result when the scrotum is half off. Flies can lay eggs, producing a mass of maggots in the wound the next day, often when you've nearly forgotten about the band. I sincerely believe the other two methods are far more humane and just as easy.

Clamping or "Pinching" This is my choice in castrating. It is bloodless. There is no open sore at any time to become infected or pick up tetanus organisms. It is easy to do and very inexpensive if your veterinarian does it. The cords and blood vessels are simply crushed, and the testicles slowly atrophy and shrink up. They do not drop off.

To use this method, beg, borrow, or buy a Burdizzo emasculatome. I've seen too many "slips" from imperfect imitations. There are different sizes. For kids, get the smallest one, designed for use on lambs. The larger ones will work, but are a little heavy and clumsy to handle. Have an assistant hold the kid, or an older buck can be tied short and held against a wall or partition. The operator then grasps the scrotum and identifies one testicle. Feeling upward, he should identify the cord. The Burdizzo is placed across the cord. Care must be taken that the center division is not included, or serious trouble may arise later. The handles of the Burdizzo are then closed and held closed for a few seconds. The same procedure is repeated on the second testicle. The same method may be used on all bucks, regardless of size or age.

Surgical Castration This is a sure and quite safe operation for the animal. I would advise a tetanus antitoxin injection following this procedure, just to be safe, but I've never known a goat to get tetanus when operated on in a clean manner, when the incisions were large enough. Once in a while bleeding is a problem, but this can generally be averted if care is taken.

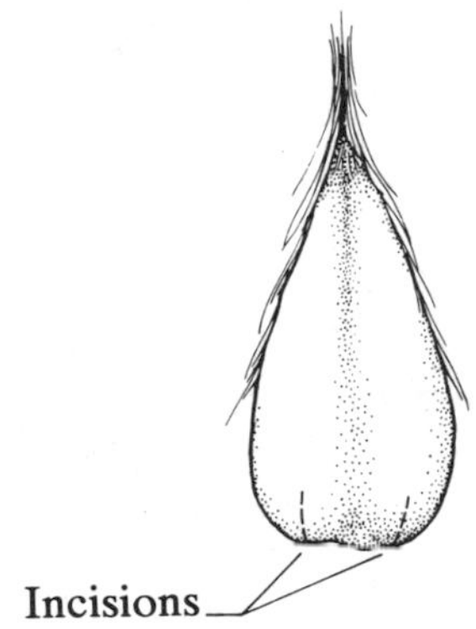

Site of Incisions for Surgical Castration

Very young kids are easiest to do, and the operation is safer for them at this time. An assistant holds the kid on his lap while the operator works. The scrotum is washed with warm soapy water. A scalpel, razor blade, or sharp knife is used to make the incisions. The testicle is held between the thumb and fore-finger, bulging it toward the bottom of the scrotum. An incision is made at least an inch long. The testicle and tunic (the white membrane covering the testicle) are then pulled through the incision.

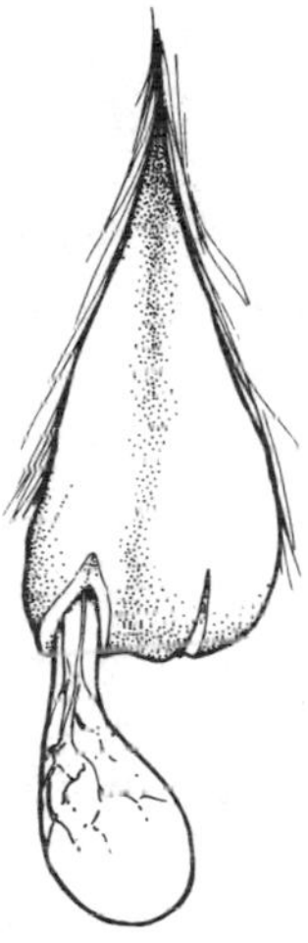

The testicle and tunic are pulled out of the scrotum.

If the buckling is fairly small, the cord will be small, requiring no tying or crushing. The testicles can be pulled out until the cord snaps. There is little if any bleeding, as opposed to cutting the cord with a sharp knife. If the kid is larger, the cord can be separated with a knife, but should be scraped until it breaks instead of making a sharp cut, as this will lessen the chances of bleeding. The cord and tunic should be drawn well out of the scrotum, for if the stump hangs out, incomplete healing will often result in a buildup of scar tissue known as a scirrhous cord. And it is a *mess* to repair.

When castrating large bucks by surgery, it is advisable to use an emasculator to crush the blood vessels and cord while cutting at the same time. The incisions are made and one testicle is drawn out. The emasculator is applied first to that testicle, then to the other. If an emasculator is not used, the stumps can be tied off with catgut (available through your veterinarian), but crushing is usually safer, as ligatures sometimes slip.

DEHORNING

Generally speaking, horns cause trouble when left on goats. Even the most gentle doe can accidentally swing her head around and catch a person in the face or eye. Children are often injured in this way, as they do not grasp the fact that Star could hurt them even though she loves them dearly.

Horns on bucks are a danger. True, not many bucks are mean, but horns are an invitation to trouble. All bucks play to show their good spirits and virility. This play can sometimes get a little out of hand, especially if he has a four-foot rack of horns! I know of several people injured by bucks this way. One man had his leg ripped open and required 18 stitches. And once a buck finds use for his horns, he often gets a little "pushy" or belligerent at his new-found strength and really becomes dangerous.

Goats can injure each other with horns. I lost a registered Nubian doe when her stall mate, a nice gentle but horned doe became angered over feed competition and hooked her belly, rupturing her spleen. Horns can harm the wearer too. Goats like to shove their heads through woven wire fencing to nibble on grass on the other side. Some horns will squeeze through the fence, but the goat cannot back out and can hang itself if not spotted in time. I have known goats that have died this way.

Dehorning Kids The best age to dehorn goats is when they are young kids. When done at this age, there is very little shock and less work involved. The easiest method and the best by far is the electric disbudding iron. The electric iron is inexpensive, as well as safe and sure when used properly. The procedure is as follows: 1. Restrain the kid in a "kid box," bag, or by an assistant holding it firmly. 2. Clip the hair away from the horn buds. 3. Heat the iron well—it should scorch wood. 4. Firmly apply to the first horn bud. 5. Rotate, pushing the iron firmly to the head. Don't let the kid's screaming stop you. Repeat mentally, "This may save your life" ten times. 6. Move to the next bud and repeat the process. When finished, release the kid and give it a feeding. You will be forgiven at once.

In a day or so, the scab will come off and the head will be smooth permanently, unless you cheated on the time or missed

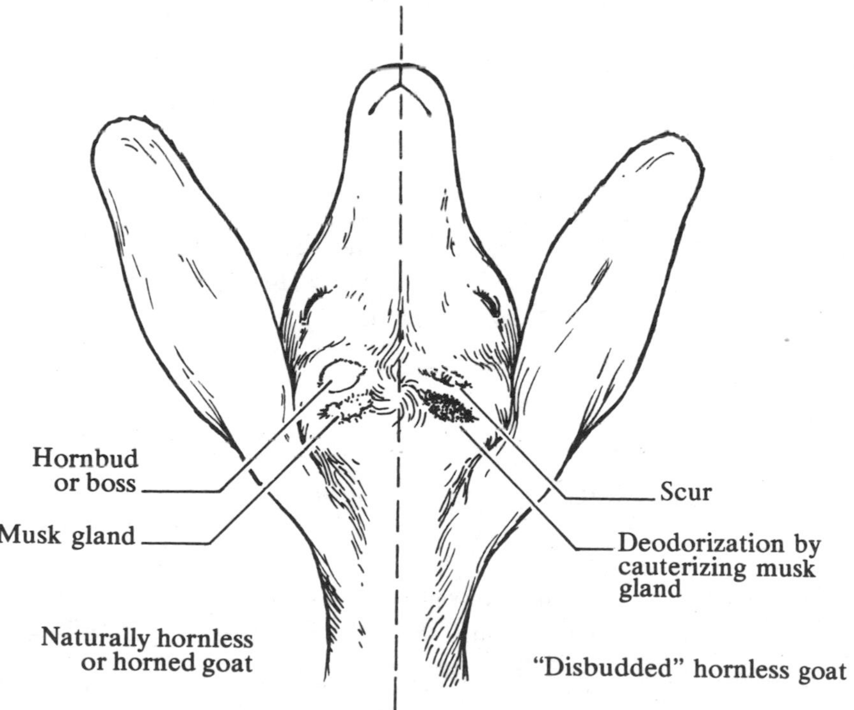

Dehorning and Descenting Goats

a small area by not rotating the iron. In this case, scurs or misshapen horns may appear. These may be removed by the iron. Just do a more thorough job!

I won't go into the use of caustic or rubber bands, as I don't like either method, especially on goats. There are too many problems. Caustic works, but you have to be very cautious about burns from the caustic ointment running onto or being rubbed on another animal or even the same one. Rubber bands are hard to place due to the wide base of the horn. They break and are lost. It *is* painful. Ask people who have used this method on milking does, and many will tell you that their does drop in milk production for a long period. When partially off, they are easily snagged on things and break, causing bleeding and more pain. Infections and tetanus are also problems.

Gougers or scoops, which are made for calves, work well on kids, but leave unsightly holes in the head, although they heal nice and smooth. The gougers have a sharp mouth which fits over the horn bud. You must have them down close to the head so there is hair taken out with the horn bud. When in position, the handles are quickly forced apart, neatly clipping out the bud. Bleeding is controlled by use of dehorning powder, if necessary. Kids with horns several inches long can be done in this way, with very little bleeding in most cases. Very few scurs result.

Dehorning Adults In dehorning adult goats, there is more technique involved and more equipment needed. A novice is advised to have his veterinarian do adult dehorning. A tranquilizer is often used, along with local anesthetic around the horn bases. I don't like using a barbiturate anesthetic unless absolutely necessary, because of the slight but ever-present danger in using it. Recently I have had excellent results with an anesthetic put out for cats, Ketamine Hydrochloride. It is a short-acting anesthetic and quite safe. The dosage is much less than that given to a cat. An adult buck will require from five to seven cc. (100 mg. per ml.). Smaller doelings and bucklings generally take one to two cc. It is given intramuscularly. (See final chapter for directions for intramuscular injections.)

A hacksaw or wire saw are the usual instruments used in dehorning an adult goat. Care must be taken to cut deep enough into the head. Done right, a band of skin and hair should be removed with the horn. There will be an unsightly bloody hole left. The holes will be larger in a mature buck than with a doe, due to the heavier base of the buck's horns. Bleeding can be controlled by pulling the arteries and use of a cautery. Do not be alarmed when blood runs in droplets from the nose or mouth. This is normal in many cases, as the blood trickles down the sinus cavities into the nose and mouth. In a very few weeks, the holes will heal smoothly. In fly season the fresh wounds should be daubed with scarlet oil or another fly repellent to prevent maggots. In goats that bleed quite a bit, place a cotton pad over each horn hole and wrap gauze snugly around the head like a bonnet. Remove after 24 hours.

DESCENTING

One drawback to owning a buck is the odoriferous musky smell he emits during the breeding season. Contrary to common opinion and old wives' tales, the odor does not have any physical connection with the sexual organs. A castrated buck does not have the odor, as the glands remain inactive when there is no longer stimulus to produce the musk. A descented buck remains virile and able to breed. He just doesn't have such a strong smell. Some think that the does aren't attracted to a nonsmelly buck, but I haven't seen this to be true.

There is some odor even to a descented buck. The major scent gland is on the head behind the horn base. Other glands are found on the legs and near the tail. They are, however, small compared to the head gland. You can feel and in many instances see the scent gland bumps on a clipped head. (Smell your hand afterwards!) A buck kid can have this gland burned at disbudding time with the electric dehorner. An electric soldering iron can also be used. The only problem is the extent of the head burned, which is unsightly and takes a while to heal.

Older bucks (and kids too) can be descented surgically. Using a tranquilizer and local anesthetic, your vet can quite easily remove the gland, leaving a fairly neat-looking head. A variety of incision patterns can be used, but the basics are generally the same. The skin is shaved and painted with antiseptic. The incision (or incisions) is made and the skin peeled back, exposing the bumpy glandular material underneath. By use of blunt dissection this is peeled away, leaving a clean head. Bleeding is controlled by a cotton pressure pack. The area is sprinkled with antibiotic powder and the skin sewn together. Some veterinarians remove the skin also, as it does contain some scent glands.

A tetanus booster or antitoxin and four days' treatment with pen-strep (penicillin-streptomycin) should be given, just to be on the safe side. No one wants to descent a buck, then have him get tetanus or an infection.

TRIMMING FEET

Goats should have regular hoof trims. Because of the type of terrain most of them travel today, their hooves do not get worn down naturally. Untrimmed hooves can lead to many problems with goats, from lameness to completely crippled front end due to contracted tendons.

While trimming feet is not a veterinary matter, if left untrimmed and allowed to grow long, they can cause trouble. There is no cut-and-dried formula as to how often the feet should be trimmed, as different ground, types of feet, exercise, or feed can all be factors in hoof growth and wear. The feet should be checked regularly, and when they begin to look a bit sloppy, they should be trimmed. The goats should be handled enough to allow their feet to be picked up with little struggle. A distraction of grain can help. While one person can easily manage to trim feet, it is helpful to have an assistant.

There are several instruments available for trimming goat feet, which range from a jackknife to special hoof nippers. As with all tools, everyone has a favorite. All will work if used properly. The main thing is to trim the wall of the toes down level with the cushion or frog. On rocky or gravel soil a goat naturally rasps down these edges, but on soft ground or with little exercise, the feet (really the wall of the claws) will grow until they are like twisted skis. This causes pain, lameness, and finally, contracted tendons and deformity. Goats with long-neglected feet can be brought back close to normality by careful and repeated correct trimming, but some are forever lame.

Diseases and Other Problems

ABSCESSES

Abscesses are fairly common in goats. They can pop up anywhere, seemingly overnight. In most instances they cause no trouble and either break and drain themselves or just quietly disappear. But they can cause trouble, especially if there are abscesses in the udder or internal abscesses.

Corynebacteria—there are many kinds, just as there are breeds of dogs—have been strongly implicated in goat abscesses, and while it is true that corynebacteria do cause abscesses in goats, so do many other bacteria. Staph, strep, *E. coli,* and many other lesser known organisms have all been isolated from goat abscesses. Therefore, no one treatment or one preventive will work in all cases.

If a goat or a herd is bothered by abscesses, the best course of action is to have your vet take a sample and send it into a lab for culture and sensitivity tests. This will not only tell just *which specific* organism is causing the trouble, but will also tell what antibiotic will take care of it. Usually a broad-spectrum antibiotic, such as oxytetracycline, pen-strep, or a sulfa combination will work, but sometimes it is an organism *only* killed by some seldom used drug. Some abscesses are so walled off that no antibiotic will help. Occasionally, an organism causing an abscess is best dealt with by use of an autogenous vaccine. This is made from the specific organisms for treatment of the condition they cause. Check with your vet to see what is available.

For the simple, once-in-a-year-or-so abscess, the treatment is easy. Isolate this animal, as an abscess that is broken drains millions of potential abscess-producing bacteria. Trim the hair around the abscess lump. Try systemic treatment (injectable antibiotics, for four days). Continue to watch the lump daily. If it does not become smaller, it will probably come to a head and break by itself. Or you can lance it when it is ready. It is a good idea to draw some fluid out of the suspected abscess with a needle and syringe before lancing it, as once in a while it is not an abscess but a hematoma (blood-filled sack). If a hematoma is lanced, an animal can bleed to death.

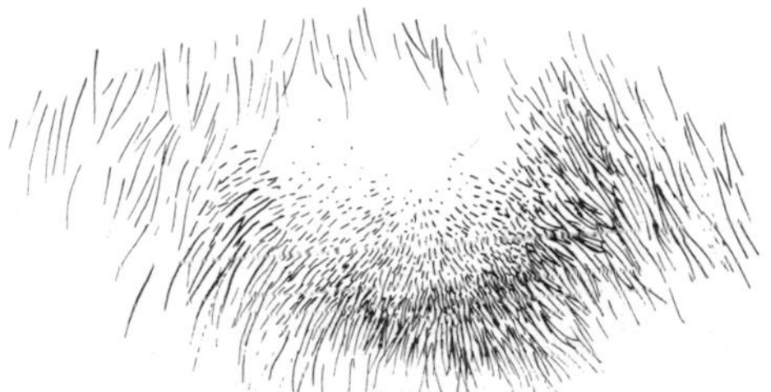

An innocent-looking bulge that has been diagnosed as an abscess.

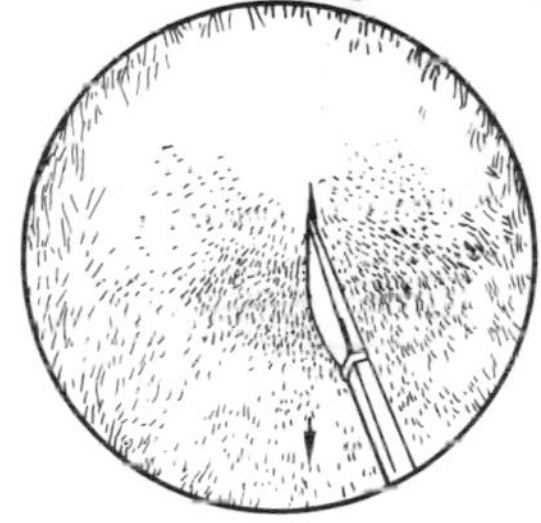

Lance the abscess quickly in a downward stroke.

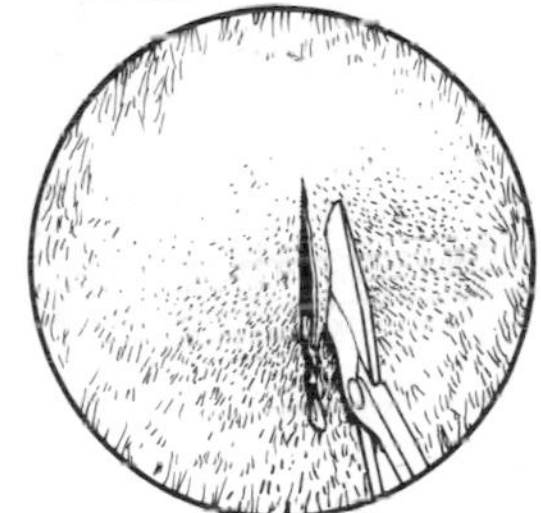

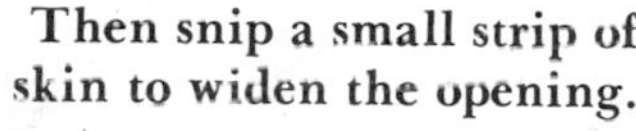

Then snip a small strip of skin to widen the opening.

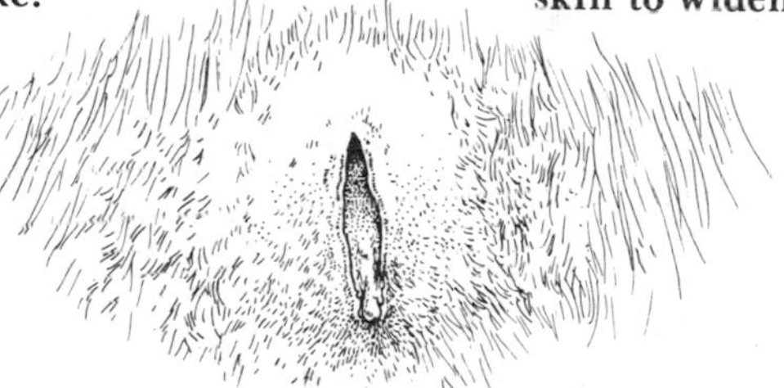

Allow the abscess to remain open after flushing and draining.

To lance the abscess, scrub the surface well with warm soapy water. Rinse and dry. Make a quick incision at the bottom of the lump. Adequate drainage is not possible if the incision is made at the top or center, as there will always be a pocket of pus left. Once the incision (at least 1½ inches) is made, clip a strip of skin off, widening the hole. This will insure that the inside heals, instead of the skin just healing together, letting the abscess re-form. Flush the pocket out with warm soapy water, rinse, let dry, then squirt in an antibiotic. (I like to squirt in the antibiotic with a mastitis tube.)

If the abscess is on the udder or is in the throat area, call your vet for sure, as there are blood vessels which can easily be cut by mistake, ending with a very dead goat. When working with an open abscess, be sure to wear plastic or rubber gloves, as some people have gotten skin infections from the drainage. Children shouldn't be allowed to play with a goat with an abscess for the same reason. An udder abscess can drain into the milk, so it's best not to use the milk from the affected side.

Caseous lymphadenitis is a term describing a serious abscess problem in goats. Here it is the lymph glands which become infected, with *Corynebacterium pseudotuberculosis,* and then abscess. As with other lymph gland diseases, it is easily spread throughout the body, many times unknown to the owner. Sometimes the first signs are a well-fed goat that just keeps getting thinner and thinner until it finally dies. If the abscesses are near the surface, the hair can be clipped and heat applied (hot packs and hot linament or ointment) to draw them to a head. When open and drained, they are packed with an antibiotic. The trouble with caseous lymphadenitis is that often internal abscesses form in addition to the external ones, which involve body organs and kill the animal. Antibiotic therapy doesn't seem to help. Because it is a serious problem, keep a suspected animal isolated. Sometimes it is best to cull such an animal rather than chance infecting the rest of the herd.

ARTHRITIS OR JOINT ILL

Sometimes related to the abscess trouble is a crippling of the joints, often the knees, known as arthritis or joint ill. As with abscesses, there is no one organism that is responsible, but many. There is often puffiness at the joints, and pain. If caught early, a veterinarian can draw off fluid from the joint to have it cultured. Antibiotic therapy can sometimes reverse this disease, but many times not. Some experimental work is being done with foreign protein therapy. Affected animals are given a subcutaneous injection daily. So far it seems to be working fairly well, but tests are not conclusive since there are not enough early affected goats on which to try this treatment.

Once severely crippled (if the joints have been damaged and the bone deformed) nothing can help. If the joint infection has been stopped and there is still trouble from bent knees, often the tendons have contracted due to disuse of the legs or misuse of the legs, forcing the goat to remain in an abnormal, half-kneeling position. This can sometimes be corrected by daily drawing the leg into as normal a position as possible without causing pain. Release and stretch again. Repeat 10 to 20 times and do it *every* day.

If this does not help, light casts can be put on if the leg can be pulled into proper position without a lot of pain. These should go from fetlock to elbow. They should be left on for two weeks, removed to check for results and pressure sores, then replaced if necessary. Also the tendons may be operated on (a tendotomy) to correct this problem. This is not a difficult operation and can be done at your vet's office under a local anesthetic. Bear in mind that if permanent damage has been done, there may be nothing that will restore full usefulness to the joints.

Be sure the feet are correctly trimmed, as a goat can grow the toes pretty long and twisting, making it painful to stand right and discouraging leg use.

Arthritis can be cut down by the following measures:
• Choose sound, good-boned breeding stock. • Keep goats where they get plenty of exercise. • Keep goats in well-bedded stalls. If cement floors are in the pens, bed very well. Banged knees

increase stress and can lead to joint infections. • Disinfect all navels at birth with iodine. This is where many joint problems originate. • Keep an iodine, salt, trace mineral supplement handy, fed free choice.

BLOAT AND INDIGESTION

Most goats bloat due to improper feeding, whether it is accidental or from ignorance. There are two types of bloat. Frothy bloat usually follows overeating lush legume pastures. In frothy bloat the gas forms in numerous tiny bubbles, which are nearly impossible to belch up. Dry bloat is usually caused by indigestion or eating too much grain, or eating grain then drinking water. Here the gas forms in pockets and is trapped. More and more of it forms and the animal is unable to belch, thus bloating.

Frothy bloat is more dangerous, as it occurs suddenly and is many times fatal. Never turn a herd of goats out into lush pasture, especially alfalfa and clover, unless they are used to it. Otherwise they will overload, and may bloat. It is safest, when turning them onto good pasture after being in the barnlot where they were fed hay, to cut a few armloads of the legume every day, increasing until a little is not eaten. Then turn them out in the afternoon of a dry day. Wet legumes bloat animals more than do dry pastures.

Even with this procedure, watch them closely the first couple of days. If bloat is noticed in one of your goats, call your vet immediately. Many times bloat can be relieved by drenching with half a pint of corn oil, peanut oil, or mineral oil. One or two teaspoonsful of turpentine added to the oil and mixed well is helpful. Kneading the bloated area will also help break up the gas. Sometimes, though, it is necessary to pass a stomach tube to relieve the pressure. *Do not use a garden hose or anything but a stomach tube.* Any other tube can slit the esophagus and kill your goat.

In an emergency, where a goat is not discovered until it is as full of gas as a balloon or is down from the pressure, it may be necessary to use a trochar and cannula to relieve the gas. The trochar is an awl-shaped instrument with a tube (the cannula) fitting over it. (See "Bloat" in the chapter on cows for illustration.) The trochar is pushed through the wall of the rumen and then pulled out, leaving the cannula in to permit the passage of gas and relieve the bloat. This is done as an emergency measure only, as some animals never really recover after being relieved in this way. The bloat goes down but the goat just doesn't do its best after being stuck. It may be that some of the stomach contents leaked into the peritoneal cavity or adhesions formed. Use a knife only to save an animal that has collapsed and appears very distressed, as the knife only makes an incision and nothing carries the gas and stomach contents through the peritoneum and on out of the body, as

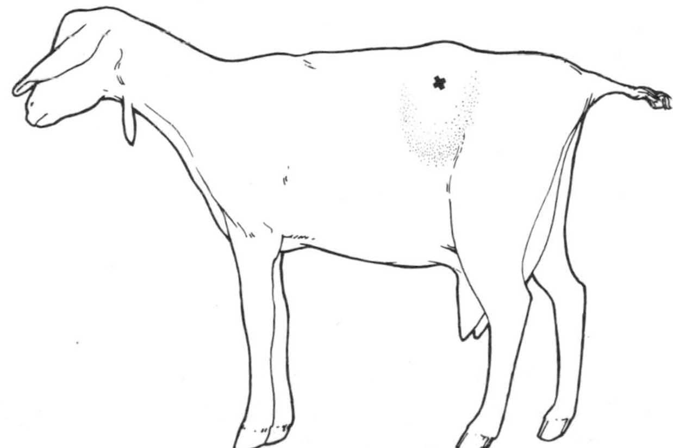

The bloated doe should be stuck at the highest point of the bloat, on the left side.

does the cannula. With the knife, all this boils into the peritoneal cavity, later to cause trouble and sometimes death.

If a goat must be stuck, mark the highest point of the bloat on the left side, just in front of the hip. A heavy gauge needle is better than a knife (14–10 gauge—three-inch). If you live a long way from the vet, it may be a good idea to invest in one, just in case you should need it. The cost is minimal.

Many goats will not bloat, but get indigestion from overeating grain or greens. They will at first appear colicky, stamping their hind feet, grunting, and biting or nosing their sides. The goat may then lie down, act generally sick, and not want to get up (but can if made to). Diarrhea usually follows. A classic example was my old Nubian doe. She was used to eating grass, hay, and garden greens. One day I took her along for a walk in the woods. I looked at the beautiful spring wildflowers—she ate them. That evening she was in misery, a good old bellyache!

In most cases, a dose or two of Kaopectate will completely clear up the problem. But in cases where the goat is in pain from gas, your vet can give it a shot to quiet the stomach cramps, and oil (as is given for bloat) orally will stop the gas buildup. It is a good idea, in the event your goats get into the grain bin and overload, to get a dose of oil into them at once. Remember, corn, peanut, vegetable, or mineral oil, not car oil! This will help move the feed through faster and usually prevents acute gastritis or bloat.

Kids are a prime target for digestive upsets, as they are fed milk, and milk can easily cause problems if fed wrong. Kids should be fed colostrum four times daily for the first three days. The colostrum acts as a laxative and also provides the kids with protective antibodies. Scours or diarrhea is many times caused by hard fecal material irritating the bowel.

Most kids are fed twice daily, but where it is possible, they have fewer problems, in my opinion, when fed less, but more often (four times daily), until they are eating hay well. Nurse does are perfect, as the kids can "snack" at will. Some does will accept several kids; the number, of course, depends on her milking ability. The amount of milk fed to kids depends on size and vigor. It can vary from half a cup to a pint at birth. Big-boned, strong, vigorous kids can handle a larger amount than kids that are smaller and somewhat "backward."

Chilled, tiny, or premature kids which don't have much nursing instinct may many times be saved, and kept scour-free, by tube feeding until the sucking instinct becomes stronger. A plastic tube (French tube or catheter) and a 12 cc. syringe are used. The milk, colostrum for three days, is fed at body temperature. Simply stick the tube into the milk, draw a full load of milk, then insert the tube slowly but firmly into the kid's mouth and down the throat. Wait until it begins to swallow, then slowly shove the tube on down. It is possible to mistakenly get the tube into the lung, but if you watch for the swallowing and work carefully, chances are slim that this will happen. If the kid coughs when the tube is down, withdraw and try again, as it could be a sign it went into the lung. The tube is inserted far enough to just reach the end of the esophagus. Eyeball it by the length of the neck. When injecting the milk, push the plunger of the syringe in slowly or the milk may churn around, making the kid squirm. This is a safe, easy method to use and the entire process—feeding and washing up the tube and syringe afterward—can be done in five minutes.

When a kid begins to munch hay, we like to get it eating Calf Manna. (Sorry, competitors, but Calf Manna is the only pelleted milk replacer that I know of *without* antibiotics, and I don't like antibiotics daily in the feed.) When they are eating the Calf Manna well, a grain mixture can be added.

When the kids are on milk, they sometimes overeat (your fault) or eat wrong (their fault). Gulping milk can lead to indigestion and diarrhea. At the first sign of loose bowels, cut the milk given at the next feeding in half. In most cases this will quickly remedy the problem. Where the diarrhea continues, you'd better see your vet for an antidiarrheal. There are two basic types: astringents and kaolin-pectin preparations. Antibiotics may be added to kill harmful bacteria, preventing irreversible scours. Give the medicine religiously. If given haphazardly or when you think of it, it won't do the job and could cost you a kid. Use exactly as directed.

BREAKS

Most broken bones occur in the legs, with goats. Accidents are commonly caused by tie-out chain becoming wrapped around legs; car accidents; getting a leg caught in fences, stall dividers, or brush; and dog bites. You can strongly suspect a broken leg if a sound goat suddenly becomes severely lame. Most broken legs dangle and the goat will not walk on all fours. Sometimes you are able to see the bone sticking up against the skin or even through the skin. If the bone is not through the skin, a plaster cast or a Thomas splint reinforced with plaster works well in most cases. Some breaks are easily repaired with the use of intramedullar pins, especially those of kids, as there is very little encumbrance after the bone is set, compared to a cast or splint.

At any rate, a broken leg or even two on a goat doesn't mean an automatic death sentence. Proper care before and after the leg is set is important. On discovering a goat with a broken leg, keep the animal quiet to prevent further damage. Leave it where it is unless it's in a dangerous or very inconvenient place, such as a swamp or a field during an electrical storm. If it must be moved, move it very slowly so that it doesn't further injure the leg. Sometimes the bone gets pushed through the skin with thrashing, which makes it easier for infection to enter.

Call your vet immediately. In some cases where a lot of shock is involved, either from the accident or pain, he may not set the leg right away, especially if a general anesthetic must be given, but will immobilize the leg with a temporary cast or splint until it is safe to do surgery.

If the leg can be set at the time of injury, it is a *must* that you check the cast or splint at least twice daily. Above the cast or below, in the event the foot shows below the cast, should be checked for swelling, dampness, and odor. These indicate possible problems, such as a too-tight cast, sores under the cast, or infection. The foot should be felt for warmth, indicating normal circulation. If it suddenly becomes cold and loses feeling—pinch or prick the skin between the claws—call your vet immediately. This indicates loss of circulation. The next step is gangrene.

The cast must be kept dry. Wet bedding, mud, rain, or swamps mean disaster to a plaster cast or plaster-reinforced splint. If the goat is turned out where there is mud or

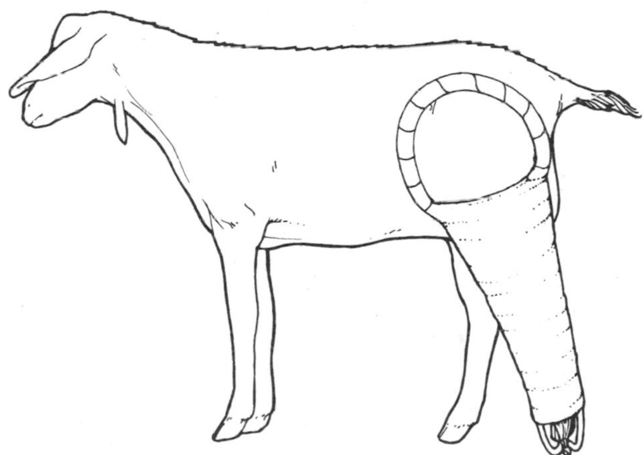

Many goats with a broken leg can be saved with a simple cast, splint, or pin.

dampness, slide a section of inner tube over the cast and tape it in place. A little car-starting fluid (ether) sprayed on the sticky side of the tape will *really* make it stick. Remove this for several hours daily to allow the cast to "breathe" and air to circulate in it.

Most casts or splints must remain on two to three weeks for kids and four to six weeks for large adults. The cast or splint may need to be taken off and replaced, if left on over three weeks.

CUTS AND MISCELLANEOUS INJURIES

The key here is for you to calmly analyze how badly the goat is hurt. Don't panic. If you think the injury is bad enough, call your vet. Describe the situation to him *exactly.* I had some people call me one day, saying their doe had broken a window and had a piece of glass in her nose. I asked how badly it was bleeding, and they replied that it bled a little, but the bleeding had stopped.

I saw in my mind a sliver of glass perhaps half an inch long. No hurry, right? Luckily I was able to go right out! That glass was two *feet* long! In fact, I don't know how she kept from breaking it when she moved. It entered one nostril and came out the other. She looked like a native with a bone in her nose. But it looked worse than it was, and there was no trouble after the "piece" of glass was removed.

Many cuts on animals heal very well with no suturing. Many times people argue for stitches, because their own doctor sewed up a half-inch cut on their hand. But many times there is quicker healing with less scarring if a cut is not sewn up. Of course, there are cuts that need suturing, but let your vet decide. Let him make his decision on a fresh cut, though. Some cuts that might have been better sewn up can't be done the next day, because the swelling, stiffness, and healing have already begun.

A clean wound, whether sutured or not, is generally a healthy wound. Try to keep it that way. Clip all the hair away from the wound. Hair is irritating at best and only retards healing, if it doesn't cause more serious trouble. Keep dirt and manure washed out of the wound with plain soapy warm water.

Animals heal quicker with the wound exposed to the air. A bandage just makes a soupy mess and is most times not necessary.

Keeping flies away from a wound is a must. Flies lay eggs on the wound and on surrounding hair. In a very short time, these eggs become maggots and enter the wound. There they begin to clean up the dead tissue. Great. But when that's gone, they begin eating live, healthy tissue. This will continue until the poor goat is alive with a seething mass of maggots. Scarlet oil or Smear 62 (don't use the latter on milking does) will keep the flies out. Apply in and around the wound.

In general, goats suffer the same type of injuries people do: bruises, strains, sprains, burns, heatstroke, etc. When in doubt, treat as you would a human with the same problem. If you can't get in touch with your vet, try a first-aid manual or even your own family doctor.

ENTEROTOXEMIA (OVEREATING DISEASE)

This is another disease caused, like tetanus, by an organism of the clostridia family, *Clostridium perfringens.* Although this problem is usually confined to young goats that are overfed, especially on grain, it can break out in any herd. Show kids being pushed for size and growth, meat animals being fattened quickly, and herds owned by an owner who just overfeeds, are all prime targets for enterotoxemia. It is usually the goats in the best appearing condition who die. The deaths are sudden, with little or no warning. Diarrhea, circling, convulsions, incoordination, and weakness are all symptoms.

As in tetanus, treatment is quite disappointing once symptoms are noticed. But vaccination is quite effective, and many people routinely vaccinate all kids and all adults every 6 to 12 months. Exercise is important for all goats. A fat goat is prone to a number of troubles, from enterotoxemia to heart attack. It's great to have those kids look growthy and mature, but being pushed just a little slower may save their lives.

EVERSION OF THE UTERUS

The uterus, in essence, is a fleshy pouch to contain the kids before birth. It is very muscular and well supplied with blood. Once in a while the doe may continue straining after the kids are born, turn this "pouch" inside out, and force it out of the body.

Eversion of the uterus can be a hereditary problem, so never knowingly buy a doeling out of a doe that has had this trouble, or a doe who herself has thrown out her uterus. Once a doe does this, 80 percent or better will do it again and again, possibly dying from it.

This is definitely an emergency situation, so call your vet immediately. There is a tremendous amount of shock involved, and some does die within 10 or 15 minutes after the uterus is fully out. Most can take more, but the sooner it is put back, the better chance the doe will have. Although the doe should not be kept for breeding, she can milk well for a full lactation and be used for meat when she dries up. In cases of a very valuable doe, be it producer or pet, she can be bred and the kids delivered by caesarean section. This requires lots of attention and bother as to the exact breeding dates and care of the doe. Some does are worth it, and some people have the time and inclination to bother plus the money for the veterinarian's surgery fee. Remember, this condition is hereditary, so the kids should not be used for breeding.

If a doe kids and continues to strain, you can sometimes prevent her throwing her uterus by standing her on a piece of plywood raised 6 to 12 inches in the back. This will take the pressure of her stomach and intestines off her uterus, which aggravates the problem. If this doesn't work, call your vet. He can give her a spinal anesthetic which will usually last until the uterus contracts back to its normal small size. Without the bulk of a large uterus, as it is just after kidding, the doe usually stops straining.

If you suddenly discover that a doe has thrown her uterus, call the vet immediately. You will recognize the uterus by the caruncles, which are the size of a hardball or smaller, and the redness. The uterus looks like a big bumpy pouch with veins. It is the size of a grocery bag when fully out. Do not confuse this with a retained placenta, which is stringy, thin, and light.

Get her rear end elevated and keep her quiet. Running around will increase the shock and the possibility of tearing it on a nail, wire, or other sharp object. A tear can mean her death. Keep a warm, moist towel on the uterus. This can not only keep it clean but greatly cut down the shock involved. Have a pail of warm water waiting for the veterinarian and a couple of towels. A bale of hay to drape with clean towels or cloth helps to rest the uterus on while he works to replace it. The uterus is heavy and sloppy, making it hard to handle, and the easier it is to handle, the quicker it can be replaced. In place of the bale of hay or straw, two people, one on each side, can support the uterus in a towel, like a hammock. But if the replacement takes any length of time, the helpers will tire and let the uterus sag, usually at a critical time, where the bale will not.

Many veterinarians use a spinal anesthetic to stop the straining both during the replacement and after, to prevent the doe from throwing it out again. Sometimes it is necessary to close the lips of the vulva. I usually do it routinely as a precaution. But this alone will not keep the uterus in if the doe really gets to straining hard. So keep her rear end elevated to cut down pressure, and keep her occupied with hay, grain, or carrots until she is past the straining. And *watch* her. If she begins to strain, call your vet. Don't wait to see if she will throw it out again because she may, and this considerably lessens your chance for having a live doe when it's all over.

FOOT ROT

Foot rot is a fungus infection that attacks the feet. Lameness is usually the first sign of trouble. The fungus gains entrance through tiny cracks in between the toes and just above the toes. Swampy ground, wet barnyards, or standing in damp bedding can chap the feet, letting the fungus enter and spread. Running goats in stubble fields or other dry, irritating grasses or brush can cause tiny scratches. The feet may swell, pus may be present, and on occasion the entire shell around the claws may slough off.

Once lameness is noticed, be sure the feet are cleaned and well trimmed, as a stone lodged in a toe can also cause severe lameness. Systemic treatment with pen-strep, oxytetracycline, or a combination sulfa usually works well. Treatment should be continued for a week. Soak the foot or feet in warm Epsom salts water, then soak with an antibiotic and/or astringent. Kopertox works well for me. With a herd problem, force each goat to walk through a foot bath of five percent formalin or copper sulfate mixture (450 grams to one gallon of water). With formalin, only use once a week. The copper sulfate can be repeated two or three times a week. Feeding an iodine supplement may help prevent foot rot in some herds—an iodized salt block is seldom enough.

Cortisone may be used to reduce swelling in the feet. Be careful with cortisone: do not use for more than four days, and use with extreme caution on does in the last month of pregnancy. It can cause abortion at this stage.

FREEZING

Due to the early kidding following the natural breeding season (August to January) of goats, many goat people are caught by unexpected births in very cold weather. It seems that it's the night when it's 35°F. below and the wind is howling that a doe decides to kid. Being damp from amniotic fluid and afterbirth, the newborn kids are prime targets for frostbite and freezing. Ears (you lucky La Mancha breeders!) and feet are most often the parts that become frozen. The doe can sometimes manage to dry off and warm a single vigorous kid born on a cold night, at least enough to keep it from freezing, but a doe who has twins or triplets can't handle all of them.

Stiff ears or unyielding feet and legs are signs of freezing. They are literally frozen! In mild freezing or frostbite, the ears or feet will swell, be tender, and feel hot to the touch. If left untreated, the swollen part will become gangrenous due to shut-off of circulation, and eventually will dry up and fall off. With ears, it is unsightly—who wants a registered Nubian with La Mancha ears or a Toggenberg with one ear? With legs and feet, freezing can be a severe handicap. A goat can survive loss of one leg or parts of two, but will hardly do as well as a goat that is sound.

Preventive measures are best. If you are in an area of subzero winters and don't have enough animals in your barn to keep the temperature above 32°F., try to have a box stall for each doe due to freshen. A heat lamp or two will usually generate enough warmth to warm the newborn kids. The stall should be square to prevent the doe from getting too far from the lamp, draft-free, and well bedded. The heat lamp should be protected by a cage to prevent accidents, and *please,* double secure it. A few extra minutes could save a lot of heartache. A fire in a barn is a terror. The doe should not be panting from the heat, so allow room for air circulation. If the stall is kept around 35°F. to 40°F., it is warm enough. After she kids, wait a day until they are all active and dry, then slowly withdraw the heat.

If you discover a doe which kidded during the night and has a kid suffering from freezing, act at once. Carry the kid to the house, fill the tub with warm water (just a bit cooler than you like your bath to be) and stand the kid in it. If the ears are frozen or frosted, soak them well. Continue for 15 minutes, warming the water as needed. Have someone warm several towels—throw them in the dryer, hang them by the oven or by the furnace. As soon as you are done soaking the kid, throw the towels on your lap, place the kid on them, and rub it dry. When it is thoroughly dry, place the kid in a box with a few rags near a source of warmth such as a register, stove, or heating pad under the box. Cortisone injected intramuscularly for four days helps; it raises blood pressure, increases circulation, and reduces swelling and pain. If the ears are caught too late, as often happens, wait until they begin to shrivel up and give a week's treatment with antibiotics to prevent infection.

FUNGUS INFECTIONS, GENERAL

To the untrained eye, there isn't much difference between a fungus infection and mange, which is caused by mites. Even a veterinarian with experience must sometimes take a skin scraping to be sure. Don't assume every bald, red spot is mange, until it has been diagnosed—by a vet, not a neighbor—for few mange remedies will touch a fungus, which can grow like mad while being incorrectly treated. On the other hand, few fungicides will kill mange mites, and left untreated the mange can spread until it becomes impossible to cure.

INFERTILITY

Much of the "infertility" in does, especially with the first-goat owner, is due to poor timing or misinformation on the owner's part. Although does can and sometimes do come into heat and conceive in the spring, the months between August and January are goats' natural breeding months. Even when does show a summer heat, many do not conceive, so it's not fair to label them "sterile."

Unless the doe owner has a buck, he should plan to leave the doe with the buck owner for at least a month. This is the safest, surest, and cheapest way to insure pregnancy. Many does are brought to the buck a day or even a few hours late. Even if the doe should stand for service, she may not conceive. Some does experience what is called a "silent heat." There are no outward signs of heat, but many times the buck will know, resulting in a successful breeding.

Abortion Abortion can be caused by many things. Injury, natural causes such as the doe's body rejecting an abnormal fetus, fatigue, bacterial infections, viruses, poisons, and so forth—all have caused does to abort. I have listed them in what I feel is the order of common occurrence. Does heavy with kid should not be allowed to jump up on things, climb, or be in a pen with rough goats. They should receive adequate exercise but not overdo it. One single abortion in a herd is usually nothing to worry about, but if it is repeated, your veterinarian should be called.

When talking about abortion, many people do not realize how small a fetus is until the last month or so before it is born. At 74 days the fetus is about the size of a baby mouse, and at 94 days about the size of a hamster. It's no wonder many does abort and no one ever knows about it! Should a doe, seemingly bred, suddenly come into heat, an abortion should strongly be suspected.

Cystic Ovaries Once in a while a doe is seen that is continually in heat. Instead of the regular 27-day cycle, she appears in heat every week or every few days. She will ride other does and accept service from the buck. Often such a doe has cystic ovaries. Positive diagnosis is difficult in many does without doing a laparotomy (surgical examination). Some does have a rectum large enough to do a rectal examination of the ovaries, but unfortunately these are in a minority. Often a veterinarian can be fairly certain, on observing the doe, that she does have cystic ovaries and he can treat her as such. Injections of chorionic gonadotropin or progesterone will often help. The doe may be bred on her first *regular* heat. In some cases there is nothing that will help, so don't feel your veterinarian doesn't know his stuff if he can't cure a doe with cystic ovaries with one shot.

Pyometra and Metritis Pyometra and metritis are similar conditions which prevent conception and often normal heat cycles. With pyometra there is more pus in the uterus, but both conditions refer basically to an infected uterus. Metritis means an inflamed uterus, but often there is a considerable amount of pus and exudate in the uterus.

There may or may not be drainage from these conditions. When there is drainage, it is good in some ways. It lets you know there *is* serious trouble present, indicates the cervix is open a little, which facilitates drainage and treatment also, and lets you begin treatment sooner because you become aware of the problem sooner. Hormone injections, which force the uterus to contract and thus expel the pus and exudate, will often help. If this doesn't work, your veterinarian may have to pass a flexible tube into the uterus to siphon off the pus and irrigate the uterus with a mild iodine preparation or antibiotic. Where the doe is running a temperature or acting sick, systemic treatment may have to be started. These conditions are often due to incomplete expulsion of afterbirth or the death of one fetus.

Retained Corpus Luteum Once in a while, a doe will not come back into heat after having kidded. She may have a retained corpus luteum, or yellow body. Of course, there are other conditions that will prevent a doe from having heat cycles, but a retained corpus luteum is quite common. It is generally easier to correct than many sterility problems, and one or two injections of estrogen, a female hormone, will often start normal heat cycles.

Vaginitis Vaginitis in itself is not a serious condition. It appears as a reddening of the vaginal walls. The lips of the vagina must be parted to see the condition, or a vaginal speculum used. Vaginitis can have various causes but is usually a bacterial or viral infection. In either case, the pH of the vagina is changed, which can kill the sperm. It is not caused by a buck but is spread by a buck, by breeding first an infected doe, then a clean doe. A doe with vaginitis will come into heat regularly but just fail to conceive.

By using artificial insemination for a while, which carries the sperm through the vagina into the uterus, or by not breeding for several weeks, the condition will often remedy itself, when caused by a virus, or can be treated successfully if caused by a bacterial infection. Douches of a mild iodine solution will often help. See your veterinarian for name brands and amount to use in solution for your does.

Fertility of the Buck So far we've neglected the buck in the discussion of infertility. This is only so because more does are seen with sterility problems, simply because there *are* more does than breeding bucks. Overuse is a common factor affecting the fertility of some bucks, especially well-bred bucks in heavy demand. Although many bucks can and do serve four or five does in a day, it is much safer to stagger breeding dates out to cut that number in half. No, I don't mean he can serve 2½ does!

A buck that is quite a bit overweight will tend to have fewer successful breedings than a buck that is in top shape. Sperm motility and the buck's potency will be greatly reduced in fat bucks. A buck should receive daily exercise. He should have an outside yard with toys, such as an old tire hanging from a tree, a sturdy crate to climb on, a basketball to push around, and another buck or a wether to play with. This play can be quite rough at times, but it is what builds muscle in a buck instead of flab from standing around all day.

Vitamin deficiencies can sometimes cut down on fertility, as can hormone imbalances. Often, vitamin injections or hormone injections may help undiagnosed causes of male infertility.

The testicles of a buck should be full and oblong. They should also be even. Shrunken, hard, or knotted testicles indicate past injury, inflammation of the testicle, or infection.

Hermaphroditism Hermaphroditism occurs fairly often in goats, often enough to discuss, at any rate. The hermaphrodite doe will generally have an enlarged clitoris, sometimes a swollen or elongated vulva, and look more bucklike than is normal for the average doe. Her neck and shoulders will be heavier, and horns, if she has them, will be larger at the base than usual. Her heat periods will not be normal, or they will be completely absent. Obviously, if she does not have ovaries, she will not come into heat. The hermaphrodite buck may appear normal, but will either not breed or will be sterile when bred.

The most frequent occurrence of hermaphroditism is in goats originating from two naturally polled (or hornless) goats that were mated. What do horns and sex have to do with each other? Not too much unless you're talking about goats. When a horned (even though disbudded) goat is mated to a naturally polled goat, the kids will nearly always be normal. But when two naturally polled animals are mated, there is a very large percentage of hermaphroditism. The rub comes when it is almost impossible to tell if a goat has been disbudded at an early age or is naturally polled. Only the goat knows, and he or she won't tell! Of course, hermaphrodites occur in horned to horned matings too, but this appears to be simply an occasional happening, as with other species of animals.

KETOSIS

Ketosis should be suspected in any strange-acting does several weeks before freshening. Ketosis shows up in several ways. A doe may act a little "dumpy" or "slow." She may stand in a corner with her head down. Later, coordination becomes poor. Weakness and staggering usually follow. The doe finally is unable to get to her feet. The entire course of the disease or metabolic disturbance often lasts for several days, from first signs to death. Ketosis generally shows up in underfed does. Not a starved doe, necessarily, but a doe not receiving enough grain and legume hay to provide adequate carbohydrates for herself and fetuses. Ketosis often shows in does carrying twins or triplets.

I haven't had much luck treating advanced cases of ketosis with drugs. In some cases, glucose fed intravenously or propylene glycol given orally with 40 units of insulin (intramuscularly) helps. Molasses drenches may help some does. Four ounces twice daily are given, diluted with warm water. When the doe is near kidding and comes down with ketosis, delivering the kids via caesarean section usually saves the doe and the kids. Consult your vet early if you suspect ketosis. If he is unfamiliar with goats, tell him it is similar to ketosis in sheep.

LICE

Lice are a real problem with goats and cattle in the winter months especially. They can bother goats and calves quicker than cows or horses because of the size of the animal. Aside from the itching and irritation, if lice are left on they can cause severe anemia and death. They are bloodsuckers, and if enough are on an animal, they can actually bleed it to death.

It pays to check several animals in a herd at random each week during the winter. With the longer winter hair for lice to hide in and the short period of sunlight, lice multiply rapidly. They look like tiny gray, oval-shaped flecks, the size of a grain of rice or smaller. They are not usually moving; they attach themselves to the goat and stay put.

Dandruff and patchy bald spots, accompanied by itching and rubbing, are signs of lice. When lice are found or strongly suspected, get a good dairy louse powder. All animals should then be dusted, whether or not lice are seen on one or two. Dust weekly for three weeks. This will kill lice as they hatch, before they can breed and lay more eggs.

MANGE

Mange is caused by mites and comes in two varieties, demodectic and sarcoptic. It can be a serious problem and is difficult to diagnose without having skin scrapings taken. It can resemble many other skin problems, such as fungus infections, staph infections, allergic reactions, or goat pox. Most mange shows on goats as baldness with small nodules, like pimples. Scabs and crusty areas follow. The skin is either itchy or extrasensitive to the touch. The skin may get thick and "stiff."

Treatment is sometimes difficult and depends on good nursing, a good mange remedy, and good luck, all following a correct diagnosis. There are many dips, sprays, powders, and rub-ons effective against mange, and the choice should be left to your vet. Some work on limited areas but are toxic if used on the whole body. Others are better used in the summer, due to the wetness of the animal if a liquid is used. Lindane is very effective but can only be used on dairy animals as a last resort, as it is absorbed into the body and then excreted in the milk for a long time after treatment. Lime-sulfur ointment often works on small lesions but is messy if used over a large area.

All hair should be clipped away from a lesion, and if it is widespread, the whole goat should be clipped. Bathing the area with hot soapy water before each treatment will help. It will remove any dandruff or loose scabs and also soften the skin, making it easier for the mange remedy to get to the mites, which burrow into the skin. A small area is very much easier to treat than an extensive area, so when in doubt on that bald red spot, call or run your goat to your vet for a check. It can spread on one goat like wildfire or spread through a herd. Always keep a suspected animal isolated.

MASTITIS

With acute mastitis the doe will act sick, running a temperature of 103°F. to 107°F. (goats can differ in "normal" temperature, so it's a good idea to know what is normal for your individual goats when they are healthy). The udder on one or both sides is usually hot and swollen hard. Mastitis means inflammation of the mammary gland, but most people think in terms of the abnormal milk that is usually present. It may be thick, chunky, watery, or like pus (smelly).

Acute mastitis is caused by a stress on the udder, which allows bacteria to multiply and cause trouble. These stresses can be anything from a bump or bang to a bee sting or a cut teat. Does with low, pendulous bags are very prone to mastitis, due to knocking them about. A doe who tangles her legs up and falls down because the teats are dragging low is a prime target. All the more reason to breed does for good udder attachments, even if they are just scrub does.

With more people going into goat dairies and milking many does, there are more goats being milked by machine. The milker must be used as an addition to your hands, not as a hired man. The machine has to be supervised closely, or it will creep up the bag, causing stress which leads to mastitis. Many does let their milk down with a bang and are completely milked out in a minute. This leaves no time to go feed kids, water the buck, or do other tasks.

Most goats milked by machine are run through a milking parlor, where there is a short milk line. However, if a long air line with several cocks is used, be sure of the vacuum on both ends. Improper vacuum puts severe stress on the udder and can cause bad flare-ups periodically.

As for treatment, the very best thing is to have your veterinarian take a sample of the milk for culture tests, thereby finding out just what bacteria is causing the trouble. This can, however, take time and can be expensive though not always —ask him. Most cases of acute mastitis respond to treatment with combination sulfas of a broad-spectrum antibiotic given systemically. I have quit using intramammary infusion (mastitis tubes) except in a few cases, as I believe you are taking a great risk of introducing other bacteria into an already stressed udder. You can't sterilize skin, and 99 percent of the tube tips that enter the teat are not sterile, even if you do soak them in alcohol. Systemic treatment goes to work in the body all through the tissues, not just on the surface of the interior of the udder. Remember, the inside of the udder looks like a sponge, not an open, hollow ball full of milk. Getting an antibiotic forced through the teat and massaged into all those little pockets where there is infection is darned near impossible.

The swelling can be taken down by use of injectable cortisone. Milking the infected quarter dry several times daily, as you would drain an abscess, will hasten recovery time.

Chronic Mastitis Once the doe has had a bout with acute mastitis, she is more easily prone to chronic mastitis. Tiny pockets of bacteria can remain, walled off by scar tissue in the udder, just waiting for an excuse (stress) to start trouble. Incomplete treatment of the acute mastitis can let chronic mastitis follow. Such incomplete treatment includes antibiotics not given for the prescribed length of time, improperly used udder infusions, or switching antibiotics.

With chronic mastitis, the doe isn't usually sick but gives chunky or abnormal milk for a day or so, then clears up. The udder may swell, but not with the hard, hot swelling of acute mastitis. There are often hard lumps, fibrous scar tissue, in the udder. She may flare up, on occasion, with acute mastitis. I seriously doubt that a doe with chronic mastitis is ever really cleared of it. As long as she is with your other does, she will be a potential source of infection for all the others.

Always milk a doe with mastitis *last* and by hand if you use a machine on the others. Then *scrub* your hands before you forget. The spray of milk that hits your hand contains millions of bacteria which can be transferred to another doe by forgetting and handling other does' bags. The mastitis doe should not run with the other milkers, as it is possible for her to drip milk and have another doe lay in it. Farfetched? Not really, when you consider the possibility of cutting six or seven years off a doe's production due to mastitis. That means a great loss in both milk and finances.

Dipping the teats after milking will help keep mastitis down. But use fresh dip for each doe and even for each teat, which is safer, as bacteria *can* live in teat dip long enough to be transferred from one doe or teat to another. The dip will not only seal the teat canal from infection, but it helps keep the teats from chapping and heals small cuts, all of which are stresses. Dipping teats will not help if the mastitis is caused by poor management practices such as high door sills to bang udders on or improper milking.

Does can be routinely tested for the presence of mastitis by using the California Mastitis Test, available through your vet or drugstore.

Gangrene Mastitis The one serious problem that can follow udder edema is gangrene mastitis. Many times this is caused by a combination of coliform bacteria and impaired circulation, as can be found with a caked bag or injury, usually a bang or bruise. If at any time the doe's bag or one side of it feels cold like a piece of meat from the refrigerator instead of warm and alive, get help. A doe can absorb enough toxin from a gangrene quarter to die in a day or so.

If the gangrene mastitis is caught quickly enough, it can sometimes be stopped, but it has a lot to do with luck. The bag may be fine and milk normally at night and be in a bad condition the next morning. Treatment consists of systemic antibiotics, cortisone, and heat applied to the bag to stimulate circulation. In severe cases, the part of the bag affected may have to be removed to save the life of the doe. If only one half is removed, she may be used as a milker in the future, as the remaining half will usually compensate. Of course, she will not ever give as much milk as before she lost half of her bag, but she can raise kids. If both halves are lost, she is usually fattened for the freezer. Once in a while a doe may be a pet or be a producer of great kids. She can be bred, but of course the kids will have to be fed by another doe or raised by hand.

MILK FEVER

Milk fever is a misnamed condition as there is no fever, but rather a subnormal temperature. It can occur just prior to kidding, but usually it occurs one to four days after. It is generally found only in high milk-producing does—I've never treated a one-quart scrub with milk fever. It is usually not found in a first freshener, unless she's an extremely good producer.

The first signs will be unsteadiness in the rear quarters, as milk fever causes an ascending paralysis. The doe will stagger, bleat, and go down. She will sometimes assume a froglike position as she tries to rise, dragging the rear legs backward. She will finally quit trying to rise and remain down. Her eyes will look glazed. She will seem not to know what is going on around her. If she is not treated, she will lapse into a coma and die.

Many times milk fever can be prevented by cutting the grain down a week or so before freshening and gradually increasing it after freshening. Don't completely milk the doe out the first few times she is milked.

In a normal freshening doe, the calcium is drawn off the bone where it is stored as milk production begins in earnest. With a doe coming down with milk fever, the glands get lazy, not drawing the calcium from the bone fast enough to replace the calcium in the blood which is going into the production of milk.

For years there have been studies done on the prevention of milk fever by feeding a high-phosphorus, low-calcium diet, or by vitamins injected daily, or in the feed. Personally, I haven't seen any great improvement in large herds. Perhaps some veterinarians have had luck with such preventive measures; it's just that I have not. Some things work fine in theory and test cases, but for some reason don't work "down on the farm."

The only practical treatment for milk fever is an injectable calcium preparation, preferably given intravenously. It can be given intraperitoneally but is absorbed slower and does not give as quick results. The calcium-magnesium preparations from your vet or drugstore are nearly always "cow size" bottles (500 cc.). Use the dosage for sheep. As soon as you notice a doe acting staggery or find her down, shortly before or after kidding, call your vet. If you wait until she gets worse, you may not be able to reach him and you may lose her.

If you are in the "boonies" and must treat your own doe, 50 to 100 cc. of the calcium-magnesium preparation is about right in most cases, depending on the size of the doe and the brand of calcium you are using. Check the label. The intravenous injection must be given slowly, as it can kill if given too fast. It should go drip, drip, drip, not glug, glug, glug! Have an assistant hold the doe still, as she may thrash after the dose has been started and begins to take effect. Be sure the needle (a 16-gauge 2½-inch needle works fine) is well into the vein and not just stuck precariously in the edge. It is easier to hit the vein the first time, with no swelling from the needle having been pulled out. Some calcium preparations are irritating to the subcutaneous tissue (that tissue between the skin and muscle) and can cause a chunk of neck to slough off if it leaks out under the skin.

Once the doe has been treated, give her a little while to get oriented before trying to get her to her feet. She can be boosted up by the use of a towel under her belly. A person on each side can lift and steady her, if necessary. There is no great rush in making her stand, however, so let her rest and munch on some grain and hay. She will also usually appreciate a drink. Most does get up unaided in a short time.

A doe can relapse with milk fever, so watch her closely for a day or so after she has had it. She should also be watched the next time she freshens, as many does will have it two or three years in a row—usually their peak production years. Her doelings have a tendency to follow in their mother's hoof prints, as they are more apt to be high milk producers than doelings out of just so-so producing dams. The more production bred into our goats, the more troubles we run into. It *is* unnatural for a goat to produce more than a quart or two daily, just as it is unnatural for a cow to milk 100 pounds a day. You've just got to take the bad with the good.

PNEUMONIA

Pneumonia or a pneumonia complex is, in my opinion, the greatest cause of death and financial loss in goats. Not only do they die from the pneumonia, but when they are left living, they are miserable and useless as far as milk or meat production goes. If too much lung surface has been damaged by the pneumonia, the animal can only stand and pant for breath. This causes a severe milk drop and weight loss.

Pneumonia can be caused by several bacteria and also viruses. It is *not* a disease found only in damp, cold, drafty barns. Pneumonia causes trouble everywhere, from spotless dairy setups to one-goat farms. As with many health problems, stress may bring it on. Stresses usually involved are:

1. Too *warm* a barn in the winter. Many goats are kept in a small building or an unused garage, which is cozy and tight. No drafts, no cold, but also no fresh air. Goats breathe, have some body moisture, and urinate. This is all moisture, which in too air tight a barn can cause dampness, chill, and stress. You can make a goat barn worse by insulating it and heating it. This makes the humidity higher, and the condensation worse. Goats can take a lot of cold, as long as it is dry cold, with plenty of shelter from wind and drafts and lots of dry bedding. The best setup for goats in the winter is loose housing, pens with protected doors so they may go in and out at will. Mine are outside in the sun, even on subzero days, as much as they are in the barn! Goats must be able to get inside, though. Goats forcibly subjected to extremes of weather will not live long.

2. Moving or shipping. Almost everyone knows about "shipping fever" or has heard of it. Simply, it is pneumonia, sometimes accompanied by diarrhea. Shipping is a stress, but it is not usually the bunch of goats moved, say, from Ohio to a new home in Michigan along with the family that gets it, but a new goat shipped and brought into the herd. The theory here is that each animal has his or her "own germs" that don't usually cause trouble, but when traded back and forth to other animals, can lead to problems. And the more hosts a disease passes through, the hotter it gets, overcoming even resistant or

vaccinated animals. This is one reason a sale barn goat can bring trouble into a herd. In a sale barn there may be several goats, all busily trading germs. Maybe one is already sick, breathing clouds of bacteria on the others. You buy one and take it home. A week later, it is sick. Two weeks later, several of your other goats are sick. POW. TROUBLE. (Let me add a note here. I'm not referring to dairy goat sales, like the Spotlight Sale for instance, which is the annual dairy goat sale held by the American Dairy Goat Association, but to the mixed livestock sales all over the country, cattle, pigs, sheep, goats, and so forth. Remember, they are being sold for a reason, and sickness has many times been one of them.)

3. Changes in the weather. Sudden severe cold snaps, rain with bad wind, hot muggy summer days, or hot days followed by icy nights are all stresses.

4. Miscellaneous stresses can include being run by dogs or motorcycles, a change in feed, moving from inside to out or vice versa, change in owners, and so on.

Pneumonia can and does start very quietly. The goat may just seem a little "off." It may lie down a little more than usual, refuse part of its grain, grunt, or not be quite as active as usual. *Please* take its temperature! Tomorrow it may be dead. Goats are quicker fatalities to pneumonia than cattle, so you must act immediately to save them.

Most goats with pneumonia will run a high temperature. The average for pneumonia is 104°F. to 106°F. If one goat has a high temperature, check the others. I've seen goats with pneumonia and a 107°F. temperature *look* okay and be eating fine. (Two had suddenly died the night before—no sign of illness, but their lungs were a mess.) Bear in mind, a goat's temperature can normally vary according to individuals or outside temperatures. A goat with a 102°F. normal temperature would be sick with a 103°F. temperature which would be normal for another goat. Know your goats' temperatures.

Goats can cough with pneumonia, but goats cough other times too so it isn't necessarily a symptom. Puffing for breath is. Don't ignore this. Isolate the sick goat. The others may come down with it, but if the sick animal is removed, there is a better chance they won't. Some pneumonias are very contagious. Others may only attack one animal in a herd. The sick animal should be in a warm, dry, draft-free place. Then call your vet. Pneumonia can kill fast and quickly destroy the productivity of a goat, so don't fool around with home cures if a vet is available.

A broad-spectrum antibiotic, such as pen-strep or tetracycline injectable or a sulfa combination, works in most cases, but in cases where a change of treatment becomes necessary, you must be careful not to change to a drug which is antagonistic to the one used first, as they may cut down each other's action. Your vet can also give you nursing hints for your particular animal. Some need to be steamed, others given injectable expectorants, cortisone, or exercise.

Once a goat has had pneumonia, it may be more apt to get it again another year, so keep an eye on it, especially in times of stress.

RETAINED PLACENTA

Most kidding does expel the afterbirth with or just following each kid. The placenta or afterbirth is a milky membrane which contains the fetus in the uterus. Once in a while a doe will not expel a placenta. Generally the condition is evident, as it will be hanging out of the vulva. But sometimes there will be no sign of it, and unless you were there and noted the absence of it at birth, the doe could become toxic and die. These "hidden" retained placentas are the ones that cause the most trouble, as the hanging ones keep the cervix open to pass drainage and pieces of afterbirth.

If a doe hasn't passed the placenta in 12 hours after kidding, call your veterinarian. The placenta can be left in longer, but some does close up too tightly to get a hand in through the cervix after 12 to 20 hours. Don't be alarmed if your vet decides to leave the placenta hanging and only gives a shot (hormones to aid in the natural release of the placenta) and places boluses in the uterus to dissolve particles and protect against infection. Sometimes this is best to insure the successful future breeding and conception of the doe.

Do not yank at the placenta to try to remove it. Caruncles, cup-shaped spongy-textured "buttons" on the uterus to which the placenta fastens, can be ripped off this way, causing fatal hemorrhage or sterility. If there is no vet available—remember, you can easily pop the doe in the back seat of the car and travel quite a distance—you can attempt to draw as much placenta as possible through the cervix to keep it open, and place two to four sulfa-urea boluses in the uterus to help dissolve the pieces and prevent infection. To try to "clean" the doe without experience is like driving a car without experience—very difficult to do right and safely.

RINGWORM

Ringworm is not a worm nor is it caused by a worm. Ringworm is so named because it shows up as a circular crusty spot, often on the face or neck. It is caused by a fungus. It most often shows up in the late winter months on goats kept inside. It is contagious, so affected animals should be isolated from other animals until it is cleared up. It is ugly, but very seldom causes much of a problem and will disappear when the goats are turned outside in the spring. It does cause trouble when it comes to selling kids, breeding stock, and milk, as it *looks* horrible.

Iodine or a fungicide available through your vet is often used for treatment. Many of the fungicides are in an oil base, which keeps the scab and crust softened for easier removal. The crust should be removed before each treatment in order to get down to the fungus. When applying iodine, soak the area in warm soapy water to soften the crust. After it is removed, pat dry, then apply the iodine, scrubbing in well with an old toothbrush. Work from the outside in, because the fungus may be spread if you rub from the inside outward. When working around the eye, always put a bland ointment such as Vaseline in the eye before applying the medicine, to prevent injury or burning.

TETANUS

Tetanus or lockjaw is fairly common in goats, as it is in people. This is not to say that goats are dying in droves from it, but it is a problem, one that is easier to prevent than cure. Eighty percent or more goats showing signs of tetanus die, even with treatment. But a yearly booster of tetanus toxoid will protect against it.

Tetanus is caused by an organism, *Clostridium tetani,* which is in the soil in many areas. It grows only in the absence of oxygen, and a deep wound or a puncture wound is an ideal incubator for the organism. The first symptoms noticed with tetanus are poor coordination, stiffness in the rear limbs, refusal (inability, actually) to eat and drink. The third eyelid becomes prominent, giving the eye a peculiar look. Bloat is often seen. Once the symptoms are noticed, the chances of recovery are poor. Massive doses of tetanus antitoxin and penicillin sometimes work, but most people cannot or will not put much money into an animal that is a poor risk.

Prevention is the cheapest and surest protection. All nails and wire should be kept away from the goat pasture. All goats should receive a yearly tetanus booster (toxoid). Any deep wounds or puncture wounds should be thoroughly washed out. Flushing the wound out well with a syringe full of warm soapy water is necessary, followed by an antiseptic such as iodine, all the way to the bottom of the wound. Although the goat has had a toxoid booster, it is still a good idea to give it an injection of antitoxin, just to be safe.

A lot of tetanus is seen in goats following dehorning or castration with an elastrator, the rubber band method, so if you use this method be sure to have all goats protected by a tetanus booster a few weeks *prior* to doing the work.

TICKS

Ticks are larger than lice and shaped differently. They more closely resemble a round, flat kernel of field corn. The body is hard. Colors range from gray through brown to nearly black. Unless disease is carried by them or they are numerous on a goat, they usually don't cause a lot of trouble. They are quite easily seen and can be removed. The longer a tick is on a goat, the larger its body gets, as it becomes engorged with blood.

Ticks can be pulled off by hand, if they are pulled off slowly. If they are yanked off, the head may break off, possibly causing infection. They may also be powdered or sprayed with an insecticide.

In tick country, goats kept clipped are bothered less than nonclipped goats. Ticks like to be hidden. There are dairy wipe-on liquids or sprays that help to repel ticks. If ticks should become a severe problem at any time, the goats can be bathed—they hate a dip—with a rotenone solution or similar preparation. Whatever you use, be sure it is safe for dairy animals. Some insecticides leave a harmful residue in the milk. I don't really like insecticides that leave strong residues unless absolutely necessary. (If you wonder why, read *Silent Spring* by Rachel Carson.)

UDDER EDEMA, CAKED BAG

This usually occurs just before freshening and just after, when there is a sudden increase in the circulation to the udder. The swelling shuts off vessels to a certain extent; thus blood is being taken into the udder faster than it is being taken out of it. Fluid seeps out of the blood vessels into the surrounding tissue. This is a "caked bag." It feels doughy to the touch, and fingerprints remain after the udder is handled. The udder may be painful to the doe.

Hot compresses, hot udder ointment, and massage all help reduce the swelling by increasing circulation. Diuretics such as Lasix have worked very well for me. These are given both in injectable and oral forms. Diuretics cause more frequent urination, drawing more fluid from the body, i.e., the udder. Usually only a couple of days of treatment are needed before the udder is normal and stays normal without further treatment. Some caked bags will just clear up naturally without treatment, as the sudden increase in circulation slows down a few days after freshening. If the udder is very badly caked, though, it should be treated, as it can be a stress, ending in mastitis, gangrene mastitis, or decreased production. Cutting the grain a week or so before freshening may help, as grain increases milk production or milk input to the bag, causing the udder to distend.

UDDER INJURIES

Being low to the ground and carrying a large bag, the doe is a prime target for snags, tears, and cuts. Goats and barbed wire are a bad mixture, as does (and bucks!) have little regard for it as a fence and will crawl through. It's very easy for the does to snag their bags on the way through. Bloody scratches or worse usually result.

If the cut is on the bag and is not deep, involving just skin, simple first aid measures are usually adequate. Rinse the injury out well with warm soapy water, to flush out any dirt. Dry, then apply an antiseptic such as sulfa powder or iodine. If the cut is deeper, gapes open, or leaks milk, it is usually best to have it sutured closed. It is also many times advisable to sew up most teat cuts, as they heal quicker and smoother when sutured than when irritated by daily milking and handling, both of which can open the wound just as it begins to heal.

When you believe an injury needs sewing up, call your vet right away. The longer an injury is left, the harder it can be to repair. Several hours after it has occurred, swelling begins to take place. Then the edges begin to dry and finally start to heal. Any dirt in the wound is now part of the animal and may cause infection. To have good healing in an older injury, the edges of the wound must be trimmed or made raw in order that they heal together, not separately. Many wounds will fill in very nicely by themselves, but udder wounds especially should be checked by your veterinarian. Scar tissue on a leg may mean nothing, but in the udder it may mean the loss of productivity of the doe.

Because the udder is the place of milk production, it is richly supplied with blood. This is why many udder wounds bleed profusely. To one not used to blood, it can be quite a shock. Don't panic. Get a clean cloth—dishtowel, diaper, anything clean and absorbent. Wipe the excess blood away, then press the cloth on the wound. Most wounds will stop or nearly stop bleeding in five to ten minutes. Don't move the cloth or remove it for a while, even if the blood has seemed to stop. A clot forms between the cut and cloth and should not be disturbed for fear the bleeding will start again.

If you plan to call your vet, don't put anything on a cut except maybe soap and water, unless it is bleeding very badly and you have some astringent powder, the kind used when dehorning. Use the powder to stop the bleeding if necessary. It is hard to examine a wound or suture it if it is caked with gobs of powder or gooey salve. And please, believe your vet about whether or not to sew up that ugly rip. He wants to do the best for your animal, not do what you'd rather he did. His judgment will be based on past experiences and will give you the best results in the long run.

WORMS

Given half a chance, goats are fairly worm-free. This is not to say goats don't have worms, but that due to their natural eating habits goats come in less contact with worm eggs and larvae than do other animals. Goats don't eat as close to the ground (and thereby pick up possible worm-infested manure) as do other stock, but prefer to nibble and browse when given a chance.

There is a big controversy among goat owners whether or not to worm regularly with a broad-spectrum wormer, which kills most of the worms goats have, or to wait until there is trouble from worms. Personally, I would recommend a routine six-month fecal exam by your vet. He can examine the manure under a microscope to determine the presence of worm eggs and minute larvae. Very seldom will any worms be visible with the naked eye. Never just assume a goat is sick and that it must be worms and proceed to worm the hapless animal. Wormers are all toxic to some extent or they wouldn't kill the worms, and this added toxicity can harm a sick goat.

There are many worms that can infect goats, and you will want to be sure your wormer kills the worms *your* goat has. It is a waste of time and money to use a wormer that is not going to help, and it can be an unnecessary risk. Wormers such as Tox-I-Ton and Thibenzole work well on most worms, and there have been some good results with Tramisol, a cattle wormer which has *not* been cleared for goats, but is being used on them. Phenothiazine works on very few worms but is very safe to use. It is worthwhile when used against those few groups.

Rotating pastures will help keep down worm infestations, as will normal sanitary measures. Keep the goats out of dirty muddy barnyards and manure piles which they love to climb! Where worms have been a problem, the pens and barnyard may be sprinkled with borax every week or so, depending on the weather. Borax, the same stuff you use for cleaning, kills worm larvae.

It is necessary for most worms to use a wormer, then repeat treatment in two weeks. This is necessary because the larvae migrate through the bloodstream, and while the wormers attack mainly the worms in the stomach and intestines, they don't always kill those in the blood or destroy the eggs. These eggs hatch, and if the goat is not wormed again in two weeks, they can completely reinfest the animal.

While at the vet's with your fecal samples, ask him to check for coccidiosis also. This is a protozoa which can cause sick and dead goats in a short time if allowed to get a start. Diarrhea and unthriftiness are the first external signs of the trouble.

SHEEP

General Care and Management

HOUSING

Sheep do not need a warm barn, except at lambing time. It must be dry and not drafty. They do need shade or shelter from the sun in the summer.

A tight woven wire fence is a must, not only to keep the sheep in but to keep dogs out and discourage coyotes. Dogs and coyotes are the worst predators on sheep. Wolves, bears and an occasional bobcat or cougar will attack sheep, but nationwide, dogs are their biggest enemies. These dogs are often someone's pets that chase sheep for the excitement of the chase. A sheep or flock of sheep runs easily, and a running sheep invites attack. This is one reason a goat or two that is used to dogs and preferably carries a good set of horns should be with a flock of sheep on pasture. It is not so much the protection the goats offer, but the fact they don't panic and run as easily as do sheep. The sheep tend to gather around the goats, and standing sheep aren't so inviting.

Parts of the Sheep

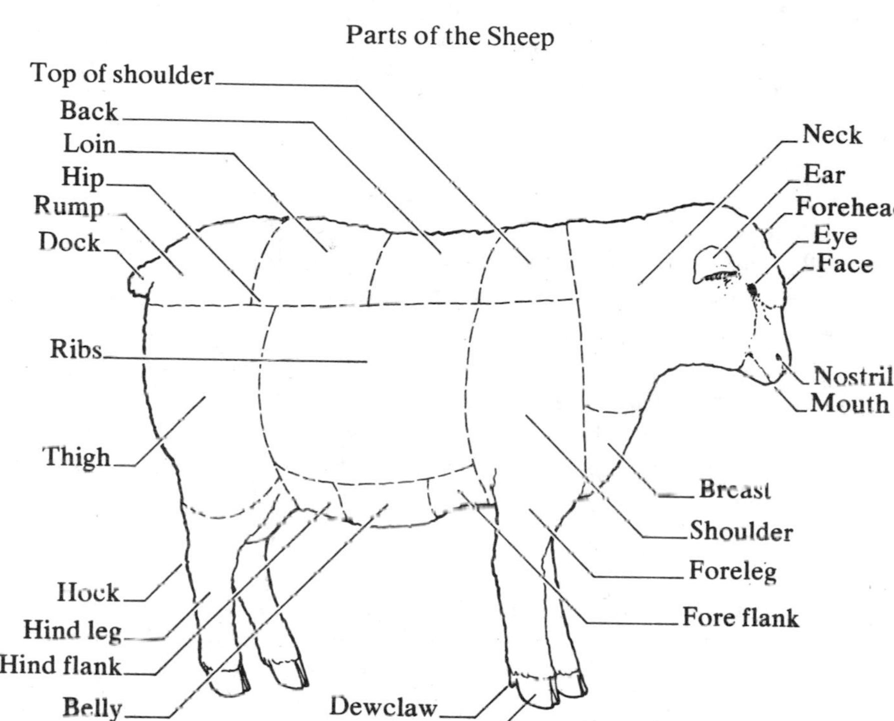

FEEDING

As sheep are found in many arid wastelands, many people get the mistaken idea they can be raised cheaply on poor pasture. This idea has caused many first-time sheep farmers to go broke. To raise sheep, you will need just as good pasture and hay as cattle require. The better your pasture and hay are, the better your sheep will be. They also need grain, or chances of losses due to ketosis or faulty nutrition will be great.

Sheep do not like a dry ground feed such as that fed to cattle. They prefer a coarser ground feed moistened with molasses. Generally, sheep on good lush pasture do not require grain.

When such pasture is not available, a good legume hay should be fed free choice, along with 1½ to two pounds of a good grade of mixed grain daily. Root crops such as turnips and rutabagas are fed to sheep with good success in many parts of the country. They should be chopped to improve palatability and to prevent choking. Corn silage can also be used to good advantage with sheep, as can many other feeds particular to an area. Your local county agent and veterinarian can help here. Bear in mind, though, that any feed changes must be gradual or digestive upsets and stress will result.

Pasture rotation is more of a must with sheep than other domestic animals, because of their susceptibility to parasites and their close grazing habits that are hard on pasture crops. Sheep should be removed from pasture when the crop is eaten down to three or four inches. Sheep pastures should never look bald.

Sheep must always be handled calmly and gently. Running or exciting sheep, especially on a warm day, can kill them. Clean water is a must at all times. And, although a creek is pretty and a handy water source, know where it comes from. If there are animals fairly close upstream, that stream can bring disease to your animals. It pays to check.

Creep Feeding Lambs Lambs will begin to munch on hay or grass and grain at two weeks of age. At first they will eat very little because they are still depending on the ewe for nourishment. But soon they will develop a taste for dry feed and be willing to nibble off and on all day. To provide an eating arrangement that allows this, yet does not let the ewes overload, it is best to provide a creep feeder. This is simply a pen in one corner of the barn or field with small openings to allow the lambs to enter and eat, but too small to admit the ewes. Grain is placed in the feed trough daily. Any leftovers

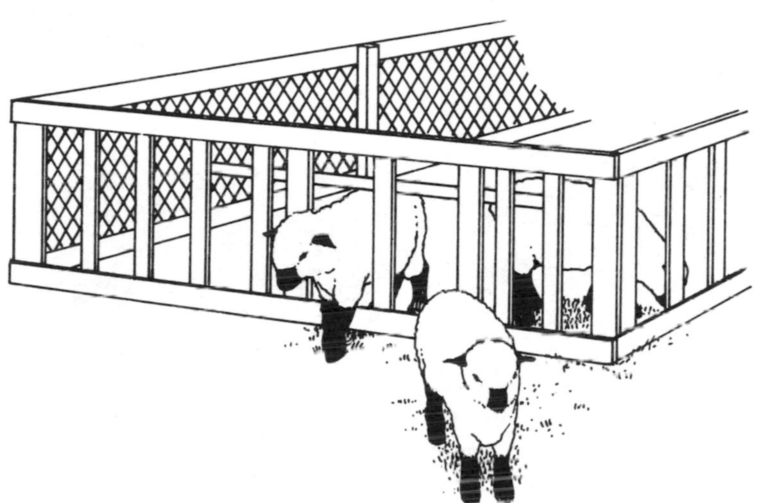

A Lamb Creep

should be cleaned up and fed to the ewes to prevent any mold or sour feed from collecting in the corners. It is a good idea to have a cover to the creep feeder if it is outside, to protect the grain from rain and wind or late snows. Lambs may be creep fed until weaning time.

RESTRAINT

When it becomes necessary to restrain sheep, either for examination or treatment, the safest method is to calmly drive the whole flock or part of it into a holding pen. It is very hard to cut out only one animal from the flock, unless you are lucky enough to own a true sheep dog, not just a dog you run with the sheep. Keep in mind that an excited sheep or flock is hard to drive. Do not yell or run. Quietly move them to the pen.

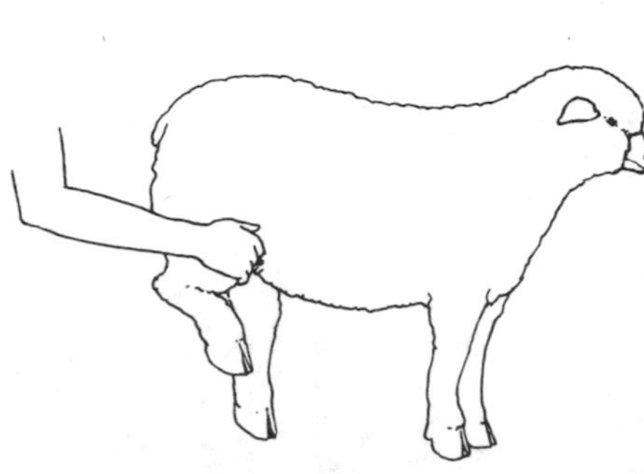

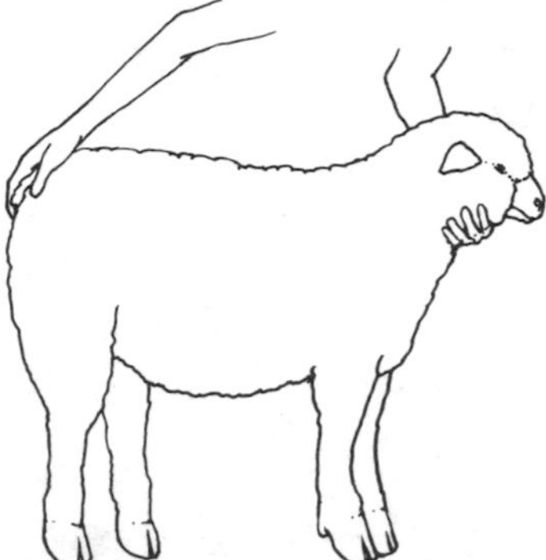

CATCHING

- Confine the animals in a small area
- Move up quietly on the desired animal after working it into a position near you
- With a swift sure movement grasp well up into the right rear flank with the right hand
- Holding firmly with the right hand, quickly grasp under the lower jaw with the left

HOLDING

- With the left hand firmly grasp a fold of flesh under the lower jaw
- Place the right hand securely over the dock; the right hand in this position can be useful in moving the animal
- As the animal quiets down the right hand may be removed

When the flock is penned, you may have to divide the pen if the flock is large. When you are ready to catch the sheep, walk toward it but don't look directly at it. When close, quickly reach out and grab the wool under the chin and tip the head upward. This will keep it off balance and make it easy to hold. Lambs are easiest caught by a hind leg.

To drench a sheep (give it liquid medicine) retain the chin hold and swing a leg over the back, straddling the animal. The drenching syringe or bottle is slipped into the corner of the mouth and over the tongue, and the liquid is slowly released. The sheep's nose should not be tipped way up, or there will be increased danger of it inhaling some of the fluid. Never squirt

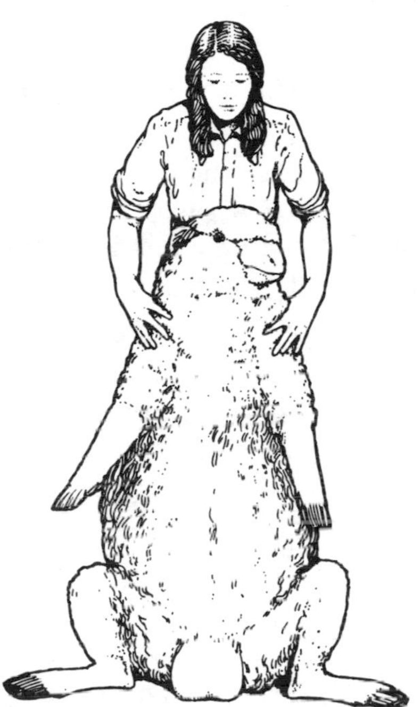

Sheep restraint achieved by it sitting down with its back on assistant's legs.

or pour it in fast, because if liquid gets into the lungs, you will have a dead sheep.

To give a bolus (large pill), you again straddle the sheep as for drenching. The bolus, dipped in grease for easy swallowing, is slipped into the balling gun. The balling gun is slipped into the mouth and over the hump in the tongue. The bolus is then quickly ejected and the head is held up, with the mouth held closed until swallowing has occurred.

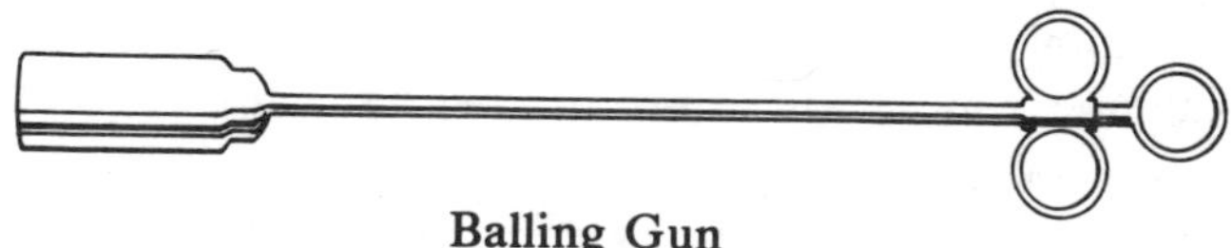

Balling Gun

Giving an intramuscular injection to a sheep can be hard if you have never done it before. How do you find the sheep under all that wool? The sheep is forced into a corner and against a wall, with a knee in the flank. Divide the wool until skin is visible. Remember, a sheep is not really fat under normal conditions, so the best place is in the thigh muscle. Slip the needle into the muscle and inject the drug. Don't go into the bone.

BREEDING

The normal breeding season is in the fall and early winter, August to December. The ewe comes into heat every 21 to 26 days. The gestation period is five months. The ewes should be bred to drop their lambs during the best month for *you*. If the barn is above freezing all winter, they can be bred in August to lamb in January. If the barn is cold or the extra care cannot be given at that time, they can be bred in November or December, to lamb in April or May.

The ram must be kept separate from the ewes unless very early lambs are desired. He absolutely must be kept from the flock if young ewes are with the flock, as ewes bred too young may have lambing trouble that may not only kill the lamb but the ewe as well. Ewes should have their first lambs when they are two years old. Ewes should be "flushed" at breeding time. This means they should be turned onto extra good pasture so they will be gaining weight when bred. One adult ram can serve 40 to 50 ewes in a breeding season, if he is in good condition—neither thin nor overly fat. A young ram can handle half that amount.

During the winter, the ewes should have good alfalfa or legume hay fed free choice, along with one to 1½ pounds of good mixed grain daily. The hay and grain, also the water and salt, should be in different areas so the ewes are forced to exercise. A month before lambing the grain may have to be increased so the ewe is gaining weight slightly as lambing approaches. Many ewes are lost to ketosis or pregnancy disease due to insufficient grain or no legume hay having been fed, which causes carbohydrate deficiency, especially in ewes carrying twins or triplets.

The ewe will usually show udder development about one to two weeks before lambing. The wool around her udder should then be clipped away to make it easier for the new lambs to find the teats.

LAMBING, NORMAL

In the week before lambing, the ewe will build up a nice full udder. It should be pink and firm, but not rock hard or bluish. She will move slower and may lie down more than usual. Her vulva will elongate and begin to relax. Approaching lambing, she may refuse feed and paw the ground. She may seek out a quiet corner, walking with head down. But don't count on such warning signs. She may just lie down and pop out twins.

Once she throws out strings of mucus, pink or tinged with blood, you will know she isn't fooling around. She will grunt and begin to strain hard. In fifteen minutes or so, a dark bulge will appear in the vulva. This is the water bag. Closely following it will appear two feet, toes pointed down. When the legs are out nearly to the knees, the nose will appear. She will usually work hard a few minutes, then the head and shoulders will be forced out. She may rest a minute, then continue labor until the rest of the lamb is expelled. Remember, lambs are born with a long tail, which is later docked.

Most ewes of good size have twins, so the second lamb will probably soon follow. The ewe will then clean both lambs until they are white and dry. Some lambs are nearly black at birth, but whiten as they get older. Within an hour they will be on their feet nursing, with their tails wagging.

LAMBING, ABNORMAL

When the ewe labors more than an hour and does not produce a lamb, she should be examined for trouble. Scrub your hands and use some liquid soap as a lubricant. Often a leg will have been deflected on the brim of the ewe's pelvis. If the head and only one leg is in the birth canal, you will have to bring up the missing leg. Be careful to get the leg belonging to *that* lamb, not a twin! It is often necessary to force the lamb back in order to gain room to bring the leg into the birth canal.

If the lamb is coming backward, it will be easily delivered in most cases unless a leg is retained, but as soon as it is born, the nose and throat must be freed of mucus and afterbirth. The lamb begins to breathe as soon as the umbilical cord breaks, which sometimes happens when the backward lamb is only halfway out. If the lamb sounds bubbly as it breathes or is not breathing, you must pick it up by the hind feet and slap its side with the flat of your hand. This forces mucus and fluid out of the throat and lungs and the new lamb will usually start breathing. The shock of the slap causes the lamb to take a deep breath. If the lamb doesn't breathe well, rub it vigorously with a warm towel, and keep wiping the fluid out of the nose and mouth.

When the front legs appear but no head, you can be almost assured that the head has been turned back inside the uterus. Here, you must push the legs back to gain room while trying to reach the head with your other hand. Often the head can be cupped in your hand and be pried around. If this doesn't work, try getting a finger and thumb in the lower jaw, like a fishhook, and draw the head around with that hold. Once the head is in position, draw head and legs out gently. Again, be sure the head belongs to the *right* twin. Two lambs cannot be born at the same time!

In the case of a lamb that is just too big to fit through the birth canal, or a lamb that has a retained head or leg that cannot be reached in a few minutes, you'd best call your veterinarian. A caesarean section may be necessary, or he may, with the use of instruments and experience, be able to deliver the lambs normally. Don't work on the ewe until she is exhausted. Exhaustion can throw a ewe into shock, and sheep die easily from shock. If you plan to take your ewe to the vet or have him out, give the ewe and the veterinarian both a chance by doing so early in the labor.

CARE OF YOUNG LAMBS

Lambing pens should be ready. Many lambs lost or rejected could have been saved by using pens. These are small (five by six feet) temporary pens, usually built by tying gates together. These wooden gates can be stacked for storage after lambing season. Their purpose is to keep the ewe from being bothered by other ewes and to keep the lambs near the mother. When a ewe is ready to lamb or has just been found with new lambs, she is put in a pen. She should be watched to be sure there are no lambing problems and that she cleans the lambs and lets them nurse. Twins or triplets are once in a while a problem, as some ewes tend to ignore one of the lambs. Sometimes it is necessary to keep shoving the one that is being ignored to her nose or even taking the other lamb away temporarily until she begins cleaning it up and mothering it. Some weak lambs must be tube fed (see "Bloat and Indigestion" in the chapter on goats). Often this can be discontinued after three or four feedings when more strength has developed. Heat is necessary here too. A heat lamp works well. Just be sure it is safely fastened so that it doesn't get knocked down, causing a fire.

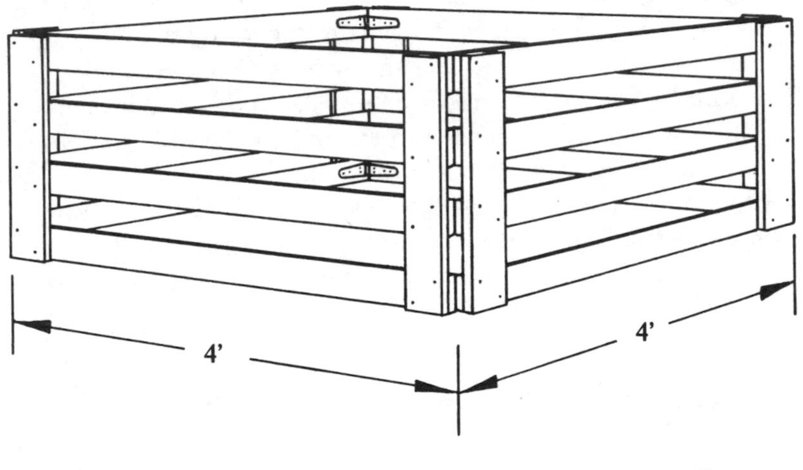

A Lambing Pen

Orphan Lambs and Rejected Lambs It is fairly common for a ewe to reject her lamb. She will completely and firmly refuse to have anything to do with it, kicking and butting it away when it tries to nurse. Sometimes these ewes can be fooled by smearing Vicks on the lamb's and the ewe's nose. She then cannot smell the lamb and may nurse it. Slipping a piece of twine around the ewe's hind legs in a figure 8 and forcing her to let the lamb nurse will eventually work. Do not tie the twine, but hold it in your hand to prevent injury.

When a ewe completely rejects a lamb or a lamb is left an orphan, you are left stuck with a lamb to raise. Sometimes another ewe with a single lamb can be persuaded to take the lamb by using Vicks on the lamb's and her nose. She cannot smell her lamb and may take the orphan. Without a foster mother, you will have to bottle feed the lamb. The lamb is placed in a warm, draft-free pen, or a cardboard box in the kitchen. For the first week after birth, the lamb should be fed at least every four hours around the clock. It will take from one to two ounces soon after birth, and can be increased gradually to an eight ounce bottleful at each meal. The lamb should be almost full, but still be eager for more milk when the bottle is empty. Goat's milk is an ideal substitute for ewe's milk, if it is available. If the lamb should develop diarrhea, cut the amount of milk per feeding in half and dose with Kaopectate. Encourage the lamb to nibble on calf pellets and mixed grain, as well as grass or good bright legume hay.

For other problems related to pregnancy and lambing see "Ketosis," "Retained Placenta," and "Eversion of the Uterus" in the section, **Diseases and Other Problems**, later in this chapter.

CASTRATION

All ram lambs not being kept for breeding should be castrated. There will be faster gain to the meat cuts in the carcass. A ram lamb will weigh as much as a wether at eight to 11 months, but the weight will not be as easily or completely utilized as meat. The lambs should be castrated young, before fly season arrives, if they are to be done surgically.

Surgical Castration An assistant can hold the lamb on his lap with the hind legs drawn up. An incision is then made on the bottom of the scrotum over each testicle. At the same time, the testicle is forced upward against the bottom of the scrotum.

The testicle and tunic—the whitish membrane surrounding the testicle—are pulled out until the cord breaks. There should be nothing hanging through the incision. When the testicle is pulled out until the cord snaps, there is very little bleeding. If the cord and tunic are cut with a sharp blade, bleeding will result. The same is done with the second testicle. If the lamb is large, the cord may have to be cut with an emasculator to prevent bleeding. This cuts and crushes the blood vessels at the same time.

With older lambs and rams, the easiest method of castration is by using a Burdizzo emasculatome. This instrument crushes the individual cords, causing the testicles to slowly shrink up. (See "Castration" in the chapter on goats.) I do not like the use of rubber bands for either castration or docking. There are just too many problems involved, from pain to tetanus and infection.

DOCKING

All lambs should be docked. Long tails harbor dampness and can encourage maggots. Some ewes are hard to breed due to the thick wool on the tail. Sheep carrying long tails are not showable, nor do they bring good prices when sold. Lambs from one week to one month are easiest to dock. Although the tail can be cut off with an axe, chisel, or knife, the best way is to use an emasculator. This quickly cuts the tail off and also crushes the blood vessels, resulting in a bloodless dock. Following docking, the stump should be dipped in an antiseptic to prevent infection. The tail should be taken off very short, leaving only an inch or so on the lamb. An injection for tetanus is advisable, just for safety. Antitoxin should be given. Lambs can be docked and castrated at the same time to save time.

Done quickly and right, there is very little shock and very little bloodshed.

Diseases and Other Problems

CASEOUS LYMPHADENITIS

This is the infection of the lymph glands by *Corynebacterium pseudotuberculosis.* On occasion, abscesses form in the lymph glands near the skin and are visible, but generally there are internal abscesses in the intestines, liver, kidneys, or lungs. This has been called "wasting disease" because most affected animals simply become emaciated or waste away.

Treatment is very unsuccessful, although if the sheep is very valuable, an autogenous vaccine may be prepared to use on the affected animal. If the lymphadenitis has progressed too far, the animal may pass the point of no return before treatment can be initiated. The sheep can be vaccinated against this problem if trouble has occurred in the flock.

ENTEROTOXEMIA OR OVEREATING DISEASE

This is a disease caused by *Clostridium perfringens* Type D, which is related to the organism that causes tetanus. Like tetanus, it cannot be successfully treated, but can be vaccinated against. It most generally is seen in show or feedlot lambs being grained heavily for fast weight gain. It often strikes the biggest lambs first. They show signs such as circling, pushing their heads against a wall, convulsions, and unsteadiness. They often die suddenly. All sheep on heavy grain should be routinely vaccinated, especially lambs from weaning to eight months of age.

EVERSION OF THE UTERUS

With an eversion the uterus is turned inside out and pushed by contractions out of the body. This is a heavy, oval-shaped, reddish mass. There are knobs every so often, looking like fleshy sponges, which serve to hold the placenta to the wall of the uterus. The pushed-out uterus must be replaced very soon, or the shock will kill the ewe. It is a definite emergency.

When the uterus has been found hanging from a ewe, call your veterinarian immediately. While waiting for him, slowly work the ewe into a small pen where she will be alone. Many ewes are lost by having other sheep walk on the uterus. It is fragile, and if torn, the ewe will very likely die. It is this fragility that makes it hard to replace. It is heavy, awkward, and slow work, and all the while the veterinarian is working, he must worry about pushing too hard and poking a hole in the uterus.

Keep the uterus clean and covered with a warm, moist towel. Get together several clean towels, a bale of hay or straw to rest the uterus on during replacement, and a pail of hot water. Many veterinarians use an injection to help shrink up the uterus to normal size. This helps to keep it in place by reducing the incentive for the ewe to strain. Even though many ewes must have their vulvas laced up to help insure that the uterus remains in place, keep in mind that the ewe can still push her uterus back out if she strains too hard. Watch her for several hours. If straining is noticed, call your veterinarian right away.

Do not plan on keeping the ewe or her lambs for breeding, as this can be an inherited weakness and will often be repeated yearly until death results.

FLIES

Sheep are more often bothered with maggots than other farm animals. This is because the dense wool covering the body makes a good hiding place, especially if the sheep has had diarrhea or a cut, which provide moisture and attract the flies. Flies lay their eggs in the cuts or damp foul wool, soiled by diarrhea or pus. Soon, sometimes in just a day, these eggs hatch out into small maggots. These maggots not only clean up any foul matter but then go on, eating the living, healthy flesh. Fly eggs are seen as tiny yellowish white specks. There can be hundreds in a small area.

This is the main reason lambs' tails are docked. The tails are heavy and hang below the rectum, gathering any loose fecal material and holding moisture. Of course, not all long-tailed sheep get maggots, but once you've seen a nice healthy sheep with the whole hind end boiling with maggots, you'll be a believer in docking. Lambs should be docked before fly season or kept inside so they can be carefully watched. Any cuts should be treated at once with a fly repellent-antiseptic, such as Smear 62 or scarlet oil.

If a sheep shows dark wool around the hindquarters, catch it and find out why. If the fleece is soiled badly with filth, you'd better either wash it thoroughly and keep the sheep up until it is dried thoroughly, or at least clip the soiled portion of the fleece off, exposing the skin to fresh air. Better to lose part of the wool than the sheep. At the same time treat diarrhea if present.

FOOT ROT

Foot rot is an infectious disease affecting the hooves of sheep. It is caused by a fungus, which gains entrance into the body through small cracks and abrasions in between the toes. Lameness is usually the first sign. The affected sheep may not eat or want to move about to graze. The toes become more inflamed until the horn of the claws separates from the skin. The feet have a bad odor. Foot rot is most often seen when the sheep are pastured in wet, swampy areas or crowded, muddy barn lots.

If the foot rot is caught early, treat with copper sulfate, or for sheep in heavy fleece, formalin may be used as it does not stain the wool. All necrotic material must be removed and the foot trimmed down well. If only one or two animals are affected, give daily soaks in hot water, then apply antibiotic and astringent. The affected animals are kept separate in dry, clean pens. The rest of the flock should be carefully checked, then driven through a five percent formalin foot bath weekly for three weeks. The flock should be moved to good, high, dry pasture where there have been no sheep for two to three weeks or longer.

The few animals not responding to treatment should be butchered, as they will remain a source of infection for the entire flock.

KETOSIS

Ketosis or pregnancy disease usually occurs in misfed ewes, from one to four weeks before lambing. There is much misunderstanding and debate about ketosis, both among researchers and sheep owners. It is not known exactly what causes the ketosis in the body. It is believed by some to be a glandular problem; others believe it is caused by insufficient carbohydrates supplied by the feed. I tend to agree with the latter idea, as ewes receiving full feed of mixed grass hay and little or no grain have had incidence of 75 percent ketosis, where with increased grain the incidence was dramatically reduced. High quality clover or other legume hay also appears to help in some flocks.

In ketosis, the ewes will begin to get dopey. They may stagger, circle, lose their balance, or just lie around. I haven't had much luck in treating ewes once they go down or get quite staggery from ketosis, and know of no one who has. The safest treatment is a caesarean section done before the ewe is in bad shape.

To check for possible ketosis, the ewes should be watched as they move daily. They may be slowly driven, or hay or grain can be fed at one end of the yard while you watch for any abnormal acting ewes. Any "slow" ewes should be cut out and penned where they can receive special attention. Extra grain mixed with molasses and even chopped raw potatoes or stale bread, fed several times daily, can sometimes relieve the symptoms.

The ewe flock should be checked for weight as they approach the eight week period before lambing. *Feel* their back and sides. Some ewes appear fat with a heavy fleece, but are in reality quite thin. The ewes should receive adequate grain before lambing and be in good flesh. Some ewes require only a pound of grain daily, but depending on the hay and the weather, they may need much more. Remember, cold weather makes the ewes eat more and they may need the extra grain to supply the body with heat. There may not be enough carbohydrates left over to nourish the ewe or her lambs.

LICE

Lice are small, grayish, soft-bodied parasites that attack sheep, most often during the winter. Due to the damage that can be done to the fleece by rubbing and scratching, it is generally best to routinely powder the flock *before* any trouble is noticed. A rotenone or pyrethrum powder is safe and effective. It is best to powder once a week for three weeks in the early winter and then again in January or February.

Lice can become so numerous before any sign of them is noticed that they can actually bleed a sheep to death. Less dramatically, they cause anemia, unthriftiness, and waste of feed, as the sheep must eat for itself and the lice.

MANGE

This is highly contagious, and treatment does not give good results. It causes high economic losses, as the fleece is usually ruined and the sheep soon becomes run-down and anemic. Large areas of crusty lesions form, which act almost as a burn, making the skin nonfunctioning. This disease is so expensive to sheepmen that it is a reportable disease, i.e., it must be reported to the area's state veterinarian, and an affected flock is quarantined.

Intense itching, followed by loss of wool in large chunks and red, crusty areas on the skin are signs of scabies. On finding a suspect sheep in your flock, call your vet right away. Isolate the affected sheep and carefully check the rest of the flock for itching or "bumpy" wool. Chances are your sheep will have something much less frightening, but take no chances. Scabies or mange is caused by tiny mites which burrow under the skin, making them very hard to kill.

PNEUMONIA

Pneumonia claims many sheep yearly and causes economic loss in sheep which do not die. After a bout with pneumonia,

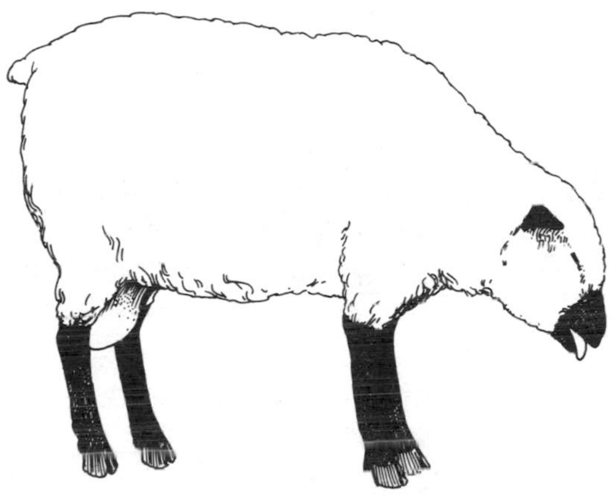

Sheep with pneumonia show signs of dejection and puffing for breath.

large amounts of scar tissue are formed on the lungs. This malfunctioning means the animal has to fight for air. It loses weight and can seldom stand a pregnancy or the added strain of raising lambs.

Pneumonia can be caused by several bacteria and viruses, the most frequent of which is the bacterial pneumonia. These bacteria grab hold following a period of stress, caused by anything from changes in the weather to being chased by dogs. The sick sheep will stand, usually puffing a bit. It may be off feed or just act a little slow. It is now that the temperature should be taken, for treatment must be started immediately if the sheep is to be saved. Sheep have the least stamina—some call it "will to live"—of any animal on the farm. Once down and sick, many seem to just refuse to live.

A sheep with pneumonia generally runs a temperature of 103°F. to 107°F. If the sick sheep was with others, take the temperatures of several others. Often there will be others not exactly looking sick, but on their way, with temperatures of

103°F. to 104.5°F. or so. Treatment should be started on these also. All sick sheep should be isolated, hopefully to check the spread of the disease. Others may be coming down with it, which means they are incubating the disease, so watch the others even though all sick ones have been removed.

Let your veterinarian advise you with pneumonia, as there are other factors besides antibiotic therapy to be considered. Sometimes an injectable expectorant must be given to break up the consolidation in the lungs. Cortisone sometimes helps, but in some cases may cause harm. Often, steaming or light exercise and sunshine will help.

Anything that can be fed to keep the sheep eating will help. Often very small amounts of chopped carrots, chopped apples, soda crackers, stale bread, lettuce, rolled oats with molasses, or other goodies will help.

RETAINED PLACENTA

After each lamb is born, the placenta or afterbirth should follow. Occasionally one of the placentas does not come away from the uterus. This is usually quite obvious, with the placenta hanging a foot or more out of the vulva. Once in a while a part rips off and the rest remains in the uterus, hidden from sight. This is the most important reason for observing the afterbirths at lambing time.

If a placenta has been retained for twelve hours, your veterinarian should be called. It is important to differentiate between a retained placenta and an eversion of the uterus. The placenta is a clear or nearly silver membrane, long and stringy. It must come away from the uterus to prevent infection due to the uterus holding pieces, while the cervix closes tightly, trapping the discharge. If it does not come away by itself, your veterinarian can either remove it manually or give an injection of hormones to encourage it to come away.

SCOURS OR DIARRHEA

Scours is most often seen in lambs from one to three weeks of age. Several bacteria can cause scours, as can viruses or just plain overeating. Milk is irritating to the intestines and when too much is eaten at once, the intestines may become raw and scouring may start. Keep watch for any lambs with wet or sticky tails. Watch closely any bottle-fed lambs, as they have the added stress of no mother to snack on. Normally, the lamb only takes a few sucks at a time, all day long, but on a bottle it gets more milk, fed only two or three times a day in most cases.

If the scouring is spotted quickly, a few doses of Kaopectate and reduced milk intake will usually remedy the problem. A small- to medium-sized lamb can take two to four tablespoonsful every four hours. If after 12 hours of treatment the stool is no firmer, consult your veterinarian. Sometimes antibiotics need to be given. The milk may have to be replaced with oral electrolytes until the body's salt balance is normal. A lamb cannot have severe diarrhea for much longer than a day without being in serious trouble.

Scours in older lambs and sheep can come from overeating grain or lush pasture. It can be a sign of allergy to a pasture plant. Coccidiosis and worms can cause scours, as can enterotoxemia, Johne's disease, and others. A general rule to follow would be to treat the animal for one day with an astringent antidiarrheal, such as copper sulfate, iron sulfate, and catechu. This will remedy simple diarrhea. If the diarrhea persists, take a stool sample (a tablespoonful or so) to your vet for a check. Let him go on from there.

SORE MOUTH

This is a very contagious disease caused by a virus which is quite hardy and transmissible to humans. It can be brought to a farm by sheep shearers or new sheep. There are plenty of signs when a flock is infected. The lips swell and scab. The scabs may extend into the mouth, and there may be scabs on the feet, between the toes, and on the nose.

Once it has broken out, no cure is possible. Feeding moist, easily mouthed foods and even drenching with gruel may be necessary to keep the animal's strength up until the virus runs its course. Antibiotics are sometimes given to prevent secondary infections. Vaccination will prevent this disease. All new sheep should be vaccinated and isolated for two to three weeks before being turned with the flock.

TETANUS

Tetanus or lockjaw is caused by an organism, *Clostridium tetani*, which is in the soil in many areas. For information about symptoms, treatment, and prevention see "Tetanus" in the chapter on goats.

TICKS

Ticks can be a problem with sheep in many geographical areas. Usually they only cause trouble as a parasite, sucking the blood, but in some areas they can spread disease. Ask your local veterinarian or county agent about ticks in your part of the country. Some places are so badly infested with ticks that sheep must be dipped several times a year. In other areas sheep only need a dip after shearing. In still other areas, there are no ticks at all.

WORMS

Here we have the biggest problem in sheep. They can become infected with many different kinds of worms, some being hard to get rid of, a few impossible to destroy. There are books written on parasites of sheep, so in no way can I adequately cover them here.

To give an idea of the variety of worms possible in sheep, here is a partial list:

Nodular worm
Bankrupt worm
Common stomach worm
Brown stomach worm
Small stomach worm
Thread-necked worm
Common tapeworm
Thread lungworm
Hair lungworm
Common liver fluke
Deer fluke
Coccidia (not a worm but a parasite)

Basically, the sheep gets worms or is reinfested with worms by grazing on grass on which there are worm eggs, small worms, or snails (carriers for some parasites). The grass is swallowed, and soon the sheep is parasitized. This is why pasture rotation is so important in sheep. They tend to graze close, thus picking up more parasites. If the pasture is long, and the sheep are not kept on it for long periods, the chances of contamination will be less. Even though sheep are wormed routinely, they are never completely worm-free under farm or range conditions, and thus reinfestation is always possible.

Worms and other parasites make trouble by causing anemia, unthriftiness, and sometimes death. Lambs are infected through the bloodstream and may die soon after birth. Stress, such as being chased by dogs or a cold winter, will kill heavily parasitized sheep.

Worm Control There is no one worm medicine that is effective against all parasites. Therefore it is best to take a fecal sample to your veterinarian or ask his opinion when suspecting worms or other intestinal parasites. It is best to know what worms your sheep have before treating, to save the sheep and your money.

A phenothiazine-trace mineral salt mix put in the pasture after lambing, ten pounds phenothiazine to 100 pounds of salt, will greatly help keep down the worm problem, but bear in mind it does not kill all worms. The sheep should still be wormed with a broad-spectrum wormer (drench or bolus) in the early summer and late fall, unless your sheep are found to have a worm which requires a different wormer. At any rate, follow your local veterinarian's recommendations. He is familiar with the types of parasites commonly found in sheep in your area.

Liver Fluke This parasite is a deadly one, infesting the liver. Sheep can pick up flukes from infected deer and snails. Much liver fluke damage is seen in sheep grazing on marshy or swampy ground. The liver fluke destroys the liver of the affected animal. There is no preventive, other than keeping the flock out of low pasture land. Treatment is very toxic and should be left to your veterinarian.

Coccidia Coccidia cause stunted growth, diarrhea (sometimes bloody), and unthriftiness. They can kill sheep. Coccidia are protozoa, one-celled parasites. Crowding, damp bedding, and foul barn lots all help coccidia get a start. If spotted in time, it can be controlled by use of nitrofurazone or sulfas, but be sure it is for coccidiosis, as there are many different sulfas, some ineffective against coccidia. Coccidiosis is more often seen in crowded feed lot lambs, as opposed to sheep on open pasture.

HORSES
(and ponies, donkeys, and mules)

General Care and Management

HOUSING

A horse is a sturdy animal, and more are overhoused than underhoused. That is, many horses are kept in all winter and even during the summer, when they would be healthier and happier outside. Horses need shelter from cold, rain, driving wind, and heavy snows. But they also need exercise and sunshine.

The very best arrangement is a box stall with a door outside to the pasture. Even in the winter they will run, play, and wander about. If this is impossible there should be a fenced area on the south side of the barn where the horses can be turned out each morning. There will be shelter provided by the barn, and the horses can be brought inside during the night or in bad weather. A box stall is best for a horse. It should be 14 by 14 feet or larger. This gives some exercise and allows room for the horse to lie flat out, if it wants to. Contrary to popular belief, most horses do not prefer to sleep standing, although they can do it. Given a chance, most will lie down to sleep, catching a snooze in between times while standing.

Bedding can be straw, sawdust, old but not moldy hay, or moss. Dried moss, available in some areas, is great for bedding and makes the manure dandy compost for the garden! In the box stall, the bedding should be deeper toward the sides, as horses can get cast or stuck if there is a low spot by the stall wall. The bedding should be four inches deep with a gravel or clay floor, six inches on wood, and eight inches on cement.

Lacking box stalls, horses can be kept well in tie or standing stalls. These stalls are five feet wide by eight to ten feet long. The horse is tied to a manger in which it has a supply of hay and a box for grain. The disadvantages to a tie stall are:

- The horse must be exercised daily.
- There is more danger of it becoming cast.
- The stall must be cleaned and bedded daily. With a box stall, you can cheat, just throwing clean bedding in daily, and cleaning it thoroughly every three days.

The sides of the tie stall should reach higher than the underside of the horse's belly and be constructed of 2 by 6 lumber, preferably hardwood. The sides should be solid, or at least have spaces in between no larger than two inches. The manger should be similarly constructed, and the section to which the horse is tied should be hardwood and very solidly built.

It is the snap that usually breaks when horses are tied. A ¾-inch nylon rope 2½ to three feet long, with a bull snap, should be used to tie the horse. To use a longer rope is to invite injury. Leave this rope tied in the stall, using a lead shank to lead the horse outside. *Always* use a lead shank, even with a gentle horse. A shying horse can dislocate fingers or a shoulder, and no horse lives that can't be scared by something. Just think of how you jump when someone talks or touches you unexpectedly!

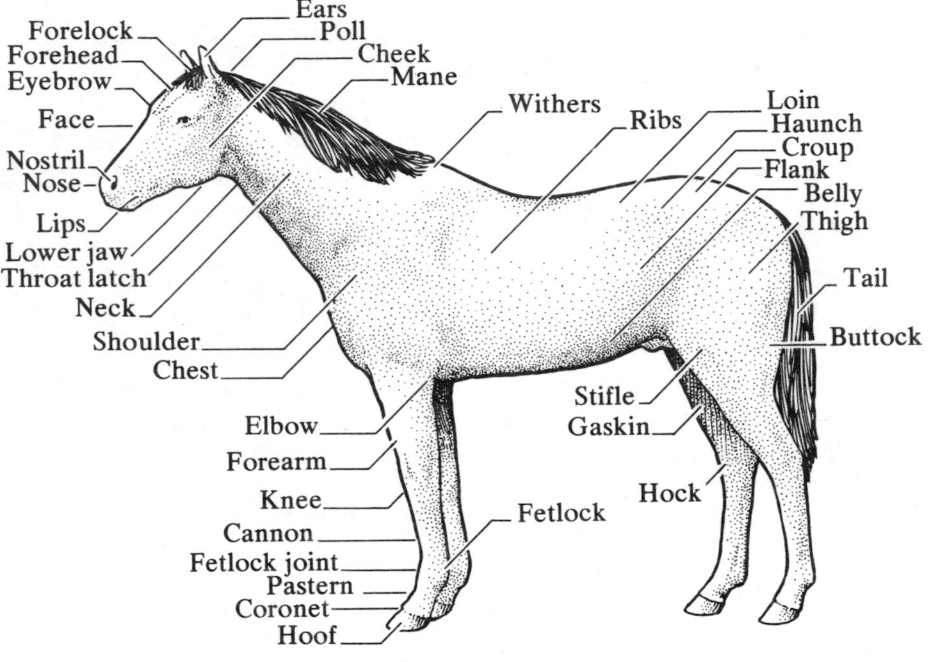

Parts of the Horse

It is a good idea to place a heel chain across the back of the stall. This can be anything from a piece of hay rope with a very heavy snap to a heavy chain and snap, strung across just below the buttocks of the horse. This will prevent the horse from backing into the aisle or another loose horse crowding in with him, causing injury to the tied horse.

FEEDING

Horses should be fed according to the amount of stress they are subjected to. The stress can range from a sunny-pastured, idle horse—near zero stress—to a horse racing regularly, under much stress from hard work, transportation, change in water, excitement, and so on.

A horse that is idle does very well on pasture only, during the spring, summer, and fall. In some locales horses can be pastured year around, but because of the poorer nutritive qualities of winter grass, it may be necessary to supplement with grain or good quality hay. In areas where there are heavy frosts and snow covers the winter grass, a good, clean, mixed hay should be fed, either free choice or twice daily if the horse tends to gain too much weight on free choice. I don't generally recommend pelleted hay, though it is nutritionally sound, for the reason that the horse quickly eats the pellets and then is bored. Cribbing, pawing, stall walking, weaving, etc., all are bad habits that can come from boredom.

The growing colt or filly, the mare heavy in foal, or the stallion at heavy service should receive grain daily. Old, sick, or thin horses also need grain, but should receive a more palatable and more fattening ration. Where most horses needing grain do well on a basic corn-oats mix, old, sick, or thin horses benefit from coarse-ground corn, steamed, rolled, or crimped oats with molasses added to improve palatability and digestion. Pelleted hay can also be fed, as the nutrition is there with less chewing effort. Old horses or horses with mouth injuries do well on ground hay. The conformation of a horse also determines the amount of feed required. A close-coupled horse of stocky build will need less feed to stay in good shape than a tall, long-backed horse.

Generally speaking, a horse doing light work daily can use about six pounds of mixed grain daily. This amount also is good for growing colts, mares in foal, and stallions at medium service. A horse worked fairly hard daily, such as pleasure training or trail riding, or a yearling, mare heavy in foal, or stallion at heavy service, can use ten pounds daily. A horse at hard work, such as showing, racing, field work, hunting, or contesting, can use up to 16 pounds or more daily, depending on the horse's conformation and disposition. A "hot" horse that worries and gets worked up easily will use more grain than a calm horse.

A salt block containing trace minerals should be available at all times, as should fresh, clean water. Although many horses survive on just eating snow during the winter, they will stay in better shape if they have access to water. Some horses do not eat enough snow to furnish their bodies with adequate water and become dehydrated. A big pailful of snow melts down to very little water. A hot, sweating horse should not be allowed to drink until it is walked or it grazes awhile and cools down. A horse that gulps water while hot will often get colic or founder, possibly even dying as a result.

EXERCISE

A horse should receive daily exercise, whether it is walking about in the pasture, turned in a paddock while the stall is being cleaned, or being worked. A horse should be built up and conditioned if it is to be worked hard. A great many horses are ruined daily from too much strain and exertion when out of condition. True, a horse *can* run for a couple of miles, but when a horse is soft (not conditioned by daily training), it's dangerous to jump on its back and tear off at a gallop. It's a sure way to kill or seriously disable it. Heaves, founder, lameness, and broken bones in the feet are only a few of the ills brought on by violent exercise. Let the TV cowboys tear around. They aren't riding your horse.

Even the stallion and brood mare heavy in foal need daily exercise. If broken to ride or drive, they can be worked daily, or exercised on a long line, or in the case of the mare, led alongside another quiet horse. Some stallions can be exercised in this manner but are generally a little hard for a beginner to safely handle.

A horse should feel hard to be in good shape. The ribs should be just barely visible as the horse moves. The backbone should be well covered and the hips rounded. The horse should not be rounded with soft fat like a beef steer. Unfortunately this is often the case, as seen in halter classes today. A horse in top condition for working or breeding is seldom plump, any more than a top athlete would be. Fat mares have breeding and foaling trouble, and fat stallions are often unwilling to breed or are less fertile than lean, well-built stallions.

RESTRAINT

Because of the horse's well-developed nervous system and power, it requires a little more knowledge to properly restrain one than it does most other livestock animals. If not properly restrained, the agitated horse can break loose and injure people or injure itself badly.

Fences Most horses are fairly easy to fence in. There is *no* 100 percent safe fence for horses, but any good, tight, well-built fence is usually quite safe for the average horse. A pole or board fence is excellent, but often expensive if used for the whole pasture. It does make a nice neat fence for a paddock or exercise ring near the barn. A stone fence or wall is also tops, but requires experience, hard work, and of course lots of stones. The most practical fence is woven wire. It is safe, easily put up, and economical. It is long lasting, but should be tightened yearly to prevent sags which some horses get their feet hung up in. The fence may have to be topped with a board or strand of barbed wire or electric wire to keep the horses from leaning over (the grass is always greener . . .) and sagging the fence.

Tight barbed wire is cheaper and just as safe in most instances. It has gotten a bad name because many horses have been badly injured by it. I've had large pastures fenced with barbed wire for years and have never had a cut animal. *Loose* barbed wire is a menace. Many horses are injured badly by getting tangled up in barbed wire that is half-buried in the grass. They panic and pull, tearing gashes all over their bodies. Barbed wire should not be used in a stallion's paddock or in a colt pasture. Colts and fillies, especially weanlings, are nervous, playful, and nosy. They may hit the fence in their play or while frightened, and get cut.

Exercise rings should not be of barbed wire. A too exuberant horse can slam into a fence while playing. Any new barbed wire fence should be shown to the horses. Lead them or ride them to it and let them study it. A few white rags will remind them if they should forget while playing. After that, they know by habit to avoid the wire. Don't turn a horse out just before dark in a newly fenced area, no matter what the fence. It's too dangerous.

Electric fence works well for horses, but should be regarded as temporary until something else is built. A single strand just above knee high on the horse is usually enough. With an electric fence, you must figure on loose horses from time to time because of shorts in the fence, breaks, too dry weather, etc. Keep this in mind if your farm is on a well-travelled road. Not only can a horse be killed on the road, but the people owning the car can sue you.

Electric fences can also cause fires. One of my horses, or a wild animal, broke down a section of electric fence in the back pasture half a mile from the house. It was during the summer and the grass was dry. When I checked the horses the next day, there was a black, fire-burned area 50 feet long, with the fence still sparking. I shudder to think of what *might* have happened, had there been any wind. An electric wire on top of a barbed wire, wood, or woven wire fence is safer all around. The fire hazard is much less, and should a short occur, the other fence will hold the animals in.

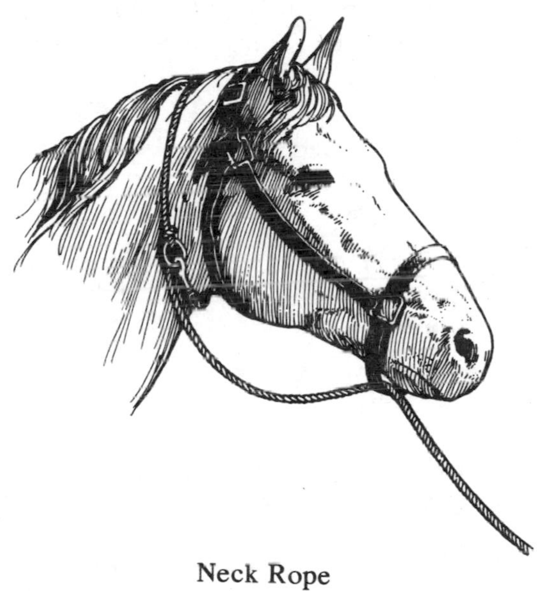

Neck Rope

Tying Safely To tie a horsc safely is an art in itself. Many gentle, well-trained horses can be tied by a light rope and halter. However, when the horse *must* stay where tied, or is fractious, stronger measures must be taken. Few halters made today will hold a horse set on breaking loose. One exception is a triple thickness flat nylon halter with good quality rings. These generally will hold. But lacking this, an ordinary halter can be made to hold any horse by use of a neck rope, which is a strong rope with a loop with a ring tied in it about two feet up from the snap. The rope is tied to a post, the snap is run through the halter and around the neck, then fastened to the ring. The horse can pull back and not break the halter, but is safe from choking.

Never tie a horse with any longer rope than it takes to let it touch the ground with its muzzle. Longer ropes invite injuries, as somehow the horse gets a foot over the rope, then panics, thrashing around. *Always* tie a horse so you can release it right away if need be. Keep in mind that a tight rope in trouble makes the knot harder to release. A jerk knot or bull snap works better as slack is not needed and the horse can be quickly released.

Cross Ties Cross ties are highly overrated in treating horses. Cross ties, which are two ropes from each side of an aisle to restrain the horse, are great for grooming, saddling, or harnessing. But they are dangerous when worming or giving injections or other treatment. In the first place, the ropes or chains are usually too light to hold the fractious horse. In the second place, a horse can back against the ties, leaping forward, hitting people, or striking out with front feet. Cross ties keep a horse from wandering, but do not restrain adequately for any procedure that upsets the animal.

Twitch The twitch is a hardwood handle with a chain loop on one end. This loop is slipped over the horse's upper lip and twisted until quite tight. It does not hurt the horse but confuses it, keeping its mind on the twitch, not the treatment. The twitch is used for many things, ranging from floating teeth to giving injections.

With a good lead rope held in the hand, and a good man or woman on the twitch, the horse can usually be handled quite safely during treatment. The person on the twitch should hang on to it, regardless of any movement the horse may make. I've been hit in the head too many times because someone became frightened and turned loose, letting the twitch become a flying missile.

Rope in the mouth You simply take a lariat, place the noose behind the ears and through the mouth. Wind tightly—don't overdo it—until the whole rope, or most of it, is in the mouth, cramming it open. This acts like a twitch, but in most instances one person can restrain and treat the horse by him or herself. There is no pain, only confusion.

Chain over the nose This is used mainly to control a pushy or rank horse. Used correctly, it will keep all but the rankest horse's front feet on the ground. Just pulling on the lead shank is of no use, and may cut the skin. The chain should be yanked, gently or quite hard depending on the horse, which brings sharp pressure on the bridge of the nose. A chain under the chin is sometimes used instead, but I don't like this, as it will often cause or encourage the horse to rear.

Hobbles There are three uses of hobbles: to keep a horse from moving off while grazing, to prevent kicking or striking, and to pass ropes through, in order to throw (cast) the horse. Simple hobbles to prevent the horse from wandering while grazing, or in some cases moving around while it is being worked on, fit around the front pasterns. Most are heavy leather, either in a figure 8 or two separate hobbles connected by a strong, short piece of chain. If the horse has never been hobbled, get an expert to work with it the first time, as some horses get panic-stricken the first time they are pulled up short by the hobbles and thrash around. The hobbles used for aiding treatment are either to prevent kicking or striking, or to cast the horse.

Front leg hobble This is only a rope or strap, placed around the doubled front leg just above the knee. This makes minor operations like cleaning a cut or clipping a flap of loose skin from a wound easier.

Breeding hobbles These can be purchased or made from a ¾-inch nylon rope. The ropes or hobbles keep a horse from kicking back, but remember that the horse can still cow kick, or kick forward. Breeding hobbles are used for rectal or vaginal examinations, artificial insemination, surgery on the tail, and service by the stallion.

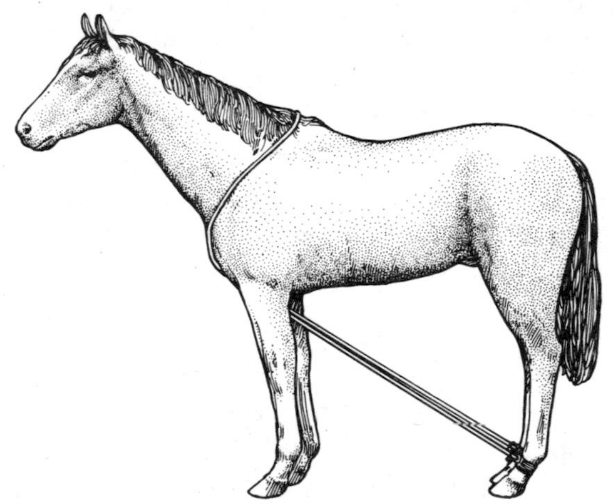

Breed Hobbles

Scotch hobble This keeps one hind leg up, making work on it easier and making the horse fairly immobile. Most horses tolerate it quite well, even when they have not been handled much. When placing the hobble on the hind foot, begin rubbing the hindquarters, then slowly

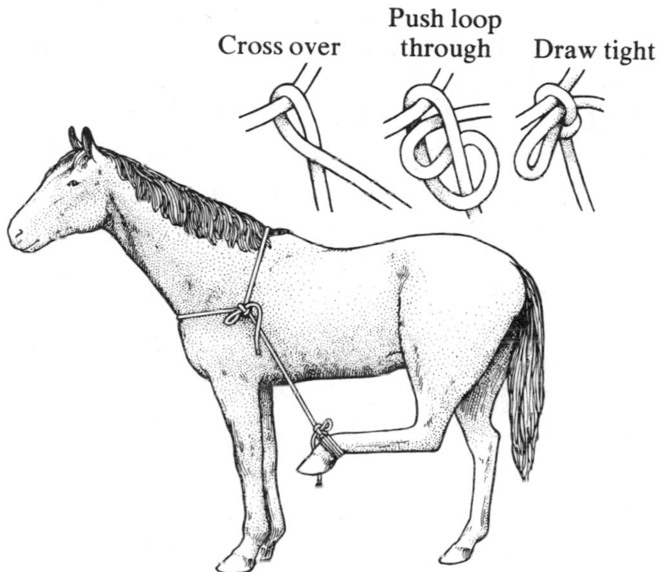

Scotch hobble using quick release knots.

but firmly work on down the leg. Touching a horse's lower leg unexpectedly is a good way to get kicked.

Throwing rig Hobbles can be placed on either front or back legs, and a rope run from one through a belly band to the other hobble, back through the band, and on to the person doing the work. Any horse can be put down safely using this rig, but it should be done by someone experienced, or else injury or unnecessary fright to the horse may occur. The down horse must also be tied correctly or it can break a leg. The legs must be tied in a completely flexed position, so that the horse cannot get enough power to put strain on the leg bones. A horse thrown correctly will not fight much, but will sort of "tip over." A panicked horse can bruise itself.

Restraining the foal A foal can usually be restrained by an arm under the neck and another behind the buttocks, as if you planned to pick it up. A larger foal or weanling can be held with nose elevated and can be kept off balance by pushing against the neck or shoulder with your hand when it attempts to move. Crowding a foal into a corner works well, but you must really crowd in, or you may get a kick or two from those fast little feet. Always watch the mare when working on a new foal. Even the gentlest mare may become a little overprotective when her offspring appears threatened.

BREEDING

Of course you mule owners must pass this one, as 99 percent of mules are sterile, being a hybrid cross between a jack and mare, whose chromosomes do not allow for fertility.

The Heat Cycle Mares come into heat every 21 to 27 days and remain in heat for two to ten days, but show the strongest signs for two to three days. A mare in heat will urinate frequently and will tease other horses. Her temperament may change. A well-trained, easily ridden mare may get nervous or temperamental. A gelding may mount her or show interest. When taken to a stallion, she will squat and urinate when teased, i.e., when the stallion is led on one side of a fence or gate, the mare on the other, and he is not permitted to mount her.

Mares begin to come into heat early in the spring, or about nine days after foaling. Many mares will continue heat cycles all year, if not bred. Others only experience heat in the spring and summer. Eleven months after conception the mare will foal, so when planning a breeding, keep the month of foaling in mind. If you show the mare in June and July, you won't want her foaling then. If your barn is not warm, you won't want the mare foaling in January or February, when many thoroughbreds foal.

Stallions Keeping a stallion is a pain! Don't, unless you are a horseman with experience and patience. A stallion is first a breeding animal. It is his instinct and purpose in life. He can never be trusted completely because of it. No matter how well trained, something can set him off unexpectedly. Most stallions regard a gelding as a stallion and will attack one at every chance. Owning a stallion means going to bed wondering if a phone call from an irate neighbor will wake you, saying your stallion broke out and is in with his mares or fighting with his gelding. It means superstrong fences, being careful of who rides in on a horse, and watching the kids. It means he will never be *all* yours. He belongs to his instincts.

Instead, take your mare to a good stallion. Let the stud owner worry about the stallion. Believe me, a fee of $50 to $200 beats the worry of being a stud owner. Besides, you don't have to feed that stallion for a whole year, which costs at least as much as the stud fee! Make arrangements in advance, as many stallion owners book their stallions ahead of time. Always plan to take your mare to the stallion. Most stallions are kept at the farm and are used to serve mares there. My own stallion is tractable and well trained. When hauled to shows, he isn't so much expecting to breed as he would be if I hauled him to mares. You don't mind a stallion hollering and dancing at home, but it's bad at a show or on the trail.

Many stallion owners want the mares to have a Coggins test for swamp fever and to be examined for vaginal or uterine infections by a veterinarian before being brought to their stallion, as one mare can bring trouble to a breeding farm. Find out ahead of time.

FOALING, NORMAL

Eleven months from the time of a successful breeding, the mare will be ready to foal. She can be pregnancy tested earlier, of course, to be sure she is in foal. Blood tests show very early, and a rectal exam is usually accurate. The mare's udder will be quite full, and a drop or two of colostrum may ooze out and harden. Just a day or two before foaling, the ligaments will slacken above the tail and her belly will drop, looking almost pointed at the bottom.

Most mares foal at night or early in the morning, so don't count on seeing the foal born unless you sleep with her! If the mare is due to foal in the late spring or early summer, the best place for her to foal is in the pasture or grassy paddock. Here it is clean and free of obstructions and booby traps for the brand-new foal. In bad weather, house the mare in a large, well-bedded box stall. Bank bedding against the wall, making it like a bird nest. This will keep the mare from lying with her rump to the wall when beginning to foal, blocking the birth. The bedding should be a foot or so deeper at the walls than in the center. Remove all feed boxes and pails soon after they are used; it's not unusual for foals to die from suffocation after being dumped into them.

Just prior to foaling, the mare may go to an isolated corner of the pasture or act restless in the box stall. She may paw or pace in the stall. Most mares will lie down to foal, and most mares foal quickly, only fifteen or twenty minutes elapsing between the times she acts restless to the time the foal is dropped. The water bag and two front feet are closely followed by the nose. Don't worry because the feet are soft and flaky; this is normal and a protection to the mare's uterus and vagina. The hooves will harden in a day.

The foal will be born in three stages. The front feet and head, the shoulders and brisket, and last, the hips and hind legs. The mare generally rests in between stages for a moment. Most often, the placenta or afterbirth will pass with the foal. This is the whitish membrane covering the fetus in the uterus. As the foal drops from the vagina, the membrane usually breaks, expelling the foal into the world. If it does not break, the mare generally takes care of this. If the mare doesn't an attendant should do it so that the foal doesn't suffocate.

The umbilical cord usually breaks, leaving a foot of cord hanging. This should be thoroughly dunked in iodine. If too much cord is left hanging, the attendant can tie it off with a nylon line and trim the cord shorter. It should then be treated with iodine. This helps prevent not only navel infection but joint ill and scours as well.

Rear Presentation With a normal rear presentation, the hind feet show first. You can tell the difference, as the toes will point up instead of down, showing the frogs and sole of the hoof. The backward foal is usually born quite rapidly and with little trouble. The one problem is that of possible suffocation or inhalation of fluids. The foal begins to breathe as the umbilical cord breaks. In a front presentation this is well and good, but in the rear presentation the foal's head is often still in the birth canal after the cord has broken.

If an attendant is present, he or she should help the mare as soon as the hips are through the vagina. Firm traction downward will hasten the birth. As soon as the foal is dropped, clean out the mouth and nostrils. If the foal is breathing irregularly or not at all, smack its chest on the side hard with the flat of your hand. It is sometimes necessary to hold the foal upside down to drain the lungs. For a normal-sized adult, the easiest way is to grasp the hind feet while squatting, back to the foal, and then stand up. This will hang the foal from your shoulders. If another helper is present, he or she can clean out the fluid as it drains. When the foal begins to struggle, let it down.

FOALING, ABNORMAL

Leg back When the mare strains, producing the head and only one foot, scrub up and check, suspecting that one knee has caught on the brim of the pelvis and has been deflected back into the uterus.

1. Locate the missing leg.
2. Get a hand over the hoof.
3. Shove back on the foal in order to gain room to slip the leg up.
4. Pull the leg up, protecting the uterus from tears by keeping the hoof covered with your hand.
5. Straighten the foal into normal birth position, and gently pull on the foal as the mare strains. Pull downward.

Head back When two feet are presented but no head, suspect that the head has been deflected back. This in my opinion is the roughest position commonly found in foaling difficulties. I'll suggest how home delivery can be done, but you really should have a veterinarian with obstetrical equipment for this one.

1. Scrub up and check the mare.
2. Locate the head.
3. Slip a rope (an obstetrical chain works better) in the shape of a noose through the mouth and behind the ears.
4. With this grip, try to work the head around. You may have to push the legs back some to gain room.

5. DO NOT use a fence stretcher, tractor, or other such equipment to try pulling the foal, or you will maim it and likely injure or kill the mare.

6. DO NOT work longer than 15 minutes without results before calling a vet. If you do, you will possibly exhaust the mare or put her into shock.

Rear presentation, leg or legs retained When the mare strains, only producing one hind foot or nothing but the water bag, suspect an abnormal rear presentation.

1. Scrub up and check the mare.

2. If both hind legs are retained, the buttocks should be pushed back with one hand while pulling up on one leg at a time. Guard each hoof with a hand to protect the uterus.

3. Once both legs are in the birth canal, firm traction will aid the mare in making the delivery, as she may be tired.

4. Treat the foal as in normal rear presentation delivery.

Abnormal deliveries requiring the veterinarian Since a caesarean section done on a mare is an awfully risky operation at best, it is important for the owner to obtain skillful help if the mare is having foaling trouble. Never attempt force, for a foal jammed into the birth canal can seldom be delivered alive, even if a vet is called. Some laymen are great in aiding a hard foaling. Such people are generally grooms who have spent their lives with horses and have gained experience helping mares foal. Do not entrust your mare to a "helpful" neighbor, unless you know he or she has had some experience.

Mares are nervous and easily put into shock, which can be fatal. They are very prone to peritonitis, caused by uterine tears or strings of afterbirth left in the uterus. If the mare cannot deliver her foal in 15 minutes, check her. If you do not feel competent to correct the problem, call the veterinarian right away. At any rate do not work more than 15 minutes without results.

The Rejected or Orphan Foal Once in a while a mare dies or is killed soon after foaling, or what is more frustrating, she just refuses to take care of the foal. Left on your hands, a foal is one of the hardest animal babies to raise. A foal is large and strong but at the same time delicate.

The best substitute for the foal's dam is another mare or jenny burro. But unfortunately, even if a nurse mare is available, many violently refuse (even when tranquilized) to accept the orphan. Rubbing camphorated oil, peppermint, or some other strong smelling substance on the mare's nose and foal's back and rump will sometimes help. Twitching or hobbling the mare may also help. If the mare seems to let the foal nurse, still keep an eye on the pair for a day or two. She may suddenly decide she's had enough of the newcomer and injure it.

Lacking a nurse mare, locate a milking doe goat, or two if one is not a good producer. Goat's milk is easier for the foal to digest than cow's milk, as the fat particles are smaller. When the foal has been without milk for several hours, dilute the goat's milk with half warm water. Feed the foal with a lamb nipple on a pop bottle. Pail feeding causes digestive upsets. The foal *must* be fed every two hours around the clock for at least two weeks and usually for a month.

Begin feeding two to four ounces every two hours. At the end of the feeding, slip a few pellets of Calf Manna into its mouth. Do *not* use a medicated calf pellet. Gradually increase the milk, giving just enough so that the foal is still hungry but almost satisfied. The first few times you give the foal pellets it may spit most of them out, but gradually it will begin to chew on them.

This is the first step to supplemental dry feeding that will let you cut out those every-two-hours-all-night feedings. As soon as the foal eats a pound a day, you can drop to two night feedings, only feeding, say, at 1 A.M. and 3 A.M. The pellets are fed free choice until the foal cleans them up rapidly. Then begin mixing a little horse feed—mixed grains with molasses, such as crimped oats, cracked corn, bran, plus vitamins and minerals—with the pellets. The foal should receive a calcium-vitamin D supplement daily to prevent rickets.

Get a bale or two of the best hay you can find and let it nibble on that. I'd stay away from alfalfa, as it can cause loose bowels and scouring in an orphan foal. If there is grass up, let it graze at will. Sunshine will really put pep into the foal, so be sure it gets lots of it. But, of course, be sure it does have access to shade and fresh, clean water.

If the foal should begin scouring, cut out the milk, feeding an oral electrolyte solution in its place. Kaopectate, an ounce or two every four hours, will help. Foals often scour briefly, a week after birth. At one time scours in foals was thought to be caused by the changes in the mare's milk when she experienced the foal heat, the heat period four to 12 days after foaling, but orphan foals experience it also. If the foal scours badly, intravenous or intraperitoneal injections of electrolytes will often help.

For other problems related to foaling see "Retained Placenta" and "Edema or Stocking" in **Diseases and Other Problems**, later in this chapter.

CASTRATION

Unless you or your groom is an accomplished horseperson, it is wisest to have any stud colts gelded, no matter how tempting it is to leave them stallions. There is too much trouble involved with keeping a stallion around. Although a colt can be castrated when quite young, most people prefer to have a little more masculinity in their geldings. Many colts gelded young do not develop the full neck and masculine build that a colt gelded as a two year old will have. If, however, the colt is acting up and is hard to handle as a yearling because he is a young stallion, it is far better to have him altered earlier than to have someone hurt by his exuberance. (Remember, however, that a colt will act full of life at that age, and gelding him will not take the life out of him if he is just naturally high-spirited.)

The horse is one farm animal that I recommend you get a veterinarian to help you castrate. In the first place, you have a large animal with very quick reflexes. He is hard to restrain sufficiently to do a decent job without an anesthetic of some kind. In the struggle to get him restrained and operated on, it is very easy for someone to become injured—including the horse.

Call your veterinarian a few days in advance of the time you would like him gelded. You wouldn't believe the people that call at lunch hour, saying they have their stallion tied up to a telephone pole and they want him castrated right now, because he just was down to the neighbors. And the veterinarian is in between calls, and running late already.

Have a couple of strong helpers on hand the day you plan to have the horse castrated. They may not be needed, but sometimes it is necessary to have someone hold a rope or sit on the head for added restraint, even with an anesthetic. Some horses move as if they were asleep and jerking their legs, under an anesthetic.

When the operation is finished and the horse has recovered, do not put him in a stall for the rest of the day, but turn him out in a paddock or small pasture instead. Standing after castration only encourages swelling. Most new geldings will graze as soon as they are up from the operation and will act fine and full of energy in a day.

HOOF CARE

The saying "No foot—no horse" is too true, so in order to preserve the usefulness and well-being of the horse, you must take particularly good care of the hooves. Good care does not necessarily mean shoeing. If the horse is not ridden on rocky, gravel, or hard surfaces, or if it is not raced, worked hard daily, or shown regularly, it may not need shoes.

Most pleasure horses need only to have their feet cleaned and checked, plus a periodic trim to keep them in top shape. Some horses, like people, have brittle nails (hooves) and have a tendency to develop cracks, splits, and chips. This can many times be alleviated by painting the hoof and frog (the triangle-shaped spongy pad on the underside of the hoof which absorbs shock while the animal is moving) with a good hoof conditioner, such as a pine tar-pine oil or lanolin preparation. Be careful you don't get a hoof black by mistake. This is only to color the hooves black for show and will not help condition them.

If the brittleness is due to a dry pasture, it sometimes helps to let the water tank run over onto a clay base which the horse stands in several times a day when going for a drink. When any abnormalities such as cracks occur, call your blacksmith at once, as it can often be taken care of quickly and inexpensively, as compared to the job a week or two of neglect will necessitate.

The hoof should be cleaned daily, especially if the horse is kept in a stall. Hooves that are not cleaned daily can pack with manure and wet bedding, becoming a perfect target for thrush, a diseased condition. When on pasture, the hooves should still receive daily inspection, as a stone or twig can become wedged between the frog and the sole of the hoof, eventually causing bruising or infection. Don't forget to check for puncture wounds in the frog and heel. Remember, a tiny puncture that doesn't cause lameness can kill the horse through tetanus.

The hooves normally grow out and require regular trimming, unless the horse is pastured on gravel. And even then it is wise to have the hooves checked for uneven wear. It is not too hard to learn to trim your own horses' feet, but at the price most blacksmiths charge, it is far better to have a professional job done. The blacksmith will not only cut off the extra growth, but trim to correct any faults in gait and help you head off any future troubles with the feet that you might overlook.

Diseases and Other Problems

BREAKS

Today many horses can and do recover well from broken legs, if given the chance. A horse can break a leg from an accident such as running into a hole, open culvert, or tangle of brush; or just break a leg turning while running in a paddock. There have been several stallions crippled while attempting to serve a mare that was unrestrained by breeding hobbles. One kick is all it takes to snap a bone. It is well worth the trouble to slip a set of hobbles on even the quietest mare before having the stallion brought out.

A horse with a broken leg will suddenly be lame. The leg will often dangle badly or flop around when the horse moves. Try to keep such a horse quiet. A broken leg will often panic a horse and this in turn can cause irreparable damage. If the horse must be moved, do so very slowly and carefully, but in most cases it is best to leave the horse where it is found until the veterinarian arrives.

Broken legs can be repaired by use of plaster casts, intramedullary pins, plates, and screws. With complicated breaks, it is usually best to send the horse to a university large animal veterinary hospital. Under normal field conditions, the sterility, equipment, and trained help are hard to duplicate. I've set broken legs out in the field, under a canvas, in a sleet storm, with only one assistant, and had the job turn out a success—but I attribute it to a lot of luck.

Fractures in the feet The foot under the hoof is not just one bone, but several small ones. Under trauma, such as stepping on a rock at a run, shock while jumping, or injury, one or more of these small bones can crack or break. Severe lameness is usually the result. With the exception of the navicular bone, many of these fractures will heal well with treatment. Navicular fractures will seldom heal. Rest, plaster casts, and splints have been used with good success. On occasion, surgery and screws or removal of bone chips are necessary. When this is done, there is the added risk of bone infection or osteomyelitis.

THE CAST HORSE

Any horse, regardless of care, can become cast. "Cast" means stuck in a down position. There are some situations that invite casting. Some horses are more clumsy than others in a tie stall, having a difficult time rising after lying down. Some horses tend to lie down in a corner of a box stall or paddock. A horse gets up by first sitting on its haunches, then throwing its neck forward to balance when the rear end lurches up. If there is no place to throw the neck forward, the horse sometimes is unable to rise no matter how strong it is.

Horses sometimes become cast on ice or in deep snow or mud. Here, obviously, the horse must be hauled off the ice or out of the mud or shoveled out of the snow. I've seen a lot of horses cast in fences. A horse often eats over a fence, getting its feet tangled. When it tries to back away, it trips, falls, and is unable to rise.

A horse can become cast when tied on too long a rope. Don't stake a horse out, because too many things can happen. A rope can become tangled around the legs, then the horse panics and falls. A horse should never be tied with a rope longer than necessary to let it just reach the ground with its muzzle. If tied just a little longer, a hind foot can get over the rope and throw the horse when it becomes unbalanced. If this happens in a tie stall the horse is in trouble, especially if it is in the middle of the night.

The bad thing about a cast horse is the panic. A horse will bang itself around, throwing its head out again and again, trying to rise. The longer down, the more battered it will become. Concussions, eye injuries, and so on are often the result. NEVER go into the stall or in close quarters with a cast horse; you could get pinned under a panic-stricken thrashing horse. Instead, climb in through the manger or hang over a partition, but keep yourself protected. It doesn't matter how much the horse likes you or how gentle it is. It is frightened like a drowning person, and like that person, it may hurt you.

Get a lead rope on the halter, then release the tie rope if the horse is tied. Then encourage it to get up, helping steady it with the lead or by boosting its hindquarters by the tail. If it is really stuck, you may have to pull it back out of the stall to enable it to rise. A come-along or fence stretcher will slowly pull it backward. A horse that weighs under 800 pounds can be pulled out by knotting the tail—but don't twist the bone—and hooking onto that. A larger horse may have to have a rope slipped across, like a breast collar and scooted back with this.

Once free of the stall, let the horse rest awhile. Keep it rolled up on its brisket, not out flat on its side. A horse left on its side for any time gives up and will die. Prop it up if need be, using a bale of hay. Feed it some hay and grain after offering it a drink

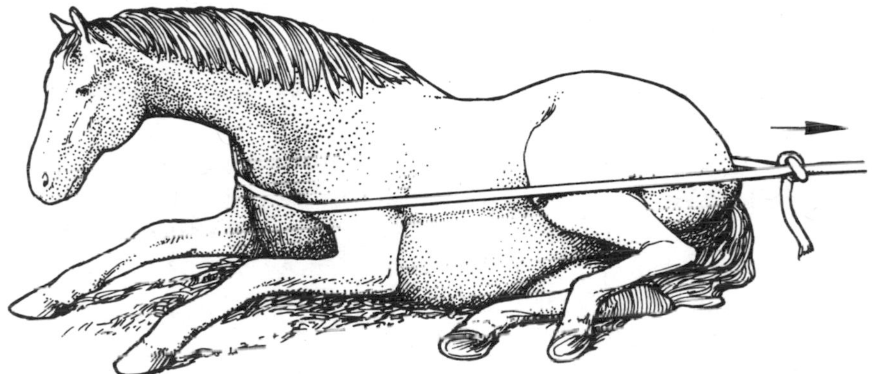

Pulling cast horse backwards from the stall.

of water. When it is rested, urge it to stand. A horse that is a bit weak benefits from a boost via the tail. Once up, let it stand a few minutes, then lead it slowly around to stimulate circulation and feeling in its legs.

COLIC

To put it simply, colic is a bellyache. It is common in horses and is quite painful, but usually is easily treated and seldom fatal. It may be caused by overeating, or eating grain then drinking large quantities of water, or drinking water while overheated. Constipation or impaction will also cause colic. The affected horse will pace about, sweat, squat, as if undecided whether to lie down or not. It may kick or look at its belly, breathe hard, and roll. The horse should be prevented from rolling or thrashing. Rolling often causes a torsion (twisting) of the bowel, which is often fatal. Thrashing can cause rupture of the bowel or stomach and external injuries, especially to the head.

If the horse is discovered down from colic in a tie stall, *never* walk in alongside it as you could be severely injured, no matter how calm the horse normally is. Pain can make the most gentle horse crazy. Instead, crawl in through the manger or from the next stall, releasing the horse and fastening a long lead shank to the halter. Then encourage the horse to get up, back it out, but do not get between it and the stall wall. A horse in pain can fall against the wall, pinning you badly. Once out of the stall, begin walking it while the veterinarian is called.

Laxatives are used in cases of impaction, which causes the blockage of the flow of normal gas. Injections to calm an overactive or cramping stomach are often given, which relieve the pain. Anyone who has horses should have an oral colic remedy in the first aid chest just for an emergency when a veterinarian is not available. But if a veterinarian is available, call him anyway. Sometimes colic is a symptom of more serious trouble, such as a severe intestinal blockage or torsion of the bowel. If let go or mistreated, you'll have yourself a dead horse.

Even after being treated, the horse should either be watched closely or walked until all pains have passed. If the horse is sweated and hot, be sure to throw a sheet or blanket over it, as it is easy for a hot horse to get chilled.

CUTS

Glass, tin, and barbed wire account for many cuts on horses. Right behind these I would list running into wooden fences or partitions, which split and gash the horse. Kicks, bites, and rips on nails also cause injury to horses. To be as safe as possible, all fences should be strong and tight. No machinery should be parked in a field containing horses, especially near a fence or in a corner where a horse can get cut up running through. No boards, junk, or brush piles should be left in the field. Any holes should be filled with rocks, then packed full of dirt. Any ragged culverts should be repaired.

In the event a cut does occur, first catch the horse, wash off the blood, and really check the injury. If the blood is running or dripping, the wound may be packed with a dry, sterile cloth. When left in place for five or ten minutes, the bleeding will usually stop. When a wound spurts blood, an artery may be cut and more pressure must be applied. A cloth may be pressed hard onto the wound by hand, or in an area where it is possible, it may be tied tightly in place with a few wraps of gauze. A wound such as this needs prompt treatment by your veterinarian, or the horse could lose enough blood to be in serious trouble.

Once the bleeding is controlled, you must decide whether or not the injury will heal better left open or sutured. If you are not experienced, ask the opinion of your veterinarian. Many wounds do heal better left alone. There is better drainage, less swelling, and often less scarring. Some wounds must have a flap of skin clipped off to make healing smoother and more complete. Small three-cornered tears or ragged cuts often benefit from being trimmed. All wounds should have the hair trimmed away from them. Hair is irritating and will very much retard healing, if not invite infection. It collects dirt and bacteria. Even with a show horse it is best to clip that hair away. The clipped hair will grow in a lot quicker than will a bald area around a wound where serum and pus have seeped.

Keeping a wound cleaned out with plain, warm, soapy water daily will greatly reduce the healing time. This is much better than smearing salve on top of salve every day. Fresh air, no bandage, and daily washing, plus systemic antibiotics, make for quick healing with no infection.

Wounds of the feet and lower leg should have the attention of your veterinarian. These wounds are especially prone to "proud flesh" or exuberant granulation. Here, scarring over produces tissue that resembles a tumor. From an inch-long cut, a mass of proud tissue the size of a basketball can form. This oozes serum, is easily injured, bleeds easily, and will continue to enlarge. When surgically removed, it often grows right back. It is best to do everything possible to prevent this problem from starting.

EDEMA OR STOCKING

A horse is said to "stock up" when it gets a doughy swelling, often in the legs. Mares often "stock up" just before or just after foaling, because the increased size of the udder shuts off circulation to some extent, causing fluid to seep out of the blood vessels and into the surrounding tissue. A gelding or stallion will sometimes have a penis that swells with edema, due to an accumulation of body secretions and dirt in the sheath.

Basically, most edema or stocking is due to something shutting down part of the circulation in an area, causing the seeping of fluid out of the blood vessels into the surrounding tissue. Edema appears swollen and feels doughy to the touch. Sprain, injury, hard or jarring work, bee sting, too tight leg wraps, and foaling all can bring on edema. Diuretics such as Lasix or Naquasone work very well to remedy the edema by stimulating the kidneys, causing more frequent urination which draws fluid from the body—in this case, the edema.

EQUINE ENCEPHALOMYELITIS (EEE-WEE-VEE)

Eastern Equine Encephalomyelitis or EEE EEE is a virus-produced disease, and although named "Eastern," it has been found in Mexico and Central and South America. It is spread from mosquitoes to birds, back to mosquitoes, then to horses and sometimes to man. Symptoms often noticed are depression, incoordination, drooping lip, high fever, pushing against a wall or fence, and being down, unable to rise. The disease is short, lasting only two to four days before the horse dies. The few horses that do live are often "dummies," having suffered brain damage from the disease.

When suspecting this disease, isolate the horse and call your veterinarian at once. Any horses living in an area or passing through an area where EEE has been reported should be vaccinated. It is a good idea for all horses to be vaccinated yearly with a EEE-WEE (Eastern Western) vaccine. With horses on the move so commonly today, encephalomyelitis could break out nearly anywhere.

Western Equine Encephalomyelitis or WEE WEE is quite similar to EEE, but is found chiefly in the West and Midwest. The symptoms are also similar but the disease is not quite as fatal, with perhaps half of the afflicted horses living. It is more often seen in man than EEE.

Being a virus, it cannot be treated with antibiotics. Good nursing will save many horses that might die otherwise. Keeping the horse standing up by means of a chute, slings, or padded stocks helps. Heavy bedding, aspirin to lower the fever—a high fever can cause brain damage—and intravenous electrolytes are often helpful. Feeding good hay and a good grain mix, by hand if need be, sometimes helps keep the horse's strength up until the disease has run its course.

Vaccination is the only preventive other than complete isolation in a "bug free" barn.

Venezuelan Equine Encephalomyelitis or VEE VEE is a fairly new disease to Americans. Most of us never heard of it until the outbreak in Mexico and along the border states a few years ago. The symptoms are similar to EEE and WEE. Although never a problem far north of the Mexican border, it is a disease to keep in mind when hauling a horse to or from this trouble area. The outbreak was stopped by strict quarantine and public awareness, but the possibility of future problems with the disease is still present.

A vaccine is available, but unless you are traveling to the Southwest, the EEE-WEE vaccine is recommended instead.

FLIES

There are several varieties of flies that bother horses. In addition to the annoyance to the horse, biting insects can spread disease in many areas. Swamp fever, equine encephalomyelitis, Rocky Mountain spotted fever, and other diseases can be spread by flies and mosquitoes.

Keeping the manure away from the stable and well spread and worked into the fields by harrowing will help prevent a lot of the stable fly problem. Draining low spots near the barn and pasture or filling them in will help keep down mosquitoes and gnats. But no matter what is done, few horses go into a pasture that is free of biting insects. If biting insects become a severe problem the only reliable course of action is to use a wipe-on or spray twice daily. Sometimes horses need additional protection, such as a noon wipe or spray, but most products have some residual effect and will last from morning to night or longer.

If your horses are shy of the sprayer, you can spray some of the insecticide on a cloth to use on the ears and face. Spraying away from the body, i.e., not touching the horse with the spray at first, will waste a little spray but will get the horse used to the sprayer's noise and the sight of the mist coming at it. Do not use force, as that will only make the horse fear the spraying.

FLOATING THE TEETH

A horse chews and grinds its food in such a way that it wears down the edges of its molars, making sharp edges at times. These points often cut the cheek or tongue, causing weight loss, indigestion, and sloppy eating. When a horse takes a mouthful of grass, or more noticeably, grain and chews with exaggerated motion, dropping gobs of half-chewed food out, suspect that it has sharp teeth.

These points should be filed down by the use of a float. This is a special file about four inches long on the end of a long handle. Many people have their veterinarian float their horses' teeth, but there is no reason why the average horse owner cannot learn to float teeth. Most veterinarians will gladly instruct you on the right way to do the work on your own horse. This frees the veterinarian to do other more pressing work.

Many veterinarians use a mouth speculum, which holds the mouth open while dental work is done, but if there is time a good job can be done by just having an assistant hold the tongue out of the mouth and to one side, and with the other hand hold the side of the halter. Some horses must be twitched to keep their attention on their nose instead of what's going on inside their mouth, as floating does make a grating sound.

You should inspect the inside of your horses' mouths twice yearly for sharp edges and points. Use a flashlight so that you can see well.

LAMENESS

There are hundreds of causes of lameness in horses, and there have been whole books written on just this subject. (I recommend *Lameness in Horses* by O.R. Adams, D.V.M., M.S., and *The Lame Horse* by Rooney.) Obviously I can only briefly touch on the subject here.

If a horse suddenly acts lame, examine the foot. Use a hoof pick to clean manure and dirt from the hoof. Work from heel to toe along the frog, to avoid injury to the heel. Check for stones or sticks wedged in between the frog and the sole. Check for slivers, glass, cuts, and punctures, which often show as black spots.

Then check to see if the shoes, if the horse wears them, are loose or are in need of resetting. Shoes can cause trouble if you don't check them daily. They must be replaced or reset every eight to 12 weeks. If the hoof grows too long, the shoes do no good and can cause lameness by forcing an unnatural angle to the pastern. Should the horse become lame soon after shoeing, have the blacksmith check for a possible nail puncture. Look for any swellings and feel for any tender spots.

After making an examination, call your veterinarian. Some forms of lameness are only temporary with treatment, but can become a permanent unsoundness if let go.

I give below, in capsule form, some of the more common causes of lameness in horses, with their symptoms and cures.

Azoturia

Appearance—after a weekend rest, still on the regular grain ration, the horse becomes lame when being worked, begins to sweat profusely, tremble, and become incoordinated. The urine may become dark, from a dark orange to almost black.

Treatment—complete rest, oral electrolytes, sodium bicarbonate, and injectable thiamine help. Most moderate cases recover.

Prevention—when resting the horse from work for a day or two, cut back the grain in proportion.

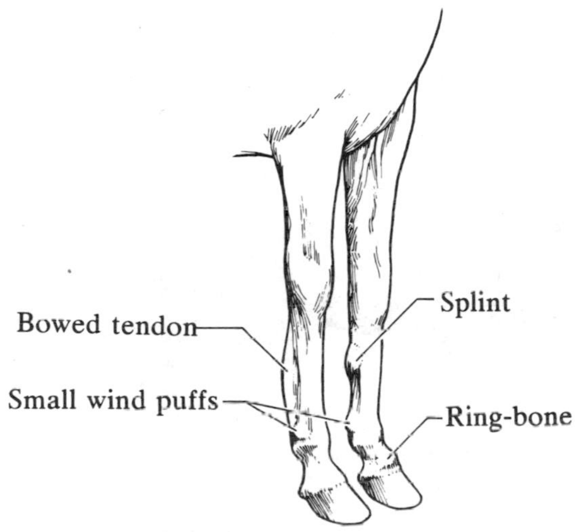

Bowed Tendon

Appearance—the tendon, often in a front leg below the knee, appears to bow outward. Soreness and severe lameness result.

Cause—severe strain or overwork.

Treatment—stand horse in cold water for at least an hour daily. A creek works well. Ice packs and complete stall rest help. An external blister (an ointment or salve rubbed into the skin to produce heat in the area, and in turn increase circulation to encourage healing) or firing (a firing pin or electrical hot point applied to the skin to achieve same effect as a blister) is sometimes used. No work for at least six months.

Capped Elbow or Hock

Appearance—lameness, large swelling which may feel full of fluid on either the point of elbow or hock.

Cause—bruising, caused by insufficient bedding or striking with toe or heel, as seen in trotters or gaited horses.

Treatment—ice packs, cortisone, mild exercise, rest from work. Antibiotics if injuries accompany bruise.

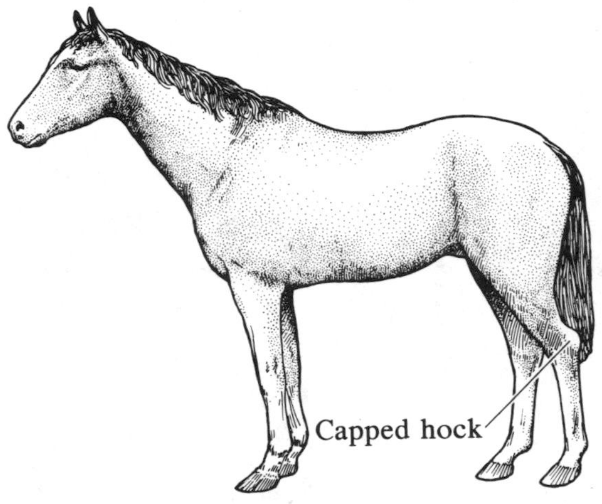

Founder or Laminitis

Appearance—reluctance to move, horse stands with feet in front of body to take weight off toes, may have an above-normal temperature. There is severe lameness.

Cause—overeating lush pasture (ponies in particular), overeating grain, drinking water when overheated, retained placenta in mares.

Treatment—injectable antihistamines, rest in well-bedded stall, standing in cold water, or ice packs. When horse begins to move around, mild daily exercise. The horse should be shod by a blacksmith who does corrective shoeing.

Navicular Disease

Appearance—horse does not "move out" but takes shorter strides and may stumble. Stands unnaturally, may point bad foot. Hooves become narrow and long.

Cause—trauma, e.g., stepping on a rock while running or jumping, hard work on unyielding surfaces, faulty conformation, forcing unnatural shock on the feet.

Treatment—none permanent. Surgery, corrective shoeing and cortisone injections help, but nothing cures the condition.

Ring-bone

Appearance—lameness, swelling, or ridges in the pastern area. At first the horse may be less lame after being worked for awhile. Then there is impairment in joint movement as calcium deposits form.

Cause—infection following injury, rickets, hard work, kicks or blows, arthritis.

Treatment—pasture rest, pull off shoes, cortisone. When inflammation subsides, the horse can be returned to light work, but must be shod by a competent blacksmith who does corrective shoeing. Some horses are never sound again, depending upon the position and size of the calcification.

Sand Crack or Quarter Crack

Appearance—cracks running up the hoof, usually up the front, from toe to nearly the coronet. Many horses have dry, cracked hooves without lameness, but when the toes grow too long, the weight of the horse can force the crack to widen. This in itself can be painful, but it also lets stones and grit work into the sensitive inner layers of the hoof. Infection and severe lameness may result.

Treatment—if it is a dry pasture, let the water tank overflow, creating a moist spot in which the horse must stand daily. Painting the hooves with a good hoof dressing helps. Be sure to get one for conditioning or softening hooves, not just a hoof black as is used for shows. Have a good blacksmith trim the feet and work on the crack. Often a groove is burned or cut across the top of the crack to stop the ascension of the crack, allowing the crack to eventually "grow out." Remember, the new horn grows down from coronet to toe, taking from nine to 14 months to completely replace the old horn. Light shoes are often used to more evenly distribute the weight and keep the crack from widening.

Splints

Appearance—lameness, small inflamed spots which later harden, due to calcium deposits.

Cause—hard work on hard or rough surfaces, blows, or injuries.

Treatment—pasture rest, liniment, surgery if extensive.

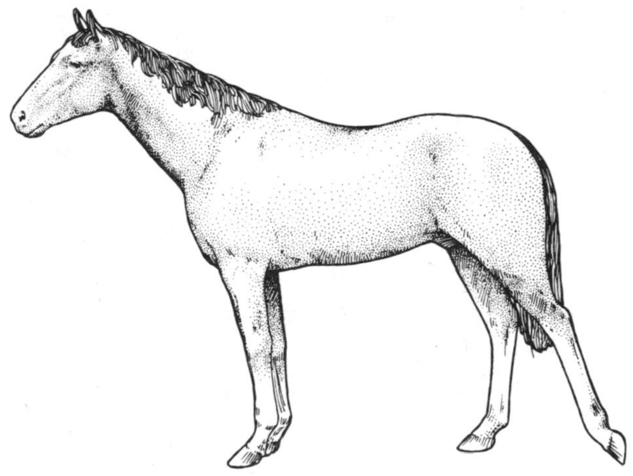

The Stifled Horse

Stifling or Luxation of the Patella

Apearance—hind leg being "stuck" straight, usually backward, when being led from a stall or being worked; sometimes seen on a young horse playing in a field.

Cause—conformation weakness, often hereditary; too straight a stifle, no angulation.

Treatment—the leg can be drawn forward by a rope running through a neck loop. This replaces the dislocation and keeps the joint from slipping apart. Blisters are often used. Rest from work is required. Treatment does not always work, and a horse that has been stifled is not a safe horse for hard work such as racing, jumping, or contesting; the condition may occur again, and if it does at any speed or on turning, the results are disastrous for both horse and rider. The horse should not be used for breeding, as the condition may be hereditary.

Thrush

Appearance—lameness and foul foot odor.

Cause—unclean or damp bedding; failure to clean out hooves properly.

Treatment—clean dry bedding; pare down any necrotic tissue (often around frog); clean hooves well. Apply astringents daily.

Wind Puffs

Appearance—puffy swellings on the lower leg and lameness.

Cause—strain.

Treatment—stand in cold running water, astringents, complete rest. In severe cases, liniment or a blister may be needed.

LICE

Lice are small, gray, soft-bodied parasites, smaller than a grain of rice. They are most often seen on the neck and chest of a horse, usually during the winter months when there is little sunlight. In addition to the intense itching and unsightly bald, moth-eaten appearing patches, the lice, if numerous enough, can actually bleed a horse to death. Horses should be thoroughly checked for these parasites weekly, from fall to spring. The hair on the neck should be parted and the skin inspected visually. Any suspicious specks can be picked off and placed on a white piece of paper for more thorough inspection.

On finding lice on your horse, purchase a good louse powder (one safe for dairy cows is safe for horses) and give the horse a thorough dusting from head to tail. This should be repeated weekly for three weeks, in order to get all the lice that hatch out after the first powder was applied. Any other horses in close contact with the infested horse should be dusted also.

MANGE

Mange is caused by tiny mites which burrow into the skin. These mites cause extreme itching, which makes the horse rub itself until bloody crusty scabs form, and these in turn are rubbed raw and the infestation spreads. Secondary infections, often a bacterial or fungus infection, can follow as the skin becomes unhealthy. If enough of the skin becomes nonfunctional, it is as if the animal had been burned badly, and the horse will die. Mange spreads quickly and will spread from one horse to another easily.

When suspecting mange, isolate the horse and call your veterinarian. He can take a skin scraping, which, when examined under a microscope, will reveal the mites. When caught early, mange is usually easily treated, but the treatment must be thorough and followed up religiously. Products such as rotenone, lindane, benzene hexachloride, and lime sulfur often work well when used properly. It is often necessary to repeat treatment weekly for three or four weeks to effect a complete cure. Be sure to follow directions, no matter what product is used.

PUNCTURE WOUNDS

Puncture wounds often occur in horses, many times in the foot because of its structure. Puncture wounds are more dangerous to a horse than to other animals, due to their susceptibility to tetanus.

When a horse begins to limp, be sure to thoroughly examine the foot from heel to toe for a puncture. This may only look like a tiny black hole. But on closer examination, you may notice soreness, pus, or blood in the area. I once took a four-inch piece of smooth wire out of the frog of a Belgian gelding. He had been limping for a week and the owner could find nothing wrong with his foot. There was only a minute black spot on the side of his frog. On probing the spot, I found the wire. I crossed my fingers and gave the horse a tetanus shot (antitoxin). After all, the wire had been rusty, covered with manure, and in the foot for a week! Luckily, the horse fully recovered.

Any puncture wound should be thoroughly flushed out with warm soapy water by means of a syringe, then soaked with iodine or another antiseptic. Remember, the antiseptic must reach to the *bottom* of the wound, not just remain on the top.

All horses should have a yearly tetanus booster, plus an injection of tetanus antitoxin when an injury has been known to occur.

RETAINED PLACENTA

Most mares throw off the placenta at the time of foaling or soon after. In case she should not, watch her closely. If she does drop it, examine it to make sure it is intact. A piece retained can cause her to become toxic and die. If after ten hours she has not released the afterbirth, call your veterinarian. The placenta should not be in the uterus more than 12 hours after foaling, or the mare may become toxic, developing founder or a septicemia, resulting in possible permanent disability or death.

The placenta which has been retained may have to be removed manually, but do not attempt to do this yourself, as one small slip can bring disaster. NEVER yank or pull on the afterbirth to remove it. Lacking a veterinarian, you may have to tackle the job yourself. Very carefully, peel the placenta away, leaving it in one piece. One hand, scrubbed and lubricated, is worked between the placenta and uterine wall, as if you were skinning. Work slowly and carefully, keeping tension on the placenta with your other hand.

SADDLE SORES

With saddle horses becoming more and more popular, horses are being bought and sold by people who do not know how to properly fit tack to the horse. And there are saddles being made that should not be used on anything but a sawhorse. A saddle that does not fit a horse—coupled with a heavy (and perhaps not too experienced) rider, plus a warm day and some hard work—will quite often cause a saddle sore.

Pressure sores on the withers are often caused by a saddle that is too low on the withers. A saddle tree built for a round-backed horse, such as a quarter horse, will not fit a high-withered horse like a saddlebred. Sores on the back are often caused by cheaply made saddles that are nailed together underneath or by debris under the saddle pad. Always check a new saddle, no matter what it costs, to be sure there are no nails underneath, and brush the back, even if there is no time to brush the rest of the horse.

When placing the saddle on the back, always lay the saddle a bit forward, then slide it back into place. This eliminates rough hair bunching up and causing sores. A saddle should always be snug on the back. A saddle sliding back and forth will cause sores, just as too large a shoe will cause blisters.

Some horses that have not been worked too much with a saddle on their back will get a gall near the elbow, where the girth passes around the barrel. The rubbing of the girth on the tender skin in the area causes a condition that is very similar to a blister on a human's heel from a pair of new shoes. To prevent this from happening, use the saddle for only short periods of time daily until the horse's skin gets toughened. While riding, check the area for any swellings or soreness, as these are the first signs of a sore.

A girth should always be kept clean, with no accumulations of mud or hair. The belly and sides of the horse should always be brushed clean before saddling the horse. After the saddle is on the back and the girth drawn tight, be sure there is no fold of skin bunched under the girth. If necessary, stretch the front legs out one at a time, as if shaking hands with the horse. This will pull the folds smooth, should there be any.

Should the horse develop a saddle sore, the quickest cure is rest from the saddle. If the horse must be ridden, ride it bareback. A horse can be used with a saddle sore by cutting a saddle pad so that nothing touches its back and by using another pad over that one. But this is not advisable, as the pads do slip with use and the sores may become worse.

SCRATCHES OR GREASE HEEL

This condition occurs most often in the summer months. It is to be suspected when sores or roughness appear on the back of the horse's pastern. It usually begins with a dermatitis which becomes infected with a fungus or bacteria. The dermatitis often begins when the skin is irritated by stubble, dry hard weeds, lime, gravel, or damp bedding. The area becomes swollen, hot, and tender. Lameness often results. The condition is often confused with rope burns or cuts from fencing. The area becomes crusted with dried serum and the hair sticks stiffly outward.

The area should be washed daily with warm, soapy water to loosen the crust. The hair should be clipped short to avoid irritation by the hair. Alternate use of an astringent and antibiotic ointment usually clears up most cases quickly. Use the astringent for three days, then the antibiotic ointment. Sometimes systemic treatment with an antibiotic and cortisone is necessary when a severe bacterial infection and swelling are present.

SPRAINS

Due to their natural activity plus the work people give them, horses are quite prone to sprains. Often the speed and strength, not to mention the weight, work against the horse, and it gets unbalanced. Like humans, the horse with a sprain will suddenly pull up lame. Heat may soon be felt in the area of the sprain. Pressure on the spot will often cause the horse to flinch or pull its leg away.

With a fresh sprain, cold is applied in the form of cold water or ice packs. Alcohol, cooling liniment, and cortisone injections are also used. Standing the horse in a cold stream or running the hose on the leg constantly for half an hour will help. Making an ice bag from a leg out of a pair of pants sewn together at the cuff works well. The bag is slipped over the hoof, up the leg, then filled with crushed ice.

Once swelling has developed, ice should no longer be

applied, but heat instead. This increases the circulation which reduces the swelling. Hot packs, heating liniment, and hot udder ointment will do well. These should be repeated twice daily at the minimum. Massage will also bring relief.

STRANGLES OR DISTEMPER

This is the so-called "shipping fever" in horses, so named because it often occurs after horses have been shipped or moved, such as to shows, tracks, or sale barns. It is very contagious. The contagion is spread by use of contaminated water tanks, hay racks, and small pastures. The affected horse will often have a heavy mucous secretion from the nose, cough, run a fever, and show enlargement or abscess of the lymph glands under and between the jaws. This is where the disease gets the name "strangles."

Any horse showing symptoms should be completely isolated. It should be kept in warm, draft-free surroundings, and not drink from any tank, pail, or pond accessible to healthy horses. There should be absolutely *no* contact of any kind with other horses. The sick horse should receive adequate feed and be watched carefully for symptoms of distress or weakness.

Once the animal shows signs of sickness, there is not much that can be done to stop the disease. Antibiotics, while not really a "cure" in this case, will help keep down secondary ailments, such as pneumonia. Good nursing is the most important. At shows or race tracks, keep your horse isolated as much as possible. Do not loan water, feed pails, or bridles to others, unless you *thoroughly* disinfect them before your horse uses them again. Remember, a horse can spread strangles before really appearing sick.

Strangles in horses is about as severe as mumps in people. Although there have been fatalities, they are rare, and the disease is more one of misery than danger. Horses can be vaccinated against strangles, but it must be done *before* they are exposed to any possible sick horses.

SWAMP FEVER—EQUINE INFECTIOUS ANEMIA (EIA)

Swamp fever is caused by a virus and is spread by biting insects or by accidentally injecting minute amounts of virulent blood, as when an old, nonsterile syringe and needle are used. The most common outbreaks occur at race tracks, breeding farms, and show stables. This is the reason many states require show and race horses to be blood tested (the Coggins test) before competing, and many breeding farms require it before accepting mares for breeding.

There are several forms of the disease: 1. *Acute,* with sudden onset, high fever, weakness, incoordination, and quick death. 2. *Subacute* is less severe and appears in a series of "attacks"—the horse may just appear to be a "poor doer." 3. *Inactive* is perhaps the most dangerous phase, as the horse usually is only sick once, then appears well for the rest of its life but remains a carrier to other horses in the area.

There is no treatment or vaccination for EIA, and it can spread very fast through a barnful of horses. Any new horses, even visitors for a week or so, should have a Coggins test before being brought to the farm. Any infected horses should be destroyed or completely isolated in an insect-proof stable.

TETANUS

Tetanus is a too-common problem in horses, as they are highly susceptible to the organism and often sustain injuries that encourage its growth. It is an anaerobic organism, one which grows in the *absence* of oxygen. A deep wound or a puncture wound provides the ideal incubator. The first signs of tetanus are usually stiffness in the limbs and refusal to eat. The nictitating membrane or third eyelid is often prominent.

Treatment is nearly useless, unless given very early in the course of the disease, usually before obvious signs are seen. Systemic treatment with antitoxin and antibiotics in massive doses sometimes works. But the real cure is prevention. Every horse should receive an annual tetanus toxoid booster, which prevents most tetanus in hidden injuries, plus an injection of tetanus antitoxin in the event of a known injury or puncture wound. All nails, wire, pitchforks, and machinery should be kept away from horses. One tiny pinprick from a nail can be the start of a terrible death for a horse. (See "Puncture Wounds" elsewhere in this section.)

WARTS

Warts are sometimes a problem on horses, and as they are caused by a virus, they are often quite contagious. They are most often seen on the muzzle and face. Although they are seldom very injurious, they can be a problem affecting the usefulness of the animal. Warts rubbed by the bridle or bit can irritate the horse to the point of making it uncomfortable. Warts, of course, also spoil the looks of a show horse. And it is at shows and fairs that many outbreaks occur. Never borrow tack or pails for water and feed. Never stable your horse next to or across from a horse with warts.

The only treatment that seems to work well on most horses is the use of wart vaccine. Often one injection will effect a cure, but sometimes a repeat injection is necessary two weeks later.

WORMS

A horse can be quite severely infested with worms and show few or no symptoms visible to the naked eye. A wormy horse can look slick and shiny and be full of spirit or it can look dopey and rough. The only sure way to know a horse is not wormy is to have your vet check a sample of its manure. When a horse is not doing well, don't just assume it must be wormy and proceed to worm it. Worm medicine is toxic and can kill a sick horse. And please, if your horse is wormy, use a wormer that will kill the worms it *does* have, not just something you got cheap at the local discount store.

There are three basic types of wormers: powders or tiny gelatin capsules to be mixed with the feed, boluses administered with a balling gun, and liquid given by drench or by stomach tube. Some are a combination that will not only kill bots but many other worms as well. Others just hit bots or one or two worms, so care must be used in choosing a wormer. Unless you have had some experience here, it would be wise to consult your veterinarian for advice.

Ascarids These are the large worms sometimes seen in the manure. They resemble bean sprouts and are from five to eight inches in length. Ascarids, or round worms, cause the most damage in young horses, mainly foals. The affected foal will not do well and may slowly go down hill, showing loss of appetite, unthriftiness, and inactivity.

Bots These are fairly large, grublike worms (actually fly larvae), which attach themselves to the stomach lining. During the summer and fall, the adult flies attach their eggs to the hairs on the legs and belly of the horse. Here they remain, tightly fastened, until they are ingested by the horse and end up in the stomach, where they attach themselves and cause their damage. They pit and scar the lining of the stomach, sometimes causing colic and perforation of the stomach which results in peritonitis, often fatal. If the horse is not wormed, the larvae are passed in the manure, settle into the ground, and later emerge as adult flies, ready to lay more eggs and continue the cycle.

To prevent a large amount of bots from entering the stomach, the bot eggs should be removed daily from the hair. Scraping the area with a razor or hacksaw blade works well and does a fast job. Then, after the first hard freeze of the fall, the horse should receive a wormer effective against bots. There are many wormers available today, some not even touching bots, so be sure the one used does kill bots.

Pinworms These worms cause intense itching around the anus, causing the horse to rub its buttocks on a fence, tree, or anything else handy. The hair across the buttocks and on the tail soon becomes scanty and rough. There may be a yellowish crust around the anus. Pinworms seldom cause much actual damage, but their presence is irritating to both the horse and the owner. Occasionally the horse will develop a secondary infection, bacterial or fungal, when the area becomes raw and irritated.

Strongyles There is a fairly large group of worms, called strongyles, that is divided into two groups—large and small strongyles. These worms are smaller than bots and less often seen in the manure than bots. They do, however, present a danger to a horse. They migrate through the bloodstream, causing scarring of the vessel walls, occasional colic, aneurysm, and thrombosis. They also cause anemia and some damage to the liver, lungs, and heart. It has been estimated that between 70 and 80 percent of all horses are infested with some type of strongyles.

Others Horses can become infected with several other intestinal parasites: tapeworms, *Habronema,* lungworm, liver fluke, and others. To be safe, the horse should receive a yearly checkup by your veterinarian. Most intestinal parasites can be diagnosed by means of a fecal examination.

PIGS

General Care and Management

Pigs have a name for being dirty animals. This is not true. In fact, given the chance, they are among the cleanest of all farm animals. It's just that they are often kept in filthy pens and are unable to remain clean. Pigs will naturally pick one area for their "toilet" and use that spot only. They will not manure in their food or lay in filth, if given anywhere else to lay.

HOUSING

Pigs are quite easy to house since all they require is a snug, draft-free dry area. They can be kept in a stall in a barn with access to an outside yard or pasture, or in an elaborate hog house complete with custom farrowing pens and slatted floors. As long as the pig is warm in the winter and cool in the summer, well fed, and has dry bedding and plenty of fresh, clean water, it will do well.

Pigs are strong animals, so when building a hog pen or fence, be sure to make it strong. One-inch lumber or plywood will not

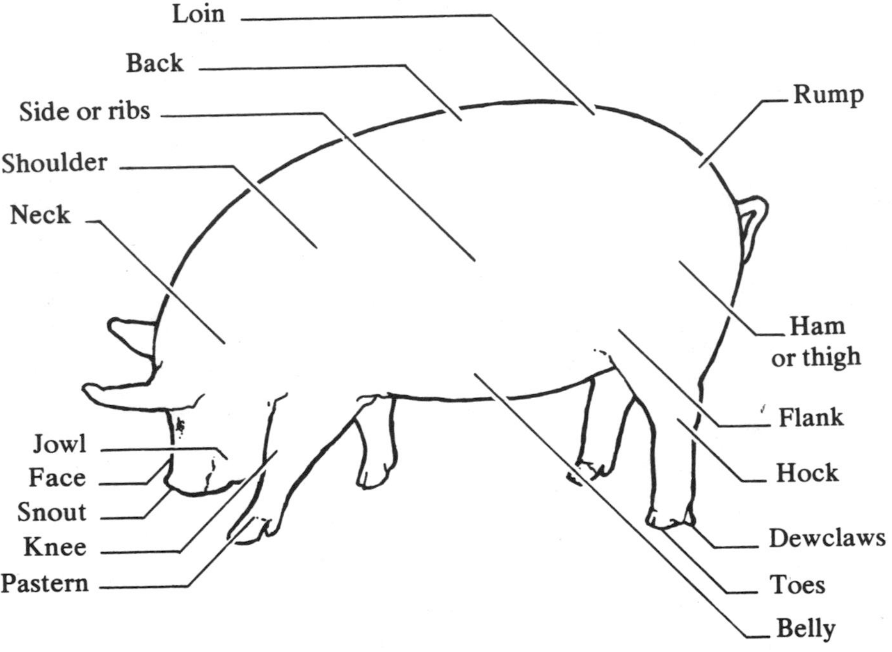

Parts of the Hog

hold a pig, nor will saggy woven wire or an old, rotten board fence. The inside pen should be built of two-inch lumber, and nailed up with 16d spikes. The boards should be nailed on the inside of the posts, as pigs are strong enough to root the boards right off the nails. All woven wire fencing should be stretched as tight as possible, with a strand of barbed wire at the top and bottom also stretched tightly.

Electric fences will contain many pigs, but they should be made of barbed wire, the two strands about 18 inches apart with the lowest strand about a foot off the ground. The pig must be "trained" to the fence by placing a pan of feed across the wire, leaving it for the pig to discover and learn the shocking power of those little wires. Board fences work well for hogs if the boards used are solid and placed on the inside of the posts. The fence will have to be three feet high; some pigs need a higher fence, as they can jump.

If the pig has a pasture area or roots his yard up badly, it will be necessary to ring it. Ringing pigs is simple. Buy a ring and ringer (both inexpensive) at a hardware or farm supply store, and place the ring in the ringer, then over the snout (the pig should be restrained). Close the ringer quickly, and the ring sinks into place. The most effective method of ringing is to place one or two rings above each nostril, on the edge of the rooter. The rooter is the hard ridge of cartilage that the pig roots with. Just be careful not to ring so deep that the bone is scraped, as this can cause infection. Movable houses are an asset, as the pigs can be moved from one pasture or yard to another, which lets the pasture recover and also helps control internal parasites.

Different sizes of pigs should not be run together. Many injuries result from this, as the larger pigs boss the smaller ones and crowd the younger pigs away from the feed and shade. A pig has a powerful jaw and a good sharp set of teeth which can cause severe damage.

FEEDING

It is true that they can be fed on garbage, but remember, the quality of the food will be the quality of the meat and the little pigs they produce. This is not to say that you can't feed your potato peelings or stale bread or apple cores to the pigs, but a balanced diet will be much more productive in the long run.

Pigs can be successfully raised on a wide variety of feeds and combinations of feeds, but the thing to remember is the value and use of each feed. Corn alone, although used for fattening hogs that are nearing the slaughter age, is not an adequate diet for growing pigs or breeding pigs. Protein is needed for growth and reproduction, carbohydrates for warmth and weight gain, plus vitamins and minerals to insure good health. Two good books to consult when looking for a balanced ration to fit your particular area are *Feeds and Feeding* by Morrison and *Hog Profits for Farmers* by McMillan.

Pigs benefit from access to good pasture. Rape, alfalfa, clover, and rye are all good choices for pasture crops. They will also eat good quality hay, especially legume hay, fed free choice. An addition of skim milk or whey is much enjoyed by pigs and very beneficial.

RESTRAINT

Pigs are often difficult animals to restrain effectively without the proper pig-handling equipment. A good pig crate with a head gate is a necessity on a farm where many pigs are kept. Where only a few pigs are raised, the occasional pig may be restrained for examination or treatment by means of ropes or gates. A fairly large pig can be restrained by slipping a rope noose around the snout, behind the tusks, then fastening it to a sturdy post about a foot or so from the ground. When tied, the

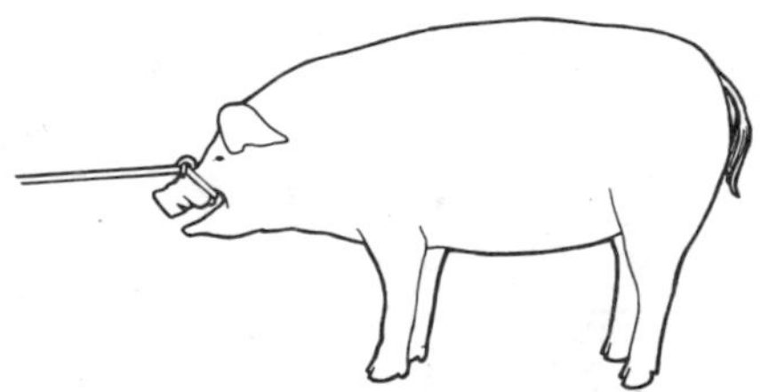

Noose on upper jaw to restrain large hog goes behind tusks for best grip. Hog pulls back, so secure well.

pig will most often back up against the rope and be held for treatment. Crowding a pig into a corner by means of a strong, portable gate about the same length and height as the pig works well for examination and treatment that is not extensive.

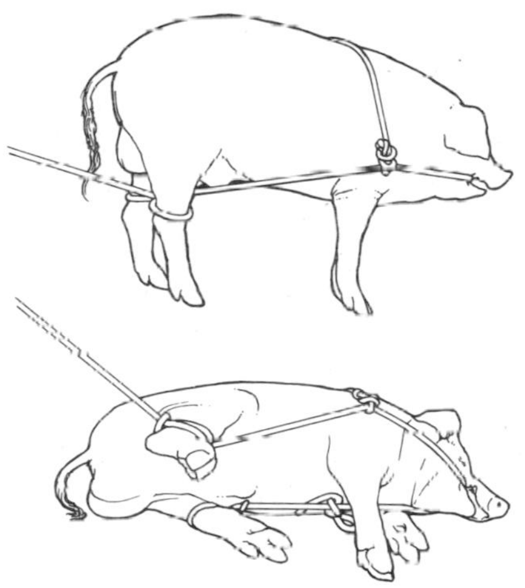

Rope Restraints of Hogs

Smaller pigs may be easiest restrained by holding them up by their hind legs with their front feet just off the ground. Operations such as rupture repair and castration can be done with the pig in this position, or laid in a V-shaped trough on its back. A pig can often be driven into a trailer by slipping a bushel basket over its head and backing it up the ramp.

A very large boar may be restrained for castration by using a 55-gallon drum. Feed is withheld for a day, with only water given. The next day, with two or three strong helpers present, the empty drum with one end cut out is carried to the boar's yard. Three or four ears of corn or a dish of ground feed is thrown in the barrel. When the boar dives in after the feed, the assistants tip the barrel up on end, leaving the boar ready for surgery or if necessary, further restraint by means of a block and tackle and ropes. Usually one person on each hind leg is enough restraint for castration.

A boar can also be restrained with hobbles—see illustration.

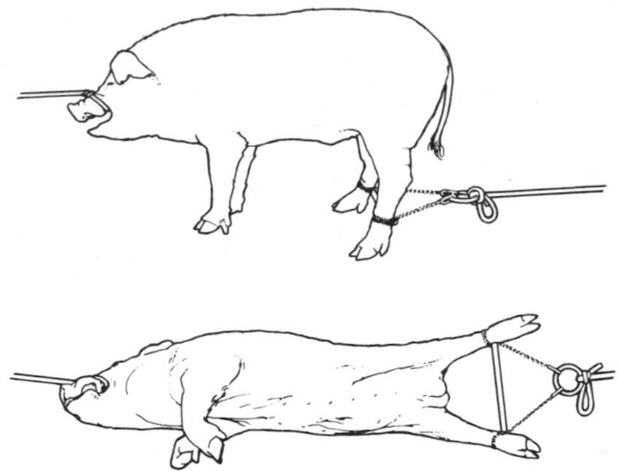

Hobble Restraint for a Boar

BREEDING

The Boar When choosing a boar, either for service or to buy, keep in mind the use your little pigs will be put to. You will want pigs with strong legs, meaty shoulders, and large hams. You will want a long hog, with plenty of lean bacon and pork chops. And you will want a gilt with at least 12 and preferably 14 functioning teats. These characteristics are passed from the boar, as well as the sow. The boar should also have a good disposition. It is no excuse to say the boar is mean "because he's a boar."

Never use a boar for breeding that has unevenly developed testicles or is ruptured (the testicles will appear extra large and quite flabby). The tendency to rupture is an inherited factor and greatly reduces the sale value of the young pigs. A boar is generally ready for light service at about seven months of age, but this depends on his development and previous care.

The Sow and the Gilt A gilt is a young female pig that has not farrowed or has just farrowed. When she is ready to have her second litter, she is no longer a gilt but a sow.

There is controversy between pig raisers as to whether it is more profitable to breed gilts, raise the litter, then sell them and buy more gilts, or to retain them and keep breeding them as sows. Gilts have fewer pigs and a little smaller pigs as a rule, but are safer mothers, as a heavy sow has a tendency to lie on her pigs, crushing or smothering them. The older sow is usually a better milker and is more predictable as far as production goes. It is easier to make a close guess as to what number of pigs she will have and the quality of them as they grow older. The gilt is often bought cheaper, farrows, and gains weight, thus increasing in value.

Whether you choose a sow or gilt, you may be able to raise two litters a year from her. In fact, if they are really pushed and taken care of, they can farrow every four or five months. Sows come into heat every three weeks, and three to five days after their litter is weaned. Sows should be flushed two weeks before breeding. This means putting them on full feed and usually lush pasture, so they are rapidly gaining weight when they are bred.

A sow shows her heat by riding other sows, grunting, frequent urination, and a red, swollen vulva. She should be taken to the boar as soon as her heat is noticed, to allow her to be settled down when she is ready to stand for breeding. After being bred, the sow should be put onto a high protein ration, at least a 13 percent supplement. She should receive all the top quality pasture or alfalfa hay she will eat. She should also receive a trace mineral-salt supplement. Plenty of fresh clean water is a must, as this will add to her condition and help make milk.

FARROWING

Three months, three weeks, and three days (114 days) after breeding, the sow will be ready to farrow. A week before she is due to farrow, she should be thoroughly cleaned off, her udders washed well with warm soapy water to help prevent parasite infestation of new pigs. She will need time to settle down in the farrowing pen in order to be ready to take care of her new pigs. Sows that eat, lie on, or disown their pigs are often sows that have been upset just prior to farrowing.

The farrowing pen should be thoroughly disinfected prior to moving her into it, and a good deep layer of fresh bedding laid down (like four to six inches of sawdust). It is a good idea to have one corner blocked off with a heat lamp hanging into it. This is a place for the little pigs to go soon after birth to keep warm, dry off, and keep out of the sow's way while she has the other pigs. Be very careful to protect the lamp from breakage, as many fires are caused by fallen heat lamps. There should be a railing around the outside edge of the farrowing pen ten inches high and ten inches away from the wall, to offer protection to the new pigs should the sow flop down in a position that would pin the pigs to the wall. The farrowing pen should be at least eight feet square for average-sized sows, and larger for very large sows. Sometimes it is better to have a longer, rectangular pen for more protection for the little pigs.

If at all possible, you should be present at farrowing time. Several clean, dry towels, a small wide-mouth jar of iodine, a pair of side cutters, a pair of scissors, and a spool of thread should be on hand.

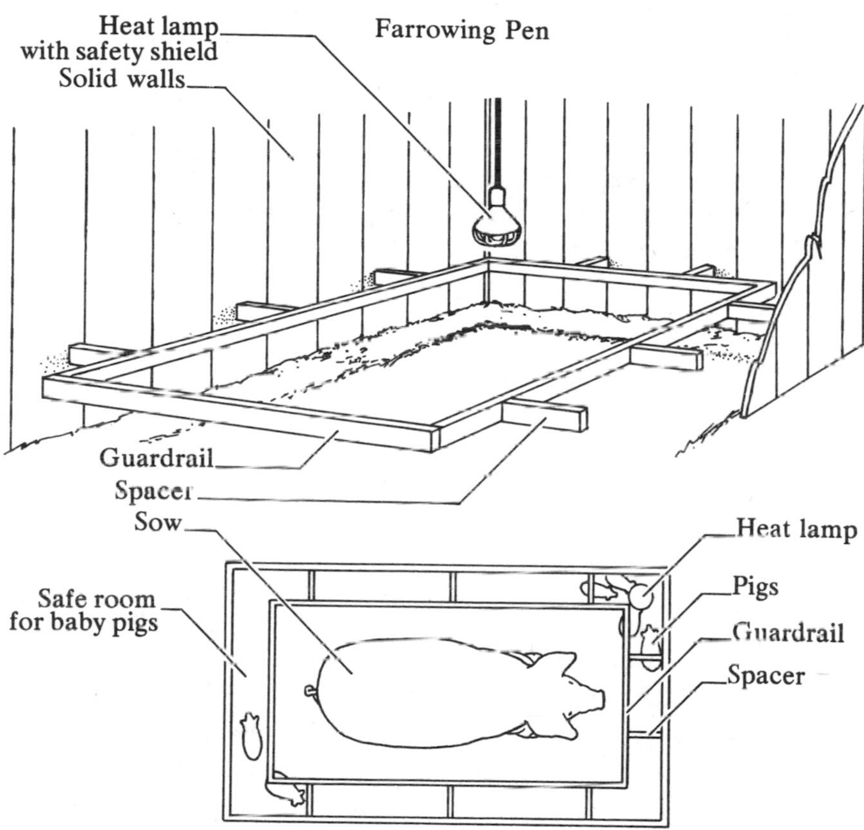

The sow will usually work for 15 to 30 minutes to produce the first pig in the litter. Most often, the following pigs will come faster. If the sow works for longer than half an hour on a pig, failing to make any progress, she should be examined. A person with a small hand should slip on a rubber glove, lubricate the glove with liquid dish soap or Vaseline, and check the progress of the pig. If it seems lodged, gentle but firm traction will often bring it out. If this does not work, call your veterinarian, as too much work on a lodged pig can exhaust the sow and cause the death of one or more pigs. Sometimes a forceps delivery is necessary, but often an injection of posterior pituitary helps the sow deliver her pigs normally.

Some sows require a tranquilizer during farrowing, as they become agitated, trying to escape their pigs, eat them, or thrash about. In such cases it is advisable to take the pigs away until the tranquilizer has worked, to prevent further excitement in the sow.

Baby Pigs As the pigs are born, it is a good idea to clean each one, dip the navel in iodine, clip the sharp needle teeth to prevent injury to the sow's udder, and place the pig under the heat lamp. If the umbilical cord is long, tie it off an inch or so from the pig's belly with strong thread, then cut off the rest, leaving a stump two inches long. Dip this in iodine.

To prevent anemia, the baby pigs should receive an iron supplement, either orally, injectable, or by painting the preparation on the sow's udder. The baby pigs should have access to a heat lamp for two weeks. At two weeks of age, they will usually begin to eat enough grain to give them a free choice creep-fed ration. (See "Creep Feeding Lambs" in the chapter on lambs.) There are pellets on the market for baby pigs that work very well for a first food. Skim milk added to a little ground pig starter will encourage week-old pigs to start nibbling at grain. At first, they will walk in it more than eat it, but soon they will be making short work of the mash and be ready to start the pellets. From the pellets, they easily graduate to a good mixed growing ration, and are ready to wean at eight weeks.

For problems related to breeding and farrowing, see "Hypocalcemia," "Anemia in Baby Pigs," "Mastitis," and "Failure to Let Down Milk After Farrowing" in **Diseases and Other Problems** later in this chapter.

CASTRATION

All pigs not intended to be saved for a service boar should be castrated between the ages of one and five weeks. At this age there is very little if any setback, and very little shock. Bleeding is either absent or minimal.

An assistant holds the pig up by the hind legs, with the belly outward. The operator stands facing the pig. The instrument needed is a scalpel, single-edged razor blade, or sharp knife. Also have on hand a pail of warm, soapy water, a bottle of antiseptic, and a towel.

The area is scrubbed with the soapy water and dried. The testicles are forced toward the belly and outward against the skin. Either one incision is made between the testicles or two incisions one at a time over each testicle. The testicle is grasped and pulled out as far as the cord will allow. In small pigs the cord can be pulled until it snaps. With larger pigs the cord must be cut very close to the body, so that when the tension is released the stump pulls back into the incision. If you cut the cord with a scraping motion instead of a clean cut, there will be less bleeding. Be sure you also remove all of the tunic—the white, tough membrane surrounding the testicle—and do not leave any of it sticking out through the incision. This causes incomplete healing and a condition called a scirrhous cord. The scrotum fills with fibrous tissue which must be dissected away from the skin and body tissue with the fingers to prevent hemorrhage. It is a finger-cramping job that no veterinarian enjoys.

After castration, be sure the incision or incisions are large enough. If too small an incision is made, the skin will close up before healing is complete, and infection or tetanus may occur. Also be sure to pour in some antiseptic after castration. If the castration is done during fly season, it may be well to use a fly repellent to prevent maggots.

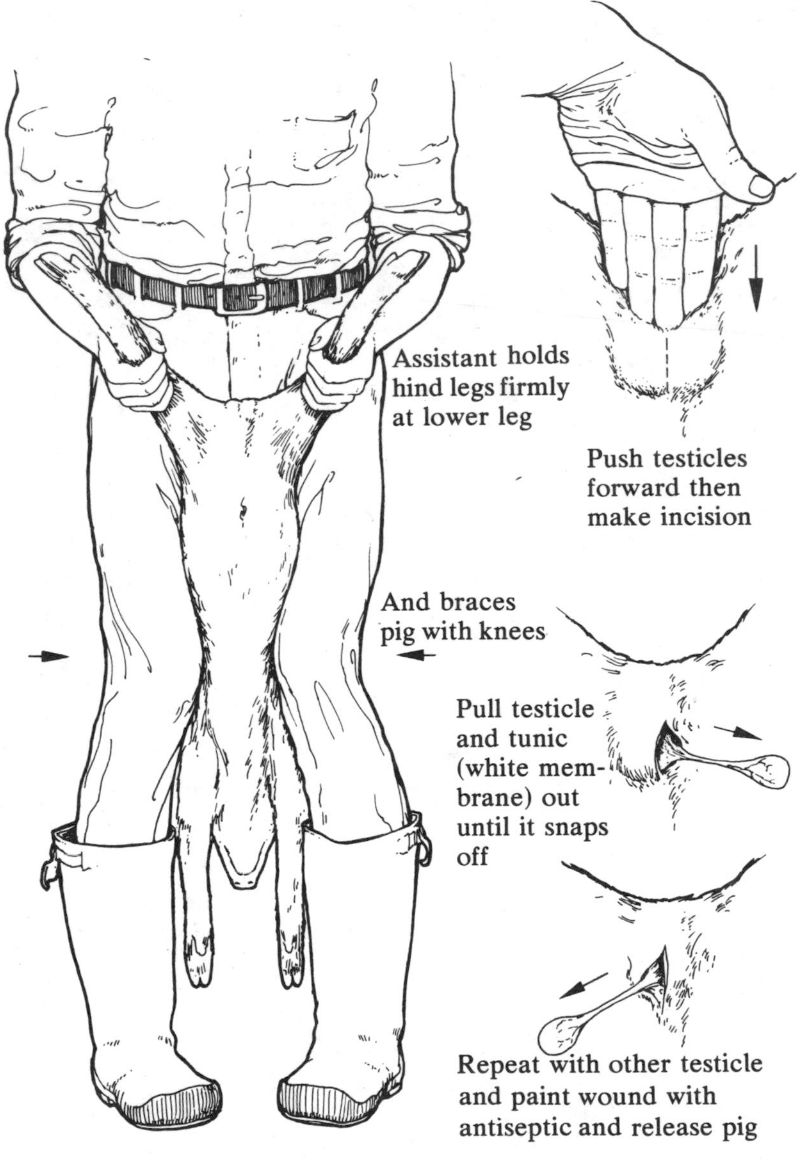
Assistant holds
hind legs firmly
at lower leg
Push testicles
forward then
make incision
And braces
pig with knees
Pull testicle
and tunic
(white mem-
brane) out
until it snaps
off
Repeat with other testicle
and paint wound with
antiseptic and release pig

The Ruptured Pig Once in a while you may run across a ruptured pig at castrating time. With a ruptured pig, often one testicle will be larger and feel softer than the other. Sometimes both testicles will appear large and sloppy. This enlargement and softness is due to the fact that there are intestines in the scrotum along with the testicle.

In cases where there is only one pig ruptured, it is often most economical to just sell the pig "as is" at weaning time. The slight knock-down you receive in market price will be less of a loss than the expense of having a veterinarian operate on the rupture. In cases where there are several ruptures, it usually does pay to call your vet. This happens frequently as rupture is an inherited defect, and where several closely related pigs are bred, there will be a greater chance of several pigs being affected.

The inguinal canal must be sewn closed after the intestines are pushed back into the body. Some hog raisers simply castrate, sewing the scrotum shut to contain the intestines. This works in some cases, but may still lower the market price, or worse, allow the strangulation of the intestinal loop, killing the pig.

Diseases and Other Problems

ANEMIA IN BABY PIGS

No matter how much iron supplement is fed to the sow, milk is low in iron, and when pigs are on mainly a milk diet, they are prone to anemia. Anemia is a costly disease, for once the pigs have become anemic, they don't gain as well as pigs that have been protected from the problem. Giving new pigs oral iron, swabbing the sow's udder daily with an iron and honey or molasses mixture, or giving injectable iron will prevent anemia. Once the pigs are on the ground or have access to green feed, the danger is greatly reduced.

Anemic pigs will at first look like the best pigs in the litter. They will look very plump and round. But unfortunately this is not fat or healthy tissue, but edema due to poor circulation.

BRUCELLOSIS

Brucellosis in pigs is caused by the organism *Brucella suis.* It not only affects pigs but can infect cattle and also man. This is not, however, the brucellosis commonly affecting cattle—that is *Brucella abortus,* causing the so-called Bang's disease in them. Both organisms cause undulant fever in man. Pigs affected with brucellosis will abort, have weak pigs which often die, show lameness, or even have hind paralysis. Some boars affected show swollen testicles. There is no treatment for brucellosis, other than slaughter. All new pigs coming to the farm should be tested or should come from brucellosis-free herds. In this respect, do not just accept the owner's word for the health status of his herd. Many brucellosis-infected herds do not show any obvious signs of the disease.

Boars should not be used on any sows or gilts brought in for service by others unless they have been found free of brucellosis nor should the boar be loaned out to other than brucellosis-free herds.

COCCIDIOSIS

While not a severe problem in swine, it can give trouble in certain locales. Coccidiosis is caused by a protozoa (a one-celled animal) which is a parasite invading the intestine. Coccidia cause unthriftiness, diarrhea, and stunting. The condition is most often seen in damp, dirty pens or hog lots. In many cases, the incidence of coccidiosis can be greatly reduced by moving the pigs to clean, dry pens and feeding a good balanced ration. Intestinal sulfas and nitrofurazone have been used to good results in treatment of coccidiosis.

ERYSIPELAS

Erysipelas can be a serious problem in young pigs in many locales. With the acute form of the disease, death may be quick, from one to four days after the first signs of illness. The infected pigs will have a high temperature, be in pain, squeal, and show diamond-shaped purple blotches on the sides, belly, and back. After the disease has ended, these diamond-shaped lesions will often slough off. Following an acute attack, some of the pigs that have lived through it will become carriers, being chronically infected with the organism which lives in the joints or heart.

If caught early, treatment is often successful. Penicillin and serum are both used, either alone or in combination. But, as in many diseases, it is safer and more economical to vaccinate against erysipelas than to gamble treating it. If there has been erysipelas in your area, consult your veterinarian about a vaccination program.

FAILURE TO LET DOWN MILK AFTER FARROWING

Some sows fail to let their milk down after farrowing, due either to excitement and stress or a hormone imbalance. If not noticed in time, the little pigs will either starve or become so stressed that they develop scours or other problems. When a sow is discovered with this problem, you should call your veterinarian at once. Very often, an injection of posterior pituitary will cause her to drop her milk down almost immediately. Once the milk flow has started, she will milk normally. If the sow has no milk, however, such an injection will not make her produce milk.

HOG CHOLERA

Due to more public awareness, along with more strict control measures, hog cholera is not the problem nationwide that it was in the past. It is the most serious hog disease, as it spreads very quickly and is most often fatal. Affected pigs are

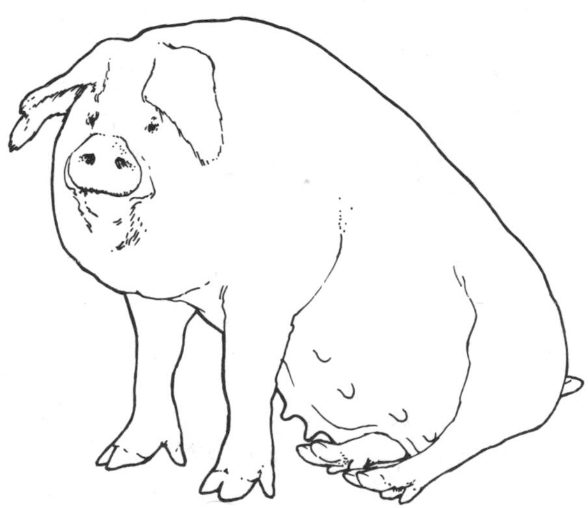

Sow with Posterior Paralysis

dull acting, have gummy eyes, diarrhea, and weakness in the hind legs. Their temperature is high, often 107°F. Any suspected cases of hog cholera should be examined at once by your veterinarian. In most parts of the country it must be reported to the state veterinarian, both for quarantine and as a warning to his office that there is a cholera outbreak in the area, enabling him to warn other hog breeders.

Before pigs have been exposed, they can be vaccinated against hog cholera. However, once exposed and possibly beginning to incubate the disease, they should receive anti-hog cholera serum. This will not help hogs sick with the disease in most cases, but will often help stop the outbreak. Consult your local veterinarian about the incidence of hog cholera in your area and the advisability of vaccination.

HYPOCALCEMIA OR POSTERIOR PARALYSIS IN SOWS

This problem is seen in heavy milking sows with large thrifty litters, usually just before or at weaning time. The pigs weigh from 25 to 30 pounds, and when multiplied by ten or 12 pigs, you may have the equivalent of a 300-plus pound pig sucking a 250-pound sow. The sow becomes thin, trying to keep milk for her pigs, and finally gets weak in the hindquarters. If not treated, she will go down in back and become completely paralyzed in the rear quarters. She will then go off feed and die.

If caught very early, just weaning the pigs will effect a cure. But once she becomes quite weak in the hind legs, she will need treatment by your veterinarian to live. Intravenous or intraperitoneal calcium, as is given in cow milk fever, often works well. Good nursing is also important, as if the sow is left in the sun without feed or water, she will give up and die, regardless of treatment. If the sow is let go too long, no amount of treatment will enable her to recover.

LICE

Lice sometimes infest pigs, often during the winter when the pigs do not have access to sunlight. Lice are small, grayish parasites that you can see with the naked eye if you look closely enough. Infested pigs will scratch, appear restless, and not do as well as they could. If infested badly enough, they can cause severe anemia and death.

On finding lice on one of your pigs, it is a good idea to thoroughly dust all pigs housed in the same building and to check any others in other buildings. There are many louse powders on the market. Be sure to read the label before buying, to make sure it is safe for pigs. Most powders made for dairy cattle are safe enough for swine. The animals should be powdered weekly for three weeks to effectively kill all the lice as they hatch and before they can reproduce.

MANGE

Mange is the most extensive external parasitic disease in swine. It leads to weight loss through irritation and intense itching. Mange is caused by tiny mites which burrow into the skin. They are not visible to the naked eye. The first sign that your pigs may have mange is when they constantly rub their backs and sides on anything available. If left untreated, the hair may be rubbed off and red, scabby areas may form.

Sows and gilts should be sprayed for mange before being bred. The pens they are put into for farrowing should be sprayed, let alone, then scrubbed with hot water and soap before the sows are moved into them. Pigs should be sprayed for mange soon after being weaned, and should they show any signs of it later, be sprayed again.

MASTITIS

Occasionally after farrowing a sow will develop one or more udders with mastitis. Injury, such as banging the udder on a low doorway, erratic milking by the little pigs, or lying on cold cement, may cause it. The udder will become hot and red, and it may be painful to the sow. She will often run a degree or two higher temperature than normal. The milk will often be abnormal. Many sows will go off feed and act sick from the mastitis.

Systemic treatment with a broad-spectrum antibiotic, along with hot packs and warm udder ointment or liniment, will help, as will massage of the affected udder and manual removal of the milk in that udder section.

NECROTIC ENTERITIS OR "NECRO"

Necrotic enteritis, caused by bacterial infection or more often by dietary deficiency, actually is the inflammation and decaying of intestinal tissue. Low protein diets, often straight corn diets, are usually the cause of necrotic enteritis. Pigs from weaning to four or five months are most often seen with it. The affected pigs have a lack of appetite, lack of energy, high temperature, and diarrhea.

To alleviate the condition, improve the diet, giving a high protein feed with vitamin B complex supplements. Giving antibiotics or sulfa drugs will help take care of any bacterial infection and also prevent secondary infections.

NECROTIC RHINITIS OR BULL-NOSE, AND ATROPHIC RHINITIS

The pig with bull-nose will quite often have a swollen snout or face. There may be a discharge from the nose, sneezing, or occasional bleeding from the nose. If the condition is allowed to progress, the tissue will decay (become necrotic), there will be foul-smelling areas, and the nasal discharge will have a foul odor. This condition is often confused with another similar condition, atrophic rhinitis. With atrophic rhinitis, there is not usually the swelling of the nose and face as seen in necrotic rhinitis, but there is the nasal discharge and sneezing. Treatment is similar.

Oral or injectable antibiotics will generally help, as will sulfa combinations. The affected pig should be kept as comfortable as possible and fed highly palatable foods that are easily eaten. Slop made of ground feed and sour milk is usually good as is raw eggs or oatmeal. When a whole herd is involved or the disease is spreading, cultures should be taken from an affected pig in order to find out the specific organism causing the trouble. The nose should be kept clean. Daily swabbing with a human nasal spray often helps.

Rhinitis is often introduced by an injury, such as bites, scrapes, or injuries caused by broken needle teeth.

PNEUMONIA

Pneumonia can be caused by a bacterial infection, virus, or inhalation of a foreign material such as dust. It can also be caused by an improperly given drench. Pneumonia causes many pig deaths, more so nationwide than a handful of diseases together. Not all pigs die from pneumonia; some become like a person with emphysema, gasping for breath at the slightest exertion, dust, or hot, humid weather. A pig in this condition cannot make decent weight gain or be a productive breeding animal. With acute pneumonia, the pig will act distressed. It may go off feed suddenly, puff or breathe hard, run a high temperature, and be reluctant to move about.

Affected pigs should be kept isolated in a dry, well-bedded, draft-free pen. Your veterinarian should be called. When caught fairly early there is a good chance of recovery, but the longer pneumonia is left untreated, the more scar tissue forms in the lungs, and the greater the chances are for death or incomplete recovery. Systemic treatment with a broad-spectrum antibiotic or sulfa combination often works well. If the pig is not coughing well enough to raise the fluid in the lungs, an injectable expectorant may be used.

TRANSMISSIBLE GASTROENTERITIS OR TGE

Caused by a virus, TGE is a highly contagious disease that has a very short incubation period. It causes diarrhea, vomiting, and severe dehydration. The mortality rate is very high in baby pigs, as they cannot take the severe diarrhea and subsequent dehydration as well as an older pig can. Older pigs can tolerate the disease better, and the mortality rate drops considerably. Weight loss is common.

Prevention is the best treatment. No new pigs should be allowed near or in the same area where other pigs are contained on the farm. All pigs should be vaccinated before any signs of trouble appear.

WORMS

Pigs are affected with several species of worms: three types of stomach worm, ascarids, strongyles, whipworms, and others. A good system of pasture rotation, plus good sanitation, routine fecal examinations by your veterinarian, and regular worming will keep these parasites to a low level. Due to the life cycle of these parasites, it is nearly impossible to have 100 percent worm-free animals, but if their numbers can be kept low there will be no economic loss from them.

Wormers such as sodium fluoride (which is administered by mixing ¾ pound of sodium fluoride thoroughly with 99 pounds of *dry* ground feed—never get the medicated feed wet or it may kill the pig—then feeding the mixture for one day only) or thiabendazole work well and are safe when used as directed.

By thoroughly washing the udders of the sow about to freshen and moving her to a clean, freshly bedded stall to freshen, then moving her and her pigs to a clean pasture that has had no pigs on it for at least a month, the little pigs will have an excellent chance of getting a worm-free start in life. Sows and gilts should be wormed before they are bred, as worming afterwards can be dangerous.

When suspecting worms in your pigs in spite of precautions, take a fecal sample to your veterinarian. He can examine it for the presence of worm eggs and minute larvae to determine just what parasites your pigs may be infested with. Some parasites need a specific wormer, which is not commonly used. Just blindly worming with any old wormer will be a waste of time and money.

POULTRY

General Care and Management

CHICKENS AND GUINEAS

Housing There are perhaps more types of housing used for chickens than any other farm animal or poultry. This housing can range from a small chicken coop in the backyard to a huge, automated laying house containing 22,000 birds. For the small farm or homestead flock, though, about the only automatic convenience available is a willing child or spouse doing chores without being nagged! So, we'll disregard the large poultry farmer here.

A chicken house should be cool and airy in the summer and warm and dry in the winter. In moderate climates this is fairly easily obtained. In cold winter areas, though, it takes a little more doing to winterize the farm flock. A double-walled construction may be needed to keep the poultry house warm enough to protect the chickens in the severest part of the winter. Double windows on the south side will not only let in sunlight, which is necessary for the health and well-being of

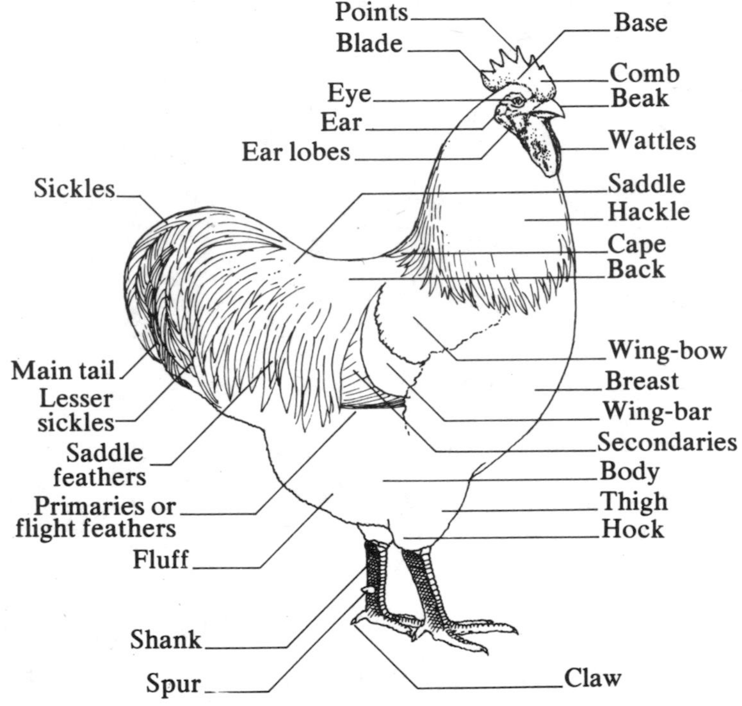

Parts of a Male Fowl

poultry during the winter, but will provide a lot of warmth. If available, a chicken house can be built into a bank of dirt. The house should face the south, with windows on the south side and the bank of dirt on the north to ward off cold winds. The birds' body heat will usually keep the coop warm enough to be comfortable, provided the building has *double* walls and *double* windows, which leaves a dead-air space insulating against the cold. *All* drafts must be plugged. An immense amount of cold air can flow through a keyhole or knothole, not to mention the crack under the door. In very severe weather a heat lamp or two may be needed to provide adequate warmth. Stacking bales of straw against the outside walls will also help block storm winds.

Note: Commercial insulation does not seem to work well in small coops. It seems to hold too much moisture, causing respiratory problems.

Plenty of dry bedding should be used, with some chopped hay scattered through it to encourage the chickens and guineas to scratch about and get exercise. They should receive warmed water twice daily during the winter and have plenty of mixed grain available. In colder houses, the chickens and guineas should receive more corn to provide needed carbohydrates for body warmth and energy.

In the summer, it is a good idea to have an outside run or pen for the birds to exercise in. If possible, two yards are best. Planting a crop in their pens, such as rape or clover, will give them some greens and also encourage exercise. Alternate yards is a large step toward poultry cleanliness and parasite control.

The best type of fencing is woven 12 to 14 gauge wire six feet high, stretched tight. Guineas can fly over this, but often will not if they are not excited and have adequate feed. If they persist in flying out, you can clip the feathers on their wings with a pair of scissors to discourage this. The woven wire is more expensive than mesh chicken wire, but will last a lot longer and will protect the birds from dogs and wild predators.

Adequate ventilation is necessary in the poultry house, as even a hundred chickens can produce a lot of stale, warm, dry air. Breathing this air over and over again is a sure way to get respiratory trouble in your flock. The temperature should not vary much between 50°F. and 70°F. year around in the poultry house.

Feeding Chickens and guineas are fed the same foods. During the summer, both can and will, if given the chance, forage for insects, grubs, and greens. In addition, they should receive free choice laying mash or mixed grain. Unless homegrown grains are available, it is usually cheaper to purchase already mixed chicken feed, due to the cost of handling and mixing small amounts of grains and concentrates. Corn, oats, wheat, barley, rice, rye, and ground buckwheat are all used in various poultry rations as a major portion of the grain mix. Rye and buckwheat may represent up to 15 percent of the grain ration, with the others making up an even higher percentage.

Cooked potatoes, milk, skim milk, buttermilk, sour milk, meat scraps, fish meal, cooked bloody eggs, soybean oil meal, corn gluten meal, and other foods are also used as part of the grain ration in different parts of the country. When formulating your own poultry ration, it is a good idea to see your county agent for assistance, as he knows the grains and supplements available in your part of the country.

Your chickens and guineas will also need minerals added to their ration. Oyster shell and limestone grit should be available for your poultry at all times. This not only provides grit needed for digestion, but also calcium carbonate for maintenance and eggshell formation. Bone meal is added to many growing rations for calcium, phosphorus, and protein. A one percent salt supplement is needed in chicken rations for palatability and digestion. Trace minerals such as iron, iodine, and manganese are also added.

Alfalfa, either green or as chopped hay, is enjoyed by chickens and guineas, and it also provides vitamins A, D, and G, plus other vitamins, protein, and minerals. Alfalfa meal is often included in poultry rations. Silage is sometimes fed to chickens. It surpasses cured or dehydrated hay or meal and is very palatable to them. A hundred hens can be fed three to four pounds of silage a day.

Chickens and guineas will also make use of waste produce from the garden. Carrots, lettuce, kale, cabbage, tomatoes, beets, squash, and pumpkins, are all enjoyed by them and provide them with necessary vitamins, protein, and minerals.

Oat, bean, and other grain sprouts are sometimes fed, but it is often difficult to get the birds accustomed to eating them.

Be sure the birds have all the water they will drink in the summer, as it does not take long for them to become dehydrated and then ill.

Incubation If you plan to raise some chicks from the farm flock, there are several methods of incubation. First, there is the old method of letting the hen lay a clutch of eggs, then incubate them herself. Then there is the method of letting one hen lay the eggs, then slipping them under a broody hen to hatch. She will sit on the eggs, then take care of the chicks after they hatch. In some locales, there are people with large incubators who do custom hatching. For a small fee they will take your eggs, incubate them, then give you back your day-old chicks. And there is the do-it-yourselfer with a small incubator that holds a hundred eggs or so.

If the hen or a setting hen is to hatch the eggs, you just have to let nature take its course, more or less. With the setting hen, you can let her sit on a couple of china eggs until you collect enough eggs to make a comfortable clutch for her to set on. Don't overload her, as she will be unable to keep too large a clutch warm.

When collecting eggs to take to an incubator or to put into your own incubator, the eggs being saved for hatching should be stored in an egg carton with the small end down. They should be handled very carefully and not be jarred. They should be stored at a temperature between 50°F. and 60°F. Cooler temperatures sometimes affect the hatchability of the eggs, and high temperatures (above 82°F.) such as occur during the late summer will not be good for hatching because of the slow development which will have occurred during storage, weakening the embryos. Eggs can be held from one week to as long as 28 days, depending on the temperature and handling. Varying temperatures will greatly decrease the hatchability after two weeks.

The best results are obtained by incubating the eggs for 21 days at a temperature of 101°F., with a humidity of about 60 percent. The hatching can be delayed by lowering the incubator temperature slightly.

When a hen is setting, she should be in a small nest box attached to a wire run. There should be plenty of food and water readily available, should she want it. As the chicks hatch, she will take over completely, keeping them warm, showing them how and what to eat, and so on.

Baby Chicks When you hatch or buy baby chicks, you have to be the "mother," and you don't have the instincts for it that a real hen does. The chicks must be kept warm and kept from straying from the heat. A large cardboard box, with the corners rounded by taping cardboard in them and a heat lamp hung in the center, will work well. The temperature should be about 95°F., with no hot spots or cold drafts. If the chicks are too cool, they will huddle together and smother. If possible, a thermostat should be used in connection with the brooder lamp to prevent accidental temperature changes. Be sure the brooder lamp is fastened well, as many fires are started every year by heat lamp accidents.

There should be fresh water available to the chicks at all times. Whenever the chicks begin to empty the waterer before it is refilled, more or larger waterers should be used. Be careful not to use too large a waterer at first, as chicks can drown in water 1½ inches deep.

Chick starter should be sprinkled on the floor the first day to encourage the chicks to peck. The second day, the feed can be placed in shallow dishes such as plastic can covers. As soon as they are eating well you can switch to regular chick feeders. Be sure you get the kind that does not allow them to stand in the feed. If they do stand in it, a lot of feed can be soiled and wasted.

The temperature of the brooder can be reduced by five degrees each week as the chicks grow older. The brooder area should also be increased in order to give the growing chicks more room, which often prevents cannibalism.

DUCKS AND GEESE

Housing Ducks and geese are more easily housed than chickens and guineas, due to their built-in down insulation. They do need shade from the summer sun, and a warm, dry shelter in the winter. Many ducks are lost or suffer damage from having their breast or keel freeze to the ground in the severe cold. Since they are sloppy with their water, there must always be adequate bedding in a duck or goose house. Sawdust or wood shavings work best, as both are very absorbent and easily replaced when soiled. Be sure the waterers are heavy enough to prevent tipping over, and always have waterers that do not allow the bird to climb into them. Bathing ducks and geese really soak the bedding.

Ducks and geese do not require roosts, as both rest lying on the floor. Nests for ducks are constructed of one-inch lumber and are 12 inches by 18 inches deep. They are made like stalls, with a four- or five-inch strip nailed across the front. Canvas can be tacked across the top to be more like a "cave." Geese nests can be similarly constructed, only larger, or they can be made out of small wooden barrels. The size depends on the breed of geese, but nests about 20 inches wide by 30 inches high are average. Geese seem to prefer single nests rather than community nests. Where best results are obtained by mating

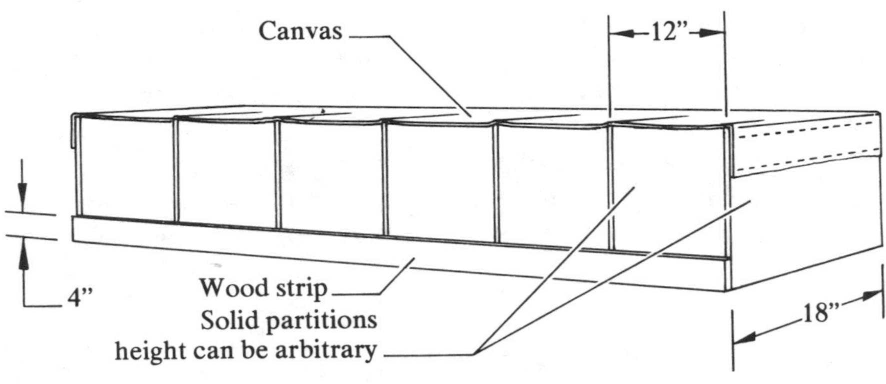

Duck Nest

one gander to two geese, a drake can mate with four or five female ducks.

The eggs should be collected daily, stored safely, then placed under the female, under a broody hen, or in an incubator. A hen can handle from three to five eggs, a goose ten to 15, and a duck seven to ten. Duck eggs are incubated as are chicken eggs, but should be kept at a slightly higher humidity at hatching time (above 60 percent). Most duck eggs hatch in 28 days, with Muscovy eggs taking 34 days. Goose eggs incubate for 20 to 35 days, depending on the breed. Smaller breeds take less hatching time than do the giant breeds.

Feeding If both ducks and geese have access to range or pasture, they will forage some of their food. They should have some mixed grain, such as oats, corn, and wheat, daily. During the laying season they should have a higher protein laying mash, where as under range conditions they get along on 18 percent protein. Breeders should never be allowed to get excessively fat. Although ducks and geese like water when they eat, the feed should not be placed near a stream or pond in the yard, as the area will soon become foul. Place waterers on higher ground. Oyster shell is necessary at all times, fed free choice.

Goslings and Ducklings Goslings and ducklings do not need heat for as long a period as do baby chicks, but for the first week or two they should be kept warm and away from dampness and drafts. Although wild ducks and geese swim with the mother just after birth, domestic ducklings and goslings should not be allowed to swim or get wet until they have feathers. They should receive a good, high-protein starter mash. Do not ever feed the ducklings and goslings dry feed when they have empty watering dishes, then water them. If you do they will quickly drink, then die from severe impaction.

Fencing Although geese and ducks can usually be contained in a two or 2½-foot fence, it is wise to use a six-foot fence made of woven wire. This will help prevent a massacre in the event a stray dog or fox wanders by.

TURKEYS

Housing More turkeys in farm flocks are lost to dampness than any other single cause. Turkeys, especially young turkeys, cannot tolerate damp bedding or dirty pens. Raising young turkeys on wire or in pens with very dry bedding is essential. Young turkeys should not be raised where chickens or older turkeys have been within several months, due to the possibility of picking up blackhead (see **Diseases and Other Problems** later in this chapter).

Turkeys need good shelter in the winter, similar to that of chickens, except their roosts must be larger and heavier. Good roosts are made with 2 by 4s. There should be more than adequate roosting space for each bird, to prevent injuries. The turkeys should not have access to their droppings under the roost.

Turkeys do well on range conditions, with portable shelters and portable roosts. The entire pasture should be fenced with at least five-foot fencing, both to keep the turkeys contained and to keep coyotes, stray dogs, and foxes from killing them. Although some people do it, I don't recommend clipping the wings to keep them from flying over fencing. It can lead to abscesses and other problems. Slipping a cloth bag over one wing and tying the drawstring snug will prevent a rogue from flying.

Feeding Turkeys are fed the same type of ration suitable for breeding chickens, only they of course consume much more of it because of their bigger size. The feed should be clean and free from mold. Breeder turkeys should have access to good clean range for access to greens, or else have alfalfa meal or freshly cut greens placed in the yard daily. There are special turkey rations made by well-known feed companies available in many parts of the country. When making your own homegrown feeds, consult your county agent for a balanced ration using concentrates and other grains available in your area.

For the first five or six weeks of life, young turkeys require a high protein ration, up to 24 percent. This diminishes by about five percent the next six weeks, then drops to around 15 or 16 percent protein. Dried skim milk, dried buttermilk, soybean oil meal, and meat scraps are all used as concentrates in turkey rations. Turkeys must have a constant supply of water, especially in the hot summer when more water is needed. A small flock of turkeys can drink a surprising amount of water in a day, so be sure to check their waterers often.

Breeding Only one male is needed for the average-sized farm flock of hens, as one male can breed ten to 15 hens. More males will only cause fighting at breeding time and possible injury. The male selected should be as close as possible to the ideal turkey you would like. When using a large male, it is a good idea to clip the sharp toenails or to protect the hens with canvas saddles. Many females are injured badly from being clawed by the males during breeding. These injuries become infected and many hens are lost this way.

Turkey eggs can be hatched by the hen herself, by a setting hen, or by an incubator. The eggs held for incubation should be kept at a temperature between 55°F. and 60°F. and can be held for as long as four to 4½ weeks, although two weeks is more reliable. Careful handling and storage (small end down in carton) keep maximum hatchability.

Turkey eggs take four weeks to hatch, and the best temperatures in the incubator during these four weeks have proven to be 100.5°F., 101.5°F., 102.5°F., and 103°F., respectively. These temperatures should be accurate and be checked several times daily for best results. The humidity should be 60 percent until the last four days before hatching. It should be raised slightly at that time. The incubator must be kept well ventilated. The eggs should be turned at least twice daily until the twenty-fourth day.

When you let a hen or hen turkey incubate the eggs, she should be left alone except for the time it takes to feed and water her. The hen should be confined in a pen and nest box until the poults are able to follow her steadily. (The chicken hen can hatch about 12 poults and the turkey hen about 20.)

Poults are a little dense at first about learning to eat. If there is no litter in the brooder, but a thick layer of newspaper and some chick starter crumbles sprinkled on the floor, they will usually begin to peck at the food. When they are eating well, you can graduate them to chick feeders. Sometimes placing a few young chicks with the poults will encourage the poults to eat, because they will attempt to mimic the chicks.

Diseases and Other Problems

ASCARIDS OR LARGE ROUNDWORMS

Ascarids are a common poultry parasite. They are most injurious to young birds due to their size and lack of resistance. They cause unthriftiness, anemia, and droopiness. Ascarids infect a bird when it eats soil or feed contaminated by worm eggs or contaminated fecal material.

Using yard rotation, spading up the empty yard and allowing several weeks' rest, keeping young birds separate from older birds, and good sanitation go a long way toward ascarid control. Worming with piperazine is effective for treatment of ascarid infestations. It is often a good idea to repeat the worming two weeks after the first treatment to insure the best possible results.

AVIAN LEUKOSIS COMPLEX

Avian leukosis is most often seen in three categories: neural (affecting the nerves), ocular (affecting the eye), and visceral (affecting the liver, kidneys, or other body organs). A bird affected can show one type, a combination of any two, or all three. It is a common problem in both large and small operations.

The bird with neural leukosis will show paralysis of the leg, neck, or wing. It can be one or both legs or wings. A bird affected in both legs will often assume a squatting position.

When one leg is affected, it will be either stretched backward or forward. If the neck is affected, the head will hang or twist to one side.

Ocular leukosis may be suspected in birds with bluish clouding or speckling of the iris and irregularities of the pupil.

Visceral leukosis may give indefinite symptoms and be difficult to diagnose unless the presence of ocular or neural leukosis accompanies it. The comb may shrivel or appear blue, and the bird may have a loss of appetite, diarrhea, and weight loss. Enlargement of the liver may be felt. On autopsy, there will often be an enlarged liver, enlarged kidneys, and hundreds of tiny, hard, pearllike tumors in the intestines.

There is no treatment.

BLACKHEAD

Although blackhead most often attacks turkeys, it can be found in chickens, also. It is caused by a protozoa which is carried by the cecal worm, which infests chickens and turkeys. Blackhead organisms can be passed directly from an infected bird by means of its droppings to a healthy bird, thus infecting it; or the organism can become encased in the egg of the cecal worm in the chicken or turkey and be passed out this way. The organism may live for several months like this, contaminating the soil for a long period of time. Poults from hatching to 12 weeks of age are most susceptible to blackhead, but older birds can become affected by it.

It is a good idea to raise poults on wire or in sanitary pens, and not let older birds or chickens have any contact with them. When older, the young turkeys should be moved often from one pasture or range to another, to avoid contamination.

Birds affected with blackhead will show droopiness, sulfur-colored diarrhea, and weight loss. There are several drugs for treatment of blackhead, available through your veterinarian or poultry supply house. Worming with phenothiazine will remove the cecal worm (the carrier), but not the organism itself. If blackhead is a problem in your area, phenothiazine mixed at low levels with the feed, or tobacco dust mixed with the feed, will often help keep the cecal worm from becoming established.

BLUE COMB

Blue comb occurs in chickens and turkeys. It is not known just what causes it, but some believe it to be a virus. Stress factors, such as hot weather, inadequate water supply, lack of shade, or a change in feed, seem to predispose a flock to the disease. Affected birds will often have a watery or pasty diarrhea, weight loss, blue comb due to cyanosis, and will be depressed. The disease may last from two weeks to a longer period in the subacute form.

Treatment consists of mixing molasses with the drinking water or mixing higher percentages of it in a wet mash. Water medicated with a broad-spectrum antibiotic such as oxytetracycline seems to work in many cases.

CANNIBALISM

Cannibalism most often occurs in young chicks that are overcrowded and bored. It often starts with toenail picking. When the toe becomes bloody, the chicks will begin to savagely attack the area, and often the injured chick will do nothing to discourage them. The sight and taste of blood will start the chicks picking at one another.

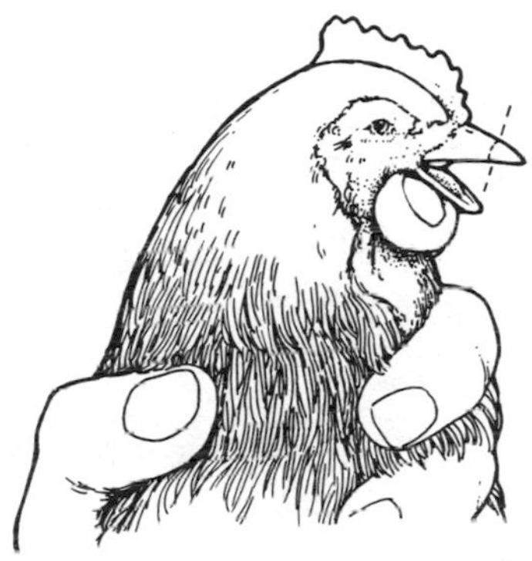

Using a dog toenail clipper, cut off one third of the beak while pushing tongue back with the point of the index finger placed in the center of lower beak

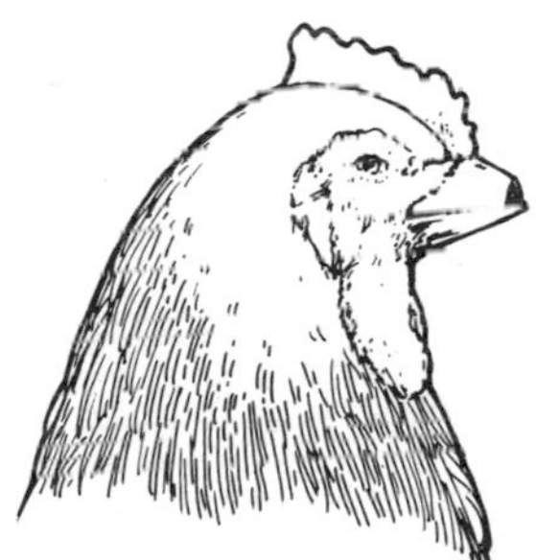

Cauterize cut end to stop bleeding

Debeaking Chickens

Moving the chicks to less crowded quarters, making sure they have a well-balanced ration, and giving them a chunk of sod or handful of grass to pick on will often help. Any injured chicks must be removed, and any that have spots of blood spattered on them should be cleaned thoroughly.

Debeaking the chicks will usually offer a permanent solution. To debeak a chick, a dog and cat toenail clipper works well. The tongue is pressed back by using a finger under the lower beak. Then the top beak is trimmed back, leaving two-thirds. Any bleeding can be controlled by cauterizing the area or by using a styptic pencil. Some people have found that pine tar, applied to the wound area as soon as bleeding is noticed, has also controlled the problem.

CECAL WORMS

Cecal worms infest the ceca of poultry, causing inflammation of the cecum and unthriftiness. The cecal worm also is the host to the protozoa which causes blackhead in chickens and turkeys.

Good sanitation, rotation and spading of yards, and keeping older birds separate from chicks will usually prevent any severe infection. Phenothiazine mixed with the feed is an effective wormer for the cecal worm.

COCCIDIOSIS

Coccidiosis is caused by a one-celled animal which is a parasite. It attacks the intestines, causing diarrhea, unthriftiness, and death. Damp, unclean quarters and mixing different aged chickens or poultry encourage the start of coccidiosis. Although coccidiosis is most often seen in chickens, it can affect all poultry.

Prevention consists of good husbandry practices and not mixing young birds with older ones. Sometimes treatment with intestinal sulfas, such as sulfaquinoxaline and sulfamethazine, is given routinely as a preventive, before trouble is noticed.

Any treatment, to be successful, must be started on the birds before they are in bad condition, before there is too much damage for anything to help. Moving the infected flock to a very warm, dry, well-lighted coop and beginning treatment with an intestinal sulfa will often work. Some coccidia have become resistant to these drugs, and more than one drug may have to be tried before results are seen. Consult your veterinarian for advice and positive diagnosis, through a fecal examination.

FOWL CHOLERA

Fowl cholera is often a fast-hitting, high-mortality disease. Many times, the first sign of trouble is dead birds. Fowl cholera should be the first disease suspected in waterfowl. Bluish combs and wattles, a fever, increased water intake, difficult breathing, head drawn back, drowsiness, and emaciation all are indicative of the disease. It may become chronic, remaining hidden in the flock, until it becomes acute in a few birds, killing them suddenly. In chronic cases there is often lameness or swollen joints, caused by the bacteria invading and settling in the joints. Positive diagnosis is made on autopsy, by culturing and finding *Pasteurella avicida.*

Cleanliness, good feeding practices, removal of any infected birds, and keeping infected flocks strictly isolated will help control the disease, and vaccination will prevent it.

FOWL TYPHOID

Fowl typhoid is caused by *Salmonella gallinarum.* It is spread by clean birds coming in contact with contaminated droppings, soil, litter, or feeding and watering utensils. It can be brought to the farm on the feet of people or animals. Wild birds can also spread the disease. Affected birds act depressed, sit with ruffled feathers, and have a yellowish or greenish diarrhea.

By means of strict sanitation, new bedding, and removal of any affected birds or suspicious birds, the disease can usually be controlled. A pullorum test will also show carriers of fowl typhoid.

GAPEWORMS

Symptoms of gapeworms are sneezing, coughing, stretching the neck out or yawning, loss of appetite, and dullness.

Chicks and young birds are most often infected when they swallow contaminated soil, litter, or feed. The young worms migrate to the lungs within a week, then move into the trachea and become imbedded. Here they cause trouble, blocking the trachea and inhibiting breathing and eating to some extent.

Feeding .1 percent thiabendazole in the feed for a period of two weeks will usually eliminate the parasites. Control of snails and slugs with an insecticide will often aid in controlling gapeworm. Not allowing young poultry onto their yard until the dew is off and the earthworms have returned to their burrows will also help, because earthworms can make the gapeworm infestation more severe, as the larvae pass through the earthworm's body.

LICE

There are over 40 species of lice that can be found on poultry. They are small grayish parasites, causing extreme discomfort to the infested bird. The lice feed on bits of feathers, skin, and blood. When severe they can cause death, especially in young birds. Lice are generally more of a problem in the winter months, but they should be kept in mind year around.

Dusting with an effective louse powder such as rotenone weekly for three weeks usually gives effective control. When treating the birds, it is well to remember the house and roosts the birds use. It is a good idea to remove the birds and spray or fumigate the entire house, paying special attention to roosts and cracks where the parasites may be hiding. The building is then closed up tight for an hour. Be sure you allow adequate ventilation for an hour before returning the birds to their house.

MITES

Mites are smaller than lice. They feed on blood and live in cracks and crevices near the roosts and in the litter where they deposit their eggs. Birds bothered by mites are anemic and appear unthrifty. Wild birds as well as domesticated birds that are moved from place to place spread the mite infestation.

The litter in the poultry house should be changed frequently. No accumulation of dirty litter should be allowed to build up. The nest boxes should be sealed yearly with varnish or paint. Roosts should be treated at least twice a year with a wood preservative. Spraying them with crankcase oil also works well. Complete fumigation of the empty house, paying special attention to the cracks and crevices, and at the same time dusting the birds well with rotenone or another similar powder will pay in more productive and contented birds.

NEWCASTLE

Newcastle is caused by a virus. It is a killer of chicks and causes economic losses due to a severe drop in egg production in laying flocks. It strikes suddenly, spreads rapidly, and can affect all poultry, even backyard and other small setups. Chicks show respiratory distress such as gasping, sneezing, and coughing. This is often followed by the development of nervous disorders, such as circling, incoordination, twisting of the neck, spasms or twitching, then death. Some may recover from the respiratory condition, but will often retain the nervous affliction.

Layers will show a sudden attack of respiratory distress, which spreads very rapidly through the flock. The birds will often quit eating, suffer a drop in egg production, and begin to show nervous disorders. The eggs that are laid are often thin shelled. The disease will run its course often without mortality, and the hens will begin to lay normally in a month. Pullets are often thrown into a molt by the disease, which delays normal egg production even further.

Chickens can be vaccinated by nasal or wing web vaccination, but there is no treatment.

PULLORUM

Pullorum has been a severe problem in poultry farming. It is now more under control, as there is more testing and eradication being done by the larger commercial hatcheries. This is one good reason for buying chicks from one of the well-known hatcheries. Most of them sell "pullorum-free" chicks which are from tested flocks.

There is certainly a chance, however, of a farm flock having this disease, as few farm flocks are pullorum tested. Pullorum appears most often in young chicks from one to three weeks of age. There is diarrhea caused by the bacteria, *Samonella pullorum,* which often sticks to the vent area. The chicks huddle together and act droopy. Adult birds may not die from the disease, but the hens will quit laying well, and those eggs that are laid will not hatch properly. Pullorum can be easily tested for, and when suspecting this disease, contact your veterinarian to arrange to have the flock tested.

Once pullorum is found in your flock, the only means of stopping it is to destroy the sick birds, and retest your flock periodically. Sulfas have helped stop the death rate, but many birds may remain carriers.

TUBERCULOSIS

Avian tuberculosis is most often seen in chickens and turkeys, but it has been found in ducks and geese as well. Avian tuberculosis is transmissible to swine and can cause reaction to a bovine TB test, although the cow does not show lesions. Poultry should not be allowed the run of the farm for this reason and should not be kept in the same pen with swine or cattle.

Tuberculosis occurs mainly in older poultry, which is the primary reason for not keeping older birds for several years. Affected birds show a weight loss and unthriftiness, or may show no signs at all until slaughtered and then examined.

Culling chickens over a year old, not allowing farm flocks to range free, and culling any suspicious birds will usually keep tuberculosis from becoming a problem.

WORMS

There are over 50 intestinal parasites affecting poultry. If you suspect that your flock is having trouble with worms, take one bird and a fecal sample to your veterinarian for examination. Many of these parasites can be easily and effectively treated, at little expense. There is no reason to take the economic loss that wormy birds cause. For specific worms see "Ascarids," "Cecal Worms," and "Gapeworms," elsewhere in this section.

RABBITS

General Care and Management

HOUSING

Rabbits are best kept in individual pens, cages, or hutches. When kept outdoors in hutches they should have shade, which can be provided by a tree, sunshade, or trellis covered by vines like squash, melons, and morning glories.

The medium-sized breeds should have a hutch at least 2½ feet by four feet, and the larger breeds a hutch three feet by six feet. In northern areas, where the winters are quite cold, the sides and back of the hutch should be solid and draft-free. Where temperatures drop below zero and winds blow, in winter it is a good idea to either move the hutches into a barn or shed, or to move them on the south side of a building for shelter, and to provide removable panels on or canvas flaps to completely shut out the blowing wind and snow. The bottom of the hutch should be made of hardware cloth, with the bottom of the nest box solid for protection from drafts and

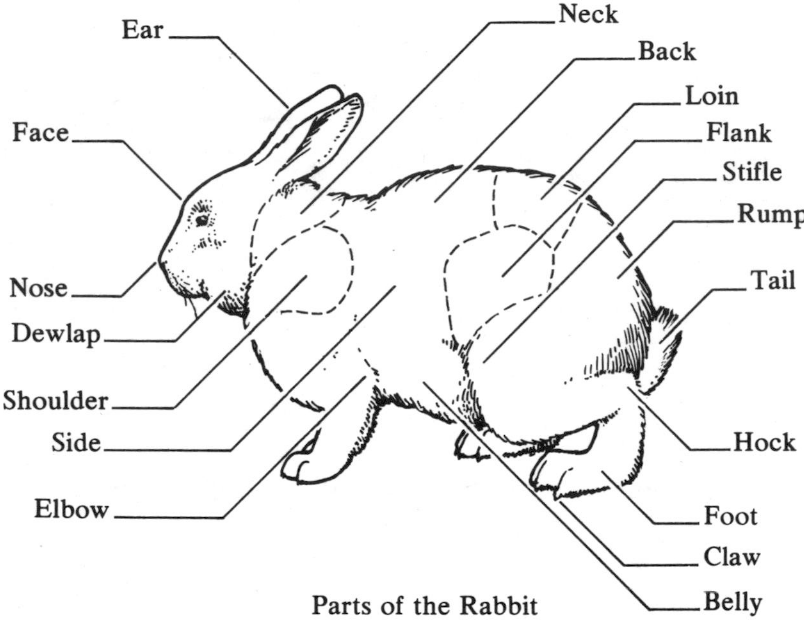

Parts of the Rabbit

winter wind. Bedding can be straw, hay, or wood shaving.

Larger rabbitries use all-wire cages to an advantage. Wooden hutches, or wooden hutches with 1-x-2-inch galvanized wire fronts (don't use poultry netting, as the rabbits chew it and attacking animals can get through it easily), are hard to keep clean and fresh smelling.

When planning to raise more than a few rabbits, it is best to visit with several rabbit breeders in your area and inspect their cages and facilities. They will usually be glad to tell you what they wish they had done differently, as well as the features they like best.

FEEDING

In most places, rabbit pellets, available through feed dealers, constitute the major portion of a rabbit diet. Rabbits can make use of other feeds, but the pellets should be used if possible, as they provide a balanced diet with all the nutrients needed. When using other feeds, especially green feeds, including garden vegetables and weeds, it is best to introduce each new feed slowly. A too sudden change in the diet can cause digestive troubles and illness. Rabbits enjoy a rack or manger filled with fresh hay. This should be kept full and not be allowed to become moldy or stale. Grains such as rolled oats, cracked corn, or wheat can be fed, but only in very small amounts until the rabbit is used to it. Garden waste such as crooked carrots, wilted lettuce, potato peelings, sunflower leaves, or beet tops all can be fed, but in limited amounts. Cabbage often causes digestive upsets, so it is best not to feed it to rabbits. Young rabbits especially are bothered by digestive problems, due to feed changes, so be particularly careful how and what you feed them.

A salt spool or block is a necessity and should be kept before the rabbits at all times, as should a supply of fresh, clean water. Automatic waterers, whether home-made or bought, are the best, as they never allow foul water in the hutch. Heavy crockery dishes are often used, but are easily contaminated by dirt and fecal material.

Rabbits, if possible, will consume a portion of their night feces. This is *not* a symptom of a nutritional deficiency but a natural occurrence, as they obtain vitamin B in this way. If they are raised on wire and don't have access to their droppings, the rabbits must have vitamin B complex supplement in their pellets.

RESTRAINT

People today are getting away from the idea that rabbits should be picked up and carried by the ears. This is a good

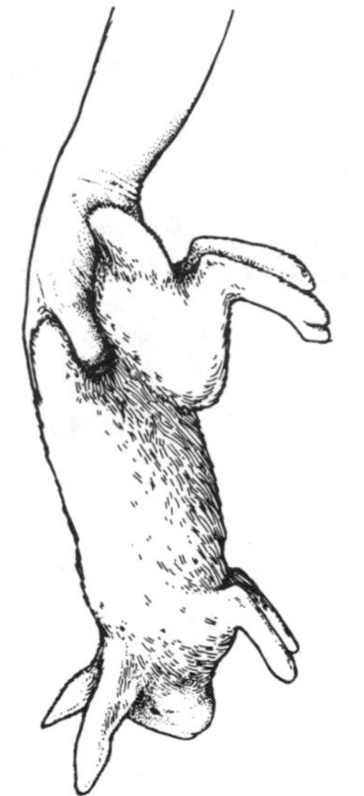

Fryers are grasped firmly over loins.

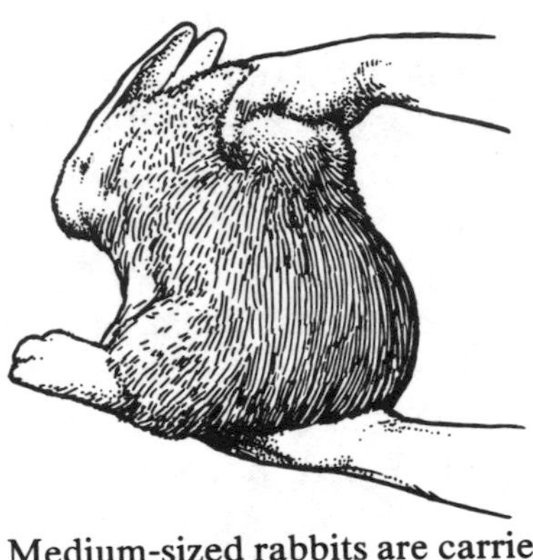

Medium-sized rabbits are carried by a good handful of neck skin and supported by a hand under the hindquarters.

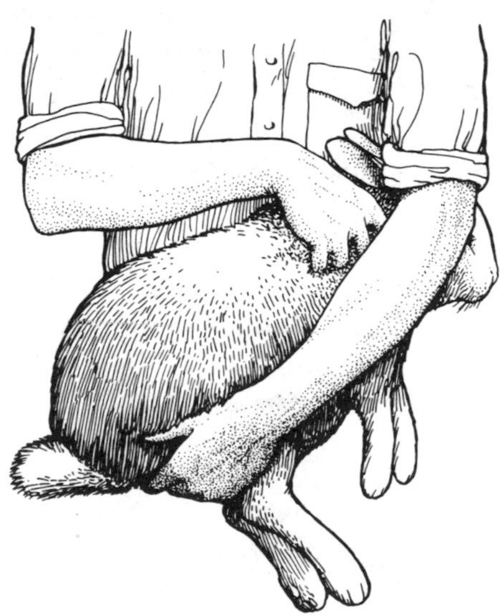

Large and giant breeds are carried by grasping neck skin fold and supported by the other arm.

thing, as handling them this way often injures them. Small rabbits are most easily carried by grasping them firmly over the loins and picking them up. Do not let go if they should struggle briefly; you can injure them if you drop them suddenly.

Larger rabbits are easiest picked up by grasping the skin above the shoulders with one hand and supporting the hind end with the other hand. Do not pick up a rabbit as you would a small dog, by lifting it under the front legs. They will often respond by kicking and scratching with their hind legs. And a rabbit can inflict some painful scratches this way!

BREEDING

Rabbits should not be bred until they reach their adult size. If the breed of rabbit you raise has an adult weight of ten pounds, you should wait until the doe reaches that size before breeding her. A few weeks is not too long to wait, when considering the extra quality you will be putting onto your doe. The doe that is bred too early will never grow to her full potential.

A doe can be bred from the age of five months (small breeds) to nine or ten months (large breeds). She should be housed fairly close to the buck's pen. When in heat, she will thump her feet, grunt, and rub her chin on her food dish, the waterer, and the edge of the hutch. When she shows these signs that she's ready to breed, put her into the buck's pen. If the reverse is done, there can be fighting, resulting in injury to the buck.

When a successful breeding has been accomplished, don't be surprised or alarmed when the buck suddenly falls backward or to the side during the breeding. This is natural, and the buck is not harmed. No more than three does should be bred to one buck in a week's time, or his fertility may become impaired.

The gestation period for a doe is about 31 days. She should be provided with an adequate nest box well in advance of her due date. Changing her nest box or moving her to another hutch shortly before kindling can cause her to reject or even eat her babies. There is no *one* cause of cannibalism in rabbits, but certainly a nervous doe will be more apt to eat her young. It is believed that cannibalism is often a warped desire to protect the young. It can be caused by a vitamin or mineral deficiency and possibly heredity sometimes can be a factor. Should the doe *not* be disturbed, and eat her young more than once, she should be culled. Some does refuse to stop this habit, once having done it.

Once in awhile a neighboring rabbit may make a doe about to kindle nervous. Bucks stamping or another doe grunting may be sufficient to cause cannibalism, as will visits to the rabbitry by a skunk, cat or dog.

The doe should be provided with nest building material, which she will add to by pulling hair from her belly to use as a lining for the nest. If the rabbits are in an area that is below freezing in the winter and the does are bred for winter litters, it will be necessary to make sure the nest boxes are very snug. Placing the nest boxes on a layer of sawdust, sandwiched between two heavy layers of cardboard and using double thickness walls for it will help cut down drafts and chill. Plenty of nesting material, such as clean straw or even cotton, will help keep the babies warm. Then tack a flap of canvas over the entrance of the box to keep in body warmth. One word of caution here: don't make it *too* warm or you will lose litters due to a damp nest box.

She will usually make her nest three or four days before kindling. Do not bother her during this time or while she is having the young. Do not disturb the nest soon after she kindles. Any such disturbance could be disastrous to the young.

Some strains of rabbits have periodic problems with kindling. Very often an injection of posterior pituitary will cause sufficient uterine contractions to allow natural birth.

The nest box can be carefully checked to be sure there are no dead babies or the litter is not too large for the doe to handle. A doe with over seven or eight young may have trouble feeding them all, and it may be necessary to cull the litter or farm some of the young out to another doe with a smaller litter. (Rubbing the doe's nose and the babies with Vicks will usually facilitate the adoption, as she will not be able to tell the scent of her own young from that of the new babies.)

Quietly check the nest after distracting the doe out of the nest by some feed, remove any dead babies, then *leave the nest alone.*

Orphan Bunnies Occasionally a doe will die, leaving you with no foster mother available. (Be sure to ask your rabbit-raising friends to see if perhaps they might have a doe that has just kindled.) If no foster mother is available you are left with two choices: to raise the litter on a bottle or to kill the young. Killing them is much easier, but, then you will not have the rewards later, having had the experience of successfully raising a nice litter on a bottle.

Young rabbits must receive a small amount (one to two cc.) of milk *every* two hours for at least the first week. This means day *and* night. They have sensitive digestive systems, and too much milk gulped down at one time will kill them. A doll bottle with a small rubber nipple is the best. An eye dropper is not good, as it gives too much milk at a time, choking the rabbits, and getting milk into the lungs, causing inhalation pneumonia.

Goat milk or regular baby formula, readily available at any grocery or drug store, will be fine for new rabbits, if the care and amount is correct.

The young must be kept warm. This is accomplished by using a small box resting on a heating pad, kept at a temperature that is just warm and cozy in the box. Feel with your own hand. A towel over the box will prevent drafts.

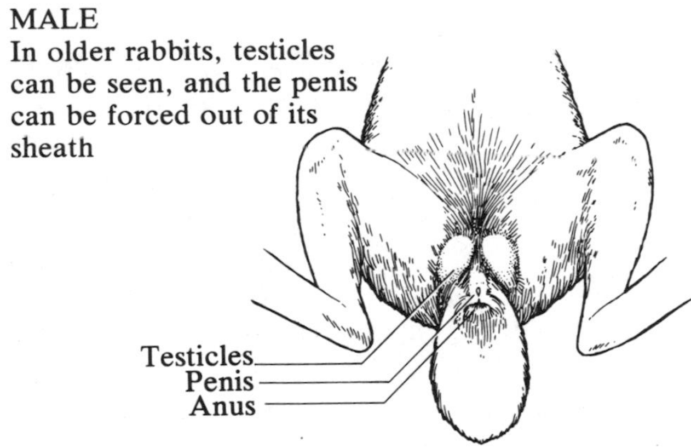

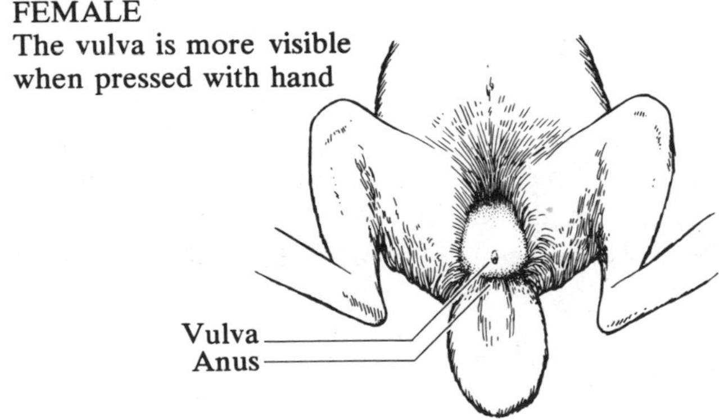

After the first week, gradually increase the amount of milk they receive until they are weaned. As soon as their eyes are opened, they will begin to nibble on pellets and soft grains. Placing a good quality green hay in with them will encourage eating solids. Giving a good vitamin-mineral supplement in the milk, and later in the water, will keep the young growing as well as their brothers and sisters who were raised by a doe.

Be sure each bunny urinates and defecates after eating. If it does not, massage the genital area with a moist warm cloth to stimulate action. When not done, the young may become constipated and die.

Diseases and Other Problems

ABSCESSES

Abscesses are often caused by *Pasteurella* (see Snuffles), although they may be caused by other organisms. These infections are often brought about by injuries such as wire tears, fighting wounds, and cuts on sharp objects in the hutch. Although an attempt can be made to treat such a rabbit, the treatment often costs more than a replacement rabbit, and it is uncertain. Use of a broad-spectrum antibiotic such as pen-strep or oxytetracycline sometimes is valuable. Applying heat to the abscess to encourage it to come to a head in order to be lanced may help. Keep in mind the contagious aspects of a *Pasteurella* abscess, and keep the rabbit isolated, wear rubber gloves, and destroy any contaminated materials used. In many cases, there is additional infection other places in the body.

COCCIDIOSIS

Liver coccidiosis and intestinal coccidiosis are both found in rabbits. Weight loss, unthriftiness, diarrhea, and weakness are all symptoms. Coccidia, which cause coccidiosis, are protozoa and are parasites of birds and animals. Animals living in poor sanitary conditions or under stress are most vulnerable. Rabbits coming in contact with oocysts, through the natural process of eating the night feces, will show signs of illness in about 30 days, depending on the amount of oocysts ingested.

Improved sanitation, moving the rabbits to wire bottom cages which give them no chance of reinfecting themselves, plus treatment with intestinal sulfas such as sulfaquinoxaline will usually clear up all but severe cases.

CONJUNCTIVITIS OR WEEPY EYE

Rabbits raised in dusty quarters, or in pens where sawdust is used regularly, are especially prone to eye irritations and infections. This is due to irritating foreign material scratching the eye or the conjunctiva. Affected rabbits will rub their eyes with their front feet and have mattered or runny eyes. Conjunctivitis can usually be stopped with a good ophthalmic ointment, especially one containing an anesthetic to cut down the itching and burning, which encourages rubbing and further irritation.

EAR MITES

With a severe ear mite infestation, the rabbit will shake its head, flopping its ears. It will scratch its ears and the backs of its ears until large scratches appear. Inside the ear there is usually a brownish, foul-smelling discharge. When secondary infections such as a fungus or bacteria attack of the irritated area get started, the infection can quickly move into the inner ear, damaging the central nervous system. Here, the rabbit may have a twisted neck or hold its head to one side, being unable to turn it to a normal position.

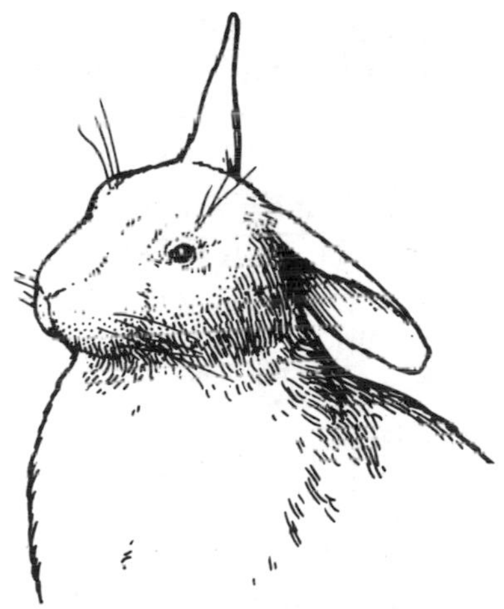

The attitude of a rabbit with ear mites with its affected ear flopped.

At the first signs of ear scratching, the rabbit should receive treatment. The brownish discharge should be cleaned away with a ball of cotton soaked in alcohol or peroxide. The ear should then be dried, and drops such as those used for cats are applied. The base of the ear should then be massaged to allow maximum coverage inside the ear, and the excess wiped off. It is a good idea to completely clean the pen and dust the rabbit with an insecticide such as rotenone.

HUTCH BURN

Rabbits kept in wooden hutches sometimes have hutch burn. This condition is caused by exposure to urine in a wet, unclean hutch. The irritated vent and genitals will be red, chapped looking, and may have brownish crusts over the area. Proper sanitation, along with the application of a bland ointment (like petroleum jelly) will hasten recovery. In some instances a bacterial infection will follow the initial irritation. In this case, systemic or topical treatment with an antibiotic is recommended.

Sometimes the infection will be spread to the nose. The same type of lesions are found on the nose as on the vent, giving the name "scab nose" to the condition. When the infection spreads to the nose there is usually a bacterial invader, so systemic treatment with an antibiotic is recommended.

IMPACTION

This condition is most often due to improper feeding. Feeding a diet lacking in roughages will predispose a rabbit to the problem. Chewing on the wood in a hutch, eating hair, or in angoras, wool, will also cause impaction. Extremely small, scanty, hard droppings are often the first sign of trouble. If not treated, the rabbit will be in pain, lying kicking on its side or stretching the hind legs out as if feeling cramps.

Mineral oil (two to eight cc.) given three times daily will often help pass the impacted fecal material or hair ball. Occasionally an enema will bring relief, but this should be tried only as a last resort, as it can produce cramps and added stress to an already stressed rabbit.

The unaffected rabbits should be given good quality hay free choice.

LICE

Although infections by lice and mange mites are rather uncommon in rabbits, those parasites should not be forgotten. Lice most often attack rabbits in hutches, especially during the winter. They can get quite a start before the rabbit gives warning of their presence by beginning to scratch. They can make the rabbit anemic and cause death. Dusting with a good louse powder is very effective in controlling lice.

MANGE

Mange is a serious problem when it occurs in rabbits, as it is so rapidly spread and difficult to treat successfully. Unless the rabbit is very valuable, it is often wisest to cull it rather than have it in the rabbitry as a potential source of infection for the other rabbits.

See your veterinarian when suspecting mange. All mange-like lesions are not mange; some bald, red spots are caused by a bacterial infection, fungal infection, or allergy. A skin scraping is the only means of positive diagnosis.

When treating mange, it is best to clip all the hair off the rabbit, as it is hard to effectively treat mange mites with matted down hair which protects them from the insecticide.

MASTITIS

Mastitis is inflammation of the mammary gland or glands. It is caused by a bacterial infection. Stress, such as a doe banging her breasts getting in and out of the nest box or scraping them on rough cage bottoms, will often cause a flare-up of mastitis just following kindling, when there is added stress on the udder due to increases in milk production. An affected doe will act listless, have hot, swollen, red mammary glands. She may run a fever.

Treating the affected doe immediately with a broad-spectrum antibiotic such as penicillin-streptomycin will usually bring about quick recovery. Sometimes the young are affected due to the severe changes in the acidity of the milk and presence of so many bacteria in it, so it is wise to remove the young, feeding them by bottle until the doe is back to normal. (See "Orphan Bunnies," earlier in this chapter.)

Check each doe daily at feeding time for any sign of abnormal breasts. Quickly finding you have trouble and treating it will save many does' productivity and many young rabbits.

MUCOID ENTERITIS

Mucoid enteritis is a frustrating disease in young rabbits from ages five to seven weeks of age. Although older rabbits can become affected, they do not often die because of it. The affected rabbits will sit humped up, act as if in pain, grinding their teeth, drooping their ears, and closing their eyes. They will often pass mucus in their droppings. There may be constipation or diarrhea.

It is not known what causes it, and there is no real cure. Feeding young rabbits medicated pellets may help in some cases. Good sanitation and husbandry may go a long way toward preventing stress, which is thought to be a factor in the disease. Treating the symptoms (i.e., antidiarrheals for the diarrhea or mineral oil for the constipation) and injecting broad-spectrum antibiotics, plus isolating affected rabbits, may help.

PNEUMONIA

Pneumonia is quite frequent in rabbits. It often follows a period of severe stress such as overcrowding, overheating, feed changes, or cold snaps. It also follows some diseases as a secondary infection. Affected rabbits will puff, show a temperature, often of two degrees or more, go off feed, and die.

Treatment with a broad-spectrum antibiotic will work well if the infection is caught in time. If left to gain strength, too much lung tissue will have been destroyed and the rabbit cannot be saved. Steaming with a human vaporizer and Vicks will often bring relief to a rabbit with pneumonia, when used in conjunction with antibiotics.

RINGWORM

Ringworm is not a worm, nor is the condition caused by a worm. It is caused by a fungus. The disease gets its name from the round, bald or crusty areas it causes on the rabbit's skin. It can be highly contagious, causing serious economic losses due to the pelt damage and damage done to saleable breeding stock. (Also, who wants to buy a rabbit from you to eat, if all the other rabbits in the hutch look mothy and scaly?)

Immediately isolate or even destroy the infected rabbit. Never attempt treatment without wearing rubber gloves. Not only is ringworm easily spread to other rabbits, but some species of fungus isolated from rabbits are contagious to people.

If you decide to try treatment for ringworm, call your veterinarian and describe the trouble. He may wish to see the rabbit to confirm your diagnosis. There are many antifungal drugs on the market, and your veterinarian will recommend one best suited to your rabbit. When applying the drug, be sure there is no hair in or around the lesion; clip it very short. When applying the medicine, work from the outside of the area to the center, for if you work from the inner area out, the infection may be spread. Weather permitting, move the cage outdoors into a sunny area, as sunshine will often aid in getting rid of the infection. Be sure, however, that there is some shade available.

SNUFFLES (PASTEURELLOSIS)

Snuffles is a common rabbit disease, whose symptoms are like the common cold in a human. The rabbit sneezes, wheezes, and coughs. The eyes will often run. The rabbit will try to wipe its nose and eyes clean, getting nasal mucus on its front feet and legs. Snuffles is caused by *Pasteurella* and is highly contagious. It most often occurs following a period of stress. A cold, damp day followed by a hot day, kindling, feed changes, and so forth, can all bring about enough stress to allow it to gain entry.

Treatment with antibiotics sometimes works, but often the disease will break out again in animals that were sick with snuffles. Proper nutrition and protection from stress will help prevent it from getting started.

SORE HOCKS

Injured, chaffed, or bruised hocks often give way to a bacterial infection in that area. Any bald, red, scabby, or swollen hocks should have prompt attention. If they become infected and the infection is not taken care of, the rabbit can develop a bloodstream infection or bone infection, either of which can kill it. Systemic treatment with a sulfa combination or broad-spectrum antibiotic, plus treating the area with an antibiotic or sulfa ointment (if the area is dry and chapped), or powder (if the area is moist), work well in most cases.

Remedy of the condition that caused the trouble in the first place is necessary to prevent any recurrence. Damp hutches should be thoroughly scrubbed and disinfected and left empty for a day in the sun to dry out. Heavy breeds of rabbits should have more support than the wire floors often give. Slats placed across the wire, or an area with a smooth board or piece of metal to sit on, will often help the condition. Rough, splintered boards on the hutch floor will often cause sore hocks.

Thumping the hind feet, such as occurs during excitement, fear, or aggression will sometimes bruise them enough to cause trouble. The rabbits should not be excited, as by prowling dogs or cats (or even children). Bucks that stamp at each other should be separated further.

WORMS

There are many species of internal parasites that can and have infected rabbits. However, because most domestic rabbits are raised on wire and are kept in individual cages or hutches, they are seldom much of a problem.

Dogs, cats, poultry, rats, mice, and wild rabbits should be kept away from the rabbit area, as many species of worms can be transmitted from one animal to another. The most common parasite transmitted in this way is the tapeworm. Contamination of the hutches, food or water dishes, or feed contaminated by cat or dog fecal material can pass tapeworm onto the rabbits. Likewise, feeding uncooked rabbit entrails to dogs and cats can infect them with tapeworm.

Signs of worms are unthriftiness, dull fur, diarrhea, cysts, and mucus or blood in the droppings. If you suspect worms may be present in a rabbit, take the rabbit and a small sample of its droppings to your veterinarian. On microscopic examination, the presence or absence of worm eggs or minute larvae will be evident.

DOGS

General Care and Management

FEEDING

Mature dogs in good health should be fed one meal a day or have free access to dry food at all times. The average dog, given free choice, will not overeat and will stay in just the right shape, providing it gets some regular exercise.

Whether self-fed or fed once daily, dry dog food of good quality is generally the best choice. It is better for the teeth than moist food, since its abrasive quality keeps them clean. Most well-known brands of dry food are a completely balanced diet, whereas many canned foods are not. An all-meat diet is not a balanced diet for a dog. In the wild, canines not only eat the muscle meat such as found in canned dog food, but the intestines, stomach contents, and bones, as well as such things as wild fruits and grasses.

Whatever food you choose, read the list of ingredients. A lot of cheaper dog foods have a very high cereal content, with very

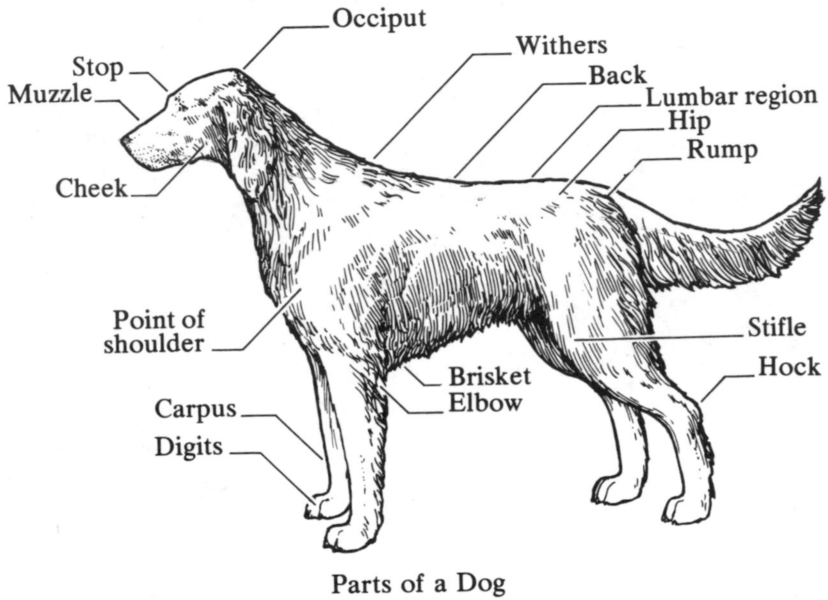

Parts of a Dog

little meat or meat by-products. If the cereal grains are listed first, chances are very high that the food is composed largely of cereal. Look elsewhere for a good food.

In addition to the dry food, the dog can have meat scraps, cooked eggs, stale bread, cottage cheese, milk, and table scraps as side dishes. It should never receive more "goodies" than dry food, however, as this is what makes a picky eater. It is like feeding a child chocolate cake, then asking him to eat his sandwich and vegetables.

The dog should receive no highly spiced, fried, or greasy foods, or foods with sharp bones such as fish, poultry, or pork chops. These all may cause digestive upsets that might lead to more serious problems. Feeding potato chips to a dog can be dangerous. Some dogs do not chew their food, and when unchewed potato chips reach the stomach, the sharp edges and points can cause so much pain that the dog can actually be thrown into convulsions. In fact, any indigestible foods can produce gas or stomach pain, which in turn can cause convulsions.

Raw meat, chopped fine or ground, can be added to dry food and mixed in well to increase consumption of the dry food. Some dogs need a bit more weight than they normally carry, for example, when under stress, and the added consumption of dry food will aid in this weight gain.

Any food not eaten during the period between feedings should be taken away. At the next feeding give a little less, until there is no food left at feeding time, but the dog is not very hungry. Never leave moist food such as dry food mixed with liquid or canned food in the dish all day. It can become sour or have high bacterial growth, and the dog may get sick should it become hungry and eat the food later.

Puppies, which have special nutritional requirements, are discussed later.

Like people, some dogs have certain foods that disagree with them and cause digestive upsets, from flatuence to diarrhea. Stay away from these foods, and find a well-balanced food that does agree with the dog. This problem is most often seen in older dogs.

DOG BEDS

No matter if your house dog sleeps on the couch or on your bed, it should have a bed or a spot of its own. Here, it can escape children, catch quick naps, and carry its bones and toys. The bed should be slightly bigger than the dog is when it's curled up. A larger bed is not as comfortable to the dog, as a dog likes to feel something around it while napping.

THE DOG HOUSE

The outside dog needs a snug dog house as protection from the elements. It should be solidly constructed, with a windbreak at the door. Except in very cold climates, it should not be insulated. Insulation sometimes allows the humidity to build up, causing condensation to form. This thoroughly chills the dog and makes it very susceptible to several illnesses.

The house should face the south and be just a bit larger than the dog is when curled up. This will let its body heat warm the house in cold weather. The roof should be flat and have a mild slope to it. Many dogs like to lie on top of their houses, but some are unable to because the owner thought a dog house ought have a peaked roof to resemble his or her own house. There should be plenty of bedding in the house in the winter, as a dog likes to curl up in a "den." Where it is unable to dig a real den, the bedding must suffice. Summer and winter, the dog must have fresh water available.

The dog house should be moved from place to place periodically. This not only keeps the area cleaner and allows the grass to regrow, but is also an aid in parasite control.

EXERCISE

The house dog should receive exercise of some type daily. A tiny dog can get exercise by chasing a ball, playing tug-of-war, or just being naturally active. A larger dog should either be turned to run in a fenced yard or taken for a walk. A dog that receives insufficient exercise is apt to become fat, develop more physical defects, and may even become neurotic. Letting a dog roam at will is not a good idea. Not only is it dangerous for the dog, but can cause trouble for you as well. An unsupervised dog is like an unsupervised child: it can get into too much trouble without half trying!

The dog that is tied or kept in a run should have regular periods of free time or exercise out of confinement. Whether it is work, such as training a hunting dog or herding stock, or just a good run in the woods, the dog will appreciate it and will not become bored. A bored dog is often a barking dog.

RESTRAINT

A dog kept outside, such as a farm dog or hunting dog, also may need special attention. Unless you live in an isolated area, they must be kept restrained by means of a run or chain, when unsupervised. Even farm dogs must be restrained, unless thoroughly trained to stay at home. Hundreds of deer and other animals, including sheep, are killed by someone's nice farm dog out "having fun." The dog does not have to be kept shut up all the time, just when there is no one around to keep an eye on it.

If you're building a dog house with a closed in run for a large dog, it should be built with a chain link or welded wire fence at least four by 12 feet in size, and six feet high. If the dog is a jumper, a top may have to be added. The easiest cleaned flooring material for the run is cement, which is also the easiest to keep parasite-free. Pea gravel or crushed rock are often used. This is better on the dog's feet than the cement, but a bit harder to keep clean. The house should be placed on the end of the run, with a hole cut in the fence for the doorway. If the house is placed in the run, the dog will use it as a jumping point, to jump out of the fence.

If the dog must be chained up, use a chain heavy enough so that it will not break when the dog gets excited. Many dogs have been hung, dragging a length of chain in the woods. The chain should be ten to 15 feet long. Strong dogs such as huskies, should have shorter chains, because when excited, they may get a foot or even their head in a loop of chain, then may run off, barking at something, and break a leg or even choke themselves. A dog that hits the end of its chain may have trouble with hematomas (large bruises) or other injuries. This may be stopped in some cases by fastening the end of the chain to an old innertube. This has enough "give" so that injuries are often prevented.

BREEDING

A female dog will come into heat roughly every six months. Smaller breeds usually begin coming into heat at six months of age, with larger breeds coming into their first heat at between eight and 12 months. It is not advisable to breed the bitch on her first heat, as she is still a puppy herself and will not be able to handle the nutritional requirements of her unborn puppies and the nutrients necessary for her growth at the same time. Thus, she may never reach the size and conformation she would have attained, had her owner waited until at least her second heat period to breed her.

The male should be chosen and arrangements made with the owner well in advance of the date the bitch is due to come into heat. The male should not be chosen on just bloodlines or looks alone, but also for temperament. The most beautiful dog in the world is of no use if it is neurotic or mean.

Special care should be taken to avoid genetic or hereditary problems. Most breeds of dogs have an undesirable characteristic that dedicated breeders are trying to weed out, for instance, deafness in dalmatians and hip dysplasia in German shepherds. A dog having any hereditary defect or having parents with these defects should never be bred, as there is too much of a chance that the puppies will pick them up.

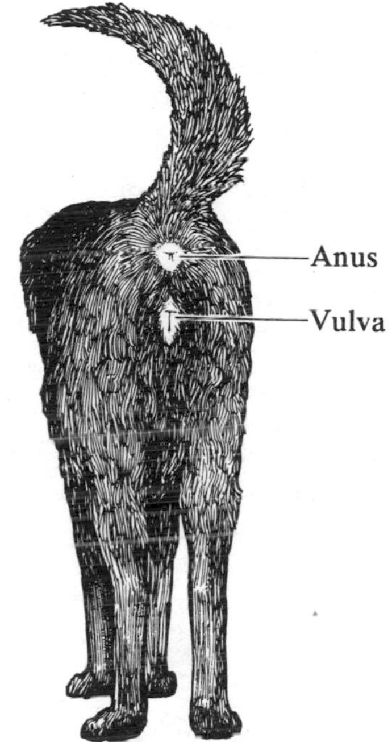

Sexing a Female Dog

Never breed a dog unless you have the time, space, and money necessary to raise the puppies until you can find homes for them. It is no solution to say, "I'll just sell the extra ones to a pet shop." There is a high percentage of pet shop puppies that never live to reach adulthood.

The bitch should be worm-free, in good physical condition (neither too fat nor too thin), free from both fleas and skin diseases, and free of any uterine or vaginal infections. The bitch will be in heat for three weeks, but will generally only accept the male from the tenth to the fourteenth day. She should be taken to the male early so that she can become accustomed to him and his surroundings. A frightened bitch may not accept the male and may even injure him.

After a successful breeding, resulting in a tie, the female can usually be taken home. Do not allow any other males near her, as a bitch can have at the same time puppies from two different males. This can be a disaster with a purebred bitch. After all, who will pay a good price for a registered Collie pup, when two of the litter mates have long, black, curly hair like the poodle next door?

The bitch will have her puppies after a gestation period of from 58 to 62 days. As the pups grow larger, she will begin to develop a ravenous appetite, and she will often eat twice what she ate before. She will need this food and also an extra protein source such as lean meat, cooked liver, or hardboiled eggs. She should receive adequate exercise. A too fat, too soft bitch will often have whelping trouble. She should not, however, have rough exercise, as it could cause abortion.

WHELPING

The bitch should be given her whelping box a week before she is due, in order for her to get used to it. Some bitches will insist upon having the pups in a closet, in the barn, or on your bed anyway, but you can try to persuade her to use the box you provide for her. The box should be in a warm, hidden location where she will not be bothered. The sides should be high enough to prevent draft and to keep the puppies in the nest. They should also be low enough so that she can escape the pups to take exercise and take care of her own needs.

You can be sure of when the bitch will have her pups by taking her temperature. It will drop from a normal one of 101°F. or 102°F. down to 100°F. or 99°F. When it falls below 99°F., she will whelp within 12 hours. When beginning labor, she will pant, dig, and push her nest material around and act restless. If she does not produce a puppy within three hours, consult your veterinarian.

Most bitches will, unaided, have their pups and take care of them. But it does pay to keep watch on her from a distance, to make sure all is well. Should a pup be born and still remain in the sac, you should break the sac and rub the pup dry with a clean towel. If this is not done, the pup may drown in the fluid.

If the bitch goes longer than half an hour to 45 minutes between pups, take her out and force her to take some mild exercise. If she does not produce another pup within half an hour after being returned to the whelping box, call your veterinarian. She may have an obstruction, or her uterus may be tired and require an injection of posterior pituitary to get things started again.

After whelping, she will have a normal discharge for several days or a week. This is most often bloody and dark and is nothing to worry about. Should it become foul smelling or look yellowish, call your veterinarian. Unless the bitch has a very large litter, she should be allowed to eat the placentas. Eating too many can cause digestive upsets and diarrhea, but eating them stimulates uterine contractions and helps to let the milk down. Should the bitch appear not to have milk, call your veterinarian. If given an injection right away, she may be forced to let her milk down. Such an injection will not, however, produce milk in a bitch that does not have milk in the first place. The bitch should be allowed free choice dry dog food during the nursing period, as this way she can more easily keep up with the terrific drain on her body that nursing a litter of pups causes. In addition, she should receive a good vitamin-mineral supplement. (See "Eclampsia" and "Metritis" in **Diseases and Other Problems**, later in this chapter.)

The Puppies The puppies will open their eyes at about two weeks, and soon after that time they can begin to be introduced to semisolid foods. At three weeks, most puppies will lick a bit of cooked, ground liver from your fingers. Then, at four weeks, you can usually put a shallow pan of baby cereal mixed with cooked liver and milk in with the pups. They will get most of it on them instead of in them the first few times fed this way, but will soon learn to lap up the gruel with relish. Don't get the food too thin, or they may get some of the fluid into their lungs.

At eight weeks, the pups will be eating considerable amounts of food and can slowly be switched to dry food fed free choice. The pups should receive an additional calcium-vitamin D supplement for proper bone growth and the prevention of rickets. If not fed free choice, the pups should be fed four times daily at eight weeks of age, three times daily at three to four months, and two times daily until nine months.

At eight weeks, they should be given their first adult distemper-hepatitis-leptospirosis vaccination and also be checked for worms. Ninety percent of puppies do have some type of worms, and it is a good idea, even if the bitch was wormed, to have the puppies checked before they go to their new homes. (See "Distemper," "Roundworms," "Hookworms," and "Tapeworms" in **Diseases and Other Problems**, later in this chapter.)

Orphan and Hand-Raised Puppies Sometimes it becomes necessary to raise a litter of puppies by hand. A bitch with mastitis, no milk, a too-large litter, or a bitch that dies may leave you with that tiring, but rewarding job.

The puppies must be fed small amounts every two hours, day and night. This has to continue for at least one week. After the week, you may drop to every three hours during the night. These amounts are about right for the average pup. Adjust as necessary by looks and feel of the pups:

Large breeds (50–75 pounds, adult dog): two to four cc. milk

Medium breeds (25–50 pounds): two to three cc.

Small breeds (10–25 pounds): one to two cc.
Feed above amounts to start with, getting pups adjusted to goat's milk or baby formula. There are puppy formulas on the market, but in some areas they are hard to get fast. After two or three days, increase the milk gradually until it is doubled in quantity. Keep increasing as the pups grow and require more food. Do not overfeed, as this will cause digestive upsets and possibly death.

The easiest way to feed pups is by the feeding tube. This is a flexible rubber tube which fits on the end of a syringe. The milk is drawn up into the syringe, where it is measured. The tube is then slowly pushed down the pup's throat. As the tube goes down, the pup will swallow it. Be sure it does, or it could go into the lungs. When down the esophagus (judge by length of neck), slowly inject the milk. If you do it too fast the milk will be sprayed and cause cramps. This method requires little experience and is fast and easy. Total time required for feeding and cleaning each pup is about two minutes.

You *must* be sure the pup urinates and defecates after each feeding. If he does not, you must massage the genital area with a moist cloth or cotton to stimulate action. This is the way the mother teaches her young to defecate, and if it is not done, the pups may become constipated and die.

NEUTERING

Spaying The decision whether or not to have the pet dog or bitch neutered is one of the major decisions that must be faced in pet ownership. The bitch especially presents a problem, as an unspayed bitch comes into heat every six months and is in heat for three weeks' time. During this time, she may spot blood on the furniture, rugs, and floor. Her scent will attract male dogs of all descriptions from near and far. There is often fighting among these males as they vie for her attentions.

There is often "helpful" advice on neutering from friends and relatives: "Don't spay her until she has had a litter, or she'll (pick one) 1. get fat, 2. not grow well, 3. get mean, or 4. act like a male." Or "Spayed dogs are all fat and lazy. She won't hunt after she is spayed." And so on. There are lots more "helpful" hints—as many hints as people that give them.

But the truth is this: the female is easiest and safest spayed before she has her first heat period. The young bitch spayed at this time will come through the surgery with little setback and be ready to hunt, play, or work in a few weeks. Spayed dogs get fat for the same reason that unspayed dogs do—people feed them too much! Spayed females do not get mean, unless treatment or temperament incline her that way. Remember, there are mean unspayed females.

Spaying consists of complete removal of the uterus and ovaries in most instances. The dog is given a general anesthetic and prepared for surgery. There are several methods of surgery, so keep in mind that the method used by your veterinarian may differ from this one in some aspects. The hair is clipped from the belly. The line of incision is scrubbed, then painted with an antiseptic. The incision is made a short distance behind the umbilical scar. (The dog is resting on her back.) The incision is carried through the skin, through the muscle, and into the abdominal cavity. The ovaries are brought up by means of a hook, one at a time. Each ovary is clamped off from the ligament and tied off to prevent bleeding. Then the uterus is clamped off, just toward the vagina from where the two horns of the uterus join (the bifurcation). This is tied off securely. Then the uterus and ovaries are removed from the body. The peritoneum and muscle layer are sutured closed, followed by the skin incision. The dog is then moved to a recovery cage to come out from under the anesthetic.

The reason this description has been included is that the average person does not have the slightest idea of what is involved in a spay and are often afraid to ask their veterinarian about it, at the risk of appearing stupid. The spay, or ovariohysterectomy, is major surgery, but when done on a young bitch in good health, there is seldom any trouble.

Castration The male dog does not present as great a problem as the female. He is most often castrated because of his wandering instincts. The male dog is usually castrated at about eight months to one year of age. This is not abdominal surgery, and thus it is often less expensive to castrate the male than spay a female.

Whether male or female, the average pet or hunting dog is often better off when neutered. The drain on a bitch from having two litters a year can severely damage her health. Breast tumors are often found on unspayed females. And in addition, the spayed female is easier on the owner. After all, the cost of feeding litters of puppies and finding them homes makes keeping her a problem. There are so many unfed, stray, unwanted pets in the country today, it is nearly immoral to just let a bitch have litter after litter when she is not contributing to improving canines in general. A top working bitch, show bitch, or brood bitch should be bred, but not even then should she be bred regularly or indiscriminately.

COAT CARE

A dog kept mostly in the house needs some special attention in certain areas of the country. As our houses are often warm and dry in the winter, many dogs shed a little (or a lot) all winter. The coat is not shiny, but dull and stiff. Even the short-haired dog needs regular grooming, not only to keep it looking good, but to keep oil in its hair and to remove dead hairs.

Short-haired dogs are best groomed with a stiff brush and chamois cloth. Be careful not to have too stiff a brush, or you may scratch a thin-skinned dog during grooming. After brushing the coat thoroughly in the direction in which the hair grows, rub a chamois a few times across it to add extra sheen to the coat. Thorough grooming of a short-haired dog, other than an occasional bath, takes only 15 minutes at most and will greatly improve the health of the dog's coat.

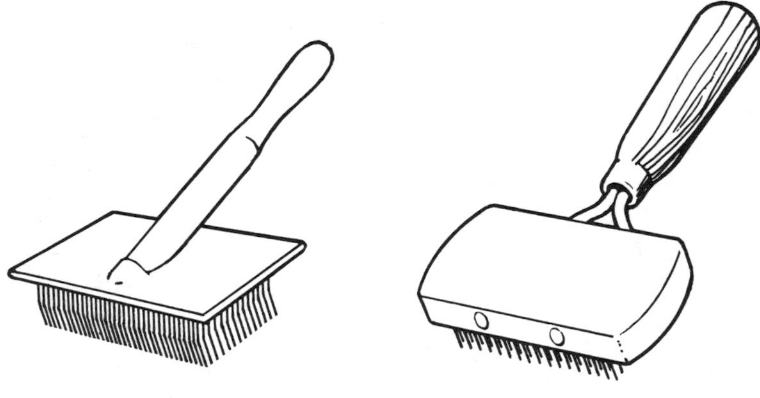

Slicker Brush—Bent Teeth **Pin Brush—Straight Pins**

A medium-coated dog such as a Chesapeake retriever should be gone over first with a slicker. This is a flat brush with bent metal pins. It is very effective for removing dead hairs and stimulating the skin. Then use the regular brush and chamois.

Long-coated dogs such as Old English sheepdogs and Afghan hounds need more frequent grooming, first using a pin brush, then a comb. Using a slicker will tear hair out, and using the comb first will cause severe pulling, should you run into mats. On long-coated breeds, always groom from the bottom of the legs upward to be sure that the coat is mat-free all the way through, not just on the top layer.

A careful watch should be kept while grooming for any fleas, ticks, or red, irritated areas. Taking prompt care of such problems will bring a faster cure and prevent further trouble.

NAIL TRIMMING

The nails should be checked periodically. Some dogs, especially house dogs, fail to wear down their nails naturally, and the nails can grow so long that they spiral until they stick into the pad. Such a condition is very painful and can bring permanent damage if not taken care of soon. The normal, well-worn-down nail is about even with the bottom pads of the foot, so that when the dog walks, the nails just brush the ground. Nails should have a blunt appearance. When they begin to develop a hook, they are too long. A nail trimmer is a handy and inexpensive purchase. With a little practice, almost anyone can keep their dog's nails trimmed and neat. When beginning, take only a little bit from each nail. There is a vein that runs down the nail, and if the nail is clipped too short, it will bleed. Should this occur, a dab with a styptic pencil will stop the bleeding.

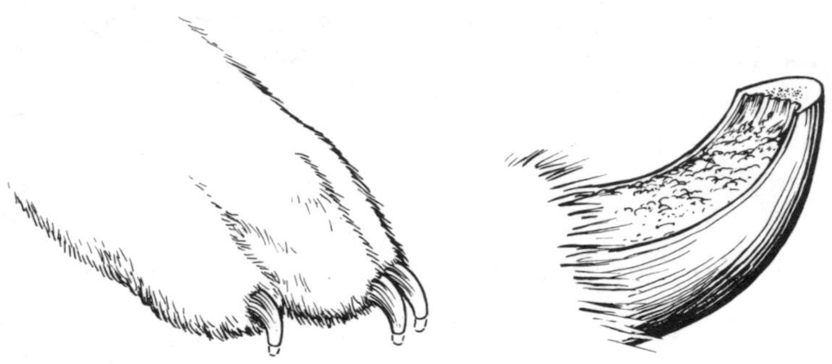

Trim the dog's nails carefully to avoid cutting into the fleshy portion of the claw called the quick.

CHECKING THE EARS

The ears should be checked at grooming time. Not only do they frequently need cleaning, especially on long-eared dogs, but they are a favorite hiding place for ticks. Should any brown discharge be present, the ears should be cleaned. Taking a ball of cotton moistened with alcohol or peroxide, remove the discharge from as deep in the ear as your finger will reach. Using a Q-tip can be dangerous if you are inexperienced or if the dog jumps, as it can puncture the eardrum. Keep a close watch on an ear that has shown a discharge. If the discharge continues, see your veterinarian, as there may be an infection or ear mites present. (See "Ear Infection" in the section, **Diseases and Other Problems**, later in this chapter.)

CHECKING THE TEETH

A dog very seldom has any dental problems, unless caused by disease or old age. Dogs very seldom get cavities. The main trouble with dogs' teeth is the diet they are fed. A soft diet, such as one consisting mainly of canned food or table scraps, does not keep the tartar cleaned from the teeth. As this builds up, it works down into the gum, often causing infection and soreness. A few hard dog biscuits or large bones to gnaw on will often prevent this trouble, as will keeping the dog on a diet of dry dog food.

Should a deposit of tartar occur, you can often remove it yourself, using a dime. Press the little rim on the coin down just beneath the edge of the gum, until it is below the tartar. Then scrape off the tartar by pressing quite firmly against the tooth. It usually comes away in a large flake. Heavy tartar deposits should be removed by your veterinarian. He should also examine your dog, should you notice any foul odor or redness in the mouth.

THE ANAL GLANDS

Every dog naturally has two glands, called anal glands, one on either side of the rectum. These are scent glands and resemble those of a skunk. A dog should have these checked at least twice a year, with smaller dogs about twice a month. Your veterinarian can show you where they are and how to express the accumulation in them that can cause trouble. Plugged anal glands can abscess, cause lameness, and even hindquarter paralysis. (See "Anal Gland Impaction and Infection" in the section, **Diseases and Other Problems**, later in this chapter.)

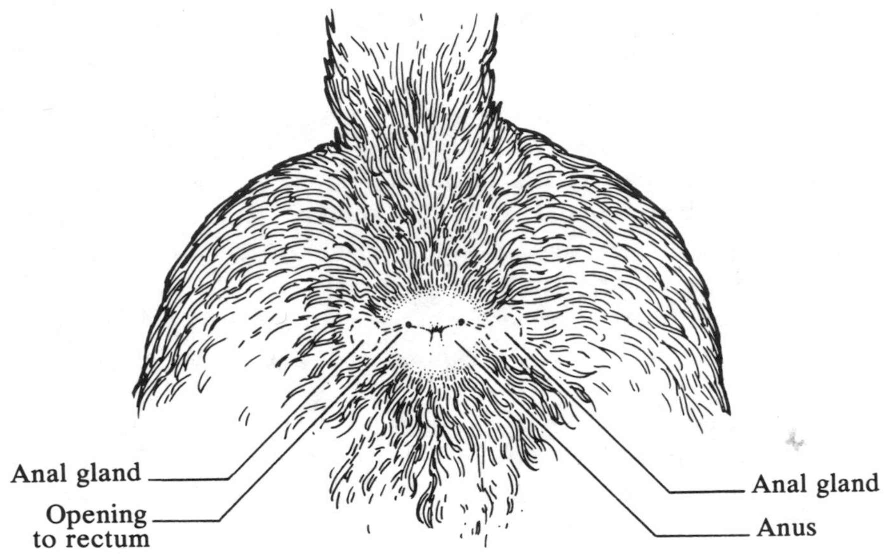

SPECIAL CARE FOR THE AGED DOG

Older dogs often need special care or attention to live out their lives in the best possible health. They may need extra dental attention as their teeth wear down. Older dogs are often fed canned foods which do not remove the deposits of tartar that accumulate on the remaining teeth. These tartar deposits work into the gums, causing sore and inflamed gums, and then infection sets in. The teeth loosen, and the dog is unable to eat.

The teeth should be checked periodically for irritation or redness. If there is any foul odor or sign of loose teeth, the dog should be taken to your veterinarian for treatment before the situation becomes worse. All tartar accumulations should be removed as they form and not be allowed to build up to thick, irritating scales.

Heart Trouble Older dogs, like people, often develop heart trouble. Overweight dogs are especially prone to this trouble. A dog in good condition that weighs 25 pounds cannot carry an added 15 pounds around in old age without having trouble. Just imagine strapping a 15-pound pack onto an aged dog's back and asking it to carry the load day in and day out with no relief! Often the first signs that heart trouble is present are coughing and enlargement of the abdomen, due to ascites. A dog with heart trouble will often have poor circulation, with fluid settling out of the blood and into the tissue. This can often be controlled by use of diuretics, which stimulate the kidneys, drawing fluid out of the body. Salt intake should be restricted. There are also oral drugs, given to strengthen the heart. These should be started under strict veterinary supervision. Your veterinarian can advise you on correct diet, which will greatly aid in maintaining the heart patient.

Urinary Incontinence Aged dogs sometimes have trouble with urinary incontinence. This means the dog cannot control urination completely and may dribble urine unknowingly. Many dogs can be helped with this problem. It is most often seen in spayed, aged females. Diethylstilbestrol is given daily, often in oral form. The dosage is gradually reduced as the dog responds, until it is kept on a low level maintenance dosage. Geriatric tablets containing vitamins and minerals often help in mild cases.

Breast Tumors Breast tumors are quite often seen on aged, unspayed females. They may or may not be malignant. With some tumors, injections of testosterone will result in regression of the growths. Spaying the female will also help in some cases. Surgery is recommended for patients in good health, while the tumors are still small in size. After they are allowed to grow large, the chances for successful surgery are greatly reduced, first because the cells may metastasize to other areas of the body such as the lung, and second because of the enormous amount of shock to the patient when removing so much tissue. When first noticed, lumps on the breast should be looked at by your veterinarian.

Arthritis Arthritis is a common problem with older dogs, again most of a bother in heavy, obese dogs. It is important that the old dog not be allowed to get fat. There is a tendency toward stiffness in old age, and the extra weight only intensifies the problem, making it crippling in many cases. Treatment with drugs, such as cortisone, aspirin, phenylbutazone, and chlorphenesin carbamate will often help dogs with periodic pain. Keeping the dog in warm, dry quarters and off of cement will aid in prevention of stiffness.

Often confused with arthritis, in older dogs especially, is lameness due to long toenails or ingrown nails. With less exercise, older dogs' nails do not wear down normally and require periodic trimming. If this is not done, the nails will grow, curl, twist, and even grow into the pad of the toe. This causes terrific pain, and the dog will be very reluctant to move about; when it does so, it will limp badly. You can very easily learn to trim the nails from your veterinarian or local dog groomer. (See "Nail Trimming" earlier in this chapter.)

Diseases and Other Problems

ANAL GLAND IMPACTION AND INFECTION

On either side of the rectum the dog has a small gland which serves mainly as a scent gland. These glands empty into the rectum during a bowel movement or at times of fright. The opening into the rectum sometimes becomes plugged with fecal material and does not allow the gland to empty. Thus, the gland fills and can become infected. A dog with a full anal gland will drag its rear end on the ground or carpet in an attempt to squeeze this accumulation out of the gland. People used to think this meant the dog had worms, and some still think so. DOGS DO NOT HAVE PINWORMS. Worming a dog with infected anal glands can be dangerous, for many times constipation goes along with the condition, and if the dog cannot get rid of the wormer, it may make it sick or even kill it.

Your veterinarian can show you where the anal glands are and how to express them yourself. If the glands are checked, and emptied if necessary, they will not be so prone to infection. Feeding a diet of dry dog food or giving several hard dog biscuits daily will often help prevent the condition, as a soft stool cannot express the glands. Feeding a diet that will give a firm stool will aid the dog in expressing the glands naturally. Exercise will usually help, too.

Should the dog have recurrent trouble with the anal glands, they can be removed by the veterinarian. The anal glands can cause other problems, such as lameness (due to pressure against the spine), itching, and tonsillitis, when infected.

BACK PROBLEMS

Some breeds of dogs are quite prone to back problems arising from the protrusion of a spinal disc. For discussion of this condition, see "Intervertebral Disc Lesions" later in this section.

BROKEN BONES

The bones most often broken on dogs are the legs, perhaps because of their long length and relative vulnerability. Car accidents, traps, blows and gunshot wounds all often result in broken limbs.

The broken leg will usually dangle in an unnatural manner. The dog is not able to place weight on it. There is extreme lameness. With a compound fracture (break in skin and bone), the end of the bone will be seen sticking through the break in the skin.

The dog with a broken leg should be kept quiet and handled gently. If the dog is in pain, a gauze muzzle may be slipped around its muzzle, to prevent any accidental bites. Where a human might groan or scream in pain, the dog will bite, no matter how much it loves you, it just can't help it.

Be careful not to cause trauma to the leg by roughness. Blood vessels can be torn by the sharp end of the bone. But, do not try to splint the leg, even for temporary protection. Many incorrectly placed splints have caused more damage to a break than the dangling leg.

The break can be set by means of an intramedullary pin, which goes up through the bone marrow (best in many breaks), plaster cast or splint. Most broken legs mend completely, with no difficulties, if the dog is given good nursing.

BRUISES

A bruise is bleeding under the skin. Since a dog's loose skin allows more bleeding to occur when it is bruised, a bruise often fills with blood causing a lump called a hematoma, discussed later in this section.

CAR ACCIDENTS

When a dog has been struck by a car the first two things you should fear are shock and internal bleeding. A broken leg or gash are minor worries, when compared to these. Check the dog's color (see if the gums are pink or pale white). A small- or medium-sized dog is best moved by first muzzling the dog, then grasping the skin behind the neck and on the back, and gently lifting the dog to a blanket or rug. Grabbing the dog around the waist or chest can stick a broken rib through a lung.

Do not try to give the dog any food or water. An injured dog is usually in shock and is not in condition to take food or water. Severe vomiting can result, which could start internal bleeding. Take the dog immediately to the veterinarian. Often an injection of a clotting drug, stimulant, or immediate surgery can save a dog that would die otherwise.

Let me make a note here. After the first twenty-four hours, there is another danger period that can last for about four days. It is in this time that an occasional dog is lost from a blood clot. The dog may be acting fine—it is active and eating—then suddenly die. (This also happens in humans.) It can be guarded against somewhat by restricting the exercise the dog takes and feeding small amounts of easily digested foods several times daily.

COCCIDIOSIS

Coccidiosis is caused by a parasitic protozoa, coccidia. It most often affects puppies, although adult dogs are often carriers and can infect younger dogs. It causes diarrhea, coughing, and dehydration. There are often secondary infections, such as pneumonia and distemper. Damp, unsanitary conditions and overcrowding help to spread coccidiosis.

Combination intestinal sulfas will usually work, and I have had good success using cottage cheese. This seems to change the pH of the intestine, killing the coccidia. I have had pups that did not respond to sulfa or antibiotic therapy clear up immediately when cottage cheese was fed as a sole diet. I know it sounds like a quack remedy (I chuckled the first time another vet told me about it), but it does usually work and causes no side effects, as sulfa drugs sometimes do in cases of dehydration.

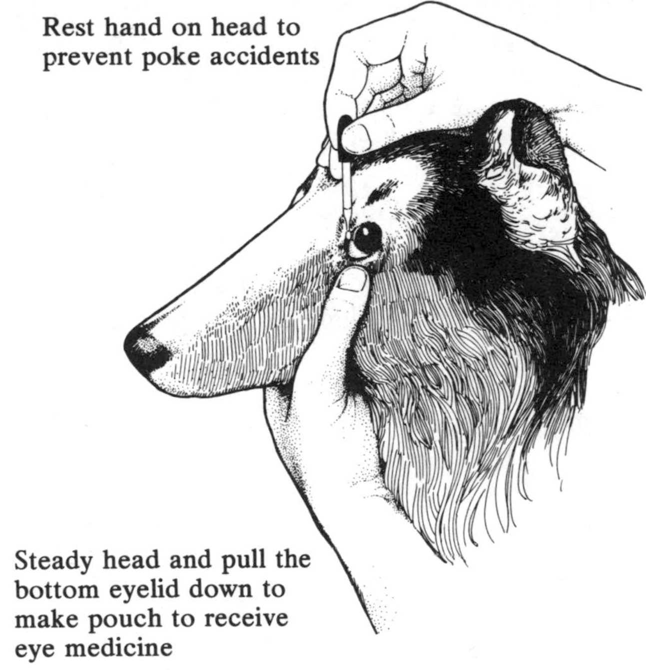

CONJUNCTIVITIS

Conjunctivitis is inflammation of the conjunctival sac next to the eye. The area will be red, swollen, and appear bloodshot.

The eye may run or stick shut. There may be pain or itching. Often there is a bacterial infection following the initial irritation. Conjunctivitis often starts with a foreign body such as dust, pollen, or weed seeds blowing into the eyes. A good way to have eye problems with a dog is to let it hang its head out the car window while someone is driving. The speed of the moving car adds great force to any grit blowing in the wind, driving it into the eye or conjunctiva.

If left untreated, the condition can get bad enough to cause blindness. Often, treatment consists of flushing the eye with a mild solution, and the application of an ointment containing an antibiotic or sulfa and an antiseptic to ease the pain and itching. Rubbing the eye only increases the injury. Dewclaws must be taped to the dog's leg to prevent the dog from scratching its eye. If it paws at the infected eye, it can hook the eye or the rim of it and cause serious damage.

CUTS AND ABRASIONS

Dogs suffer the same type of injuries humans do, including cuts, bruises, and scrapes. The same type of first aid is indicated. Stop the bleeding by means of pressure to the wound with a gauze pack or a tourniquet (loosen every 15 minutes, or gangrene may occur). Call your veterinarian unless the injury is minor. If it is, clip the hair from the edges and clean the wound gently with warm, soapy water. Use no Lysol or such disinfectant, as you may be killing more cells than cleaning them. Do not bandage the wound. Bandages retard healing and often cause infection by providing a warm, protected, moist area for bacteria to breed.

Few wounds on a dog actually require sutures. People usually prefer having a wound sewn closed, often just so they do not have to look at the ugliness. They often heal quicker and without scars if they remain open, healing from the inside. Keep an open mind when asking your veterinarian if he thinks a wound should be sutured. Some should be, of course, but certainly not all.

CYSTITIS

Cystitis is inflammation of the bladder. It is quite common in dogs, but not always diagnosed, as many times there is just a mild inflammation which causes no visible problems. Cystitis is most frequently caused by bacterial infections and calculi (stones).

A dog with cystitis often urinates frequently, vomits, dribbles urine unconsciously, and acts restless. Lifting the dog may bring yelps of pain. There is often blood in the urine. Where the cystitis is caused by a stone (a bit more trouble in males), there may be a complete blockage of the urethra. When the dog is not able to urinate, it absorbs the wastes and soon becomes toxic. Within a short time the dog is in real (and possibly irreversible) trouble.

With an infection in the bladder, medication usually brings prompt relief, but the infection must be correctly diagnosed. Surgery is the best treatment for a dog with stones, as they are usually quite large and nearly impossible to dissolve.

DIABETES

Diabetes is a disease that strikes dogs as well as people. It most often occurs in fat dogs over four years of age. The first signs are an increased thirst and frequent urination. Then there is a weight loss, quickly getting to the point of emaciation. The dog begins to act weak. In severe cases there is uncontrollable vomiting.

When caught fairly early, and when there are no complicating factors, diabetes can be controlled quite easily if the owner is willing to spend a little extra time with the dog daily. Some mild cases are controlled by diet alone. The carbohydrate intake is severely cut, and the dog is fed foods such as lean meat, boiled eggs, and boiled fish. Other cases respond well to oral medication. Still other dogs need insulin injections daily, given before meals. If given religiously, a diabetic dog can be maintained quite well with the insulin. The needle used is very small, and the injection is practically painless.

DISTEMPER

Distemper is a disease of the central nervous system, caused by a virus. Most frequent signs are running, mattered eyes, plugged crusty nose, diarrhea, and vomiting. Chorea, or twitching of a leg, one side of the body, or tail, usually develops when the disease is nearing its worst.

Distemper is often confused with rabies, also a virus. There is no similarity between them. You will not get distemper if bitten by a dog ill with distemper; you will get rabies, unless treatment is given, after being bitten by a rabid dog. A dog sick with distemper may be crabby, but biting is not a symptom of distemper. Distemper may occur year around in most areas of the country. It is highly contagious and does not even need close contact to spread. You can bring it home on your clothes, or a distempered dog can just pass through your yard and spread the virus to your dog.

Treatment, once the disease has gotten under way, is often frustrating for both the owner and the veterinarian. The sick dog may look better and have signs of recovery one day, but then get worse the next. Antibiotics will not cure the disease, as it is a virus, but they can prevent secondary infections such as pneumonia.

Treatment with antiserum or globulin can help some dogs. Good nursing is very important in this disease. Without it most dogs will die. The dog sick with distemper will not want to eat, so it must be coaxed to eat, force fed, or tube fed. The dog must be kept warm and clean. The eyes and nose must be cleaned several times daily. A dog having severe convulsions must sometimes be given drugs to combat them, so that it does not become overtired.

As with many other diseases, distemper is more easily prevented than treated. A puppy born from a dam that is immune to distemper through vaccination will have a certain level of immunity from its dam's colostrum milk. This immunity wears off, and the pup must be vaccinated in order to remain protected. This first vaccination is usually done at eight weeks of age. It is often given in a combination shot containing distemper, hepatitis, and leptospirosis vaccine. The pup must receive a booster in several weeks, followed by a yearly booster.

Puppies may be vaccinated earlier, at three weeks of age, with a temporary vaccination. Puppies not receiving their dam's milk, or those under stress, often do well with this added protection. As opposed to older belief, there is not a "permanent" distemper vaccination. To keep active immunity, the dog should receive the yearly booster.

EAR INFECTION

Dogs, especially long-eared dogs, are prone to ear infections of several types. The most common is ear mites. Ear mites burrow into the ear, creating places for bacteria and fungus to enter. The moist, dirty ear that often accompanies the mites makes a perfect breeding place for these infections, and thus, an eruption. Bacterial and fungus infections cause a lot of trouble in dogs' ears. They often get a start from irritation due to dirt and wax buildup, water or shampoo in the ear, foreign bodies, or injuries.

The dog will usually scratch at its ears with its hind feet, and rub its head on the floor or against a chair. The dog may shake its head, hold it to one side, and appear in pain. When you look in the ear, it will often appear red and swollen, have a brownish, foul-smelling accumulation inside, and be hot.

Mild cases, caused by accumulations of wax and dirt, may be taken care of at home. Dip a ball of cotton into alcohol or peroxide, and swab out the ear by using your finger and the cotton ball gently but firmly. This should be repeated for two days. There should be a great improvement, but if not, the dog should be taken to the veterinarian.

Fungus or bacterial infections in the ear should be treated by your veterinarian. Any extreme aggravation or itching should be taken care of at once, before other problems such as a hematoma (large blood blister) develop.

ECLAMPSIA

In many respects this condition resembles one called "milk fever" in cows and goats. It can occur before whelping, but is generally afterward, when the puppies are a few days old. It is often a small bitch with a fairly large litter that is affected. She will begin to pant, walk with a stiff gait, stumble, fall, and be unable to rise. She may have convulsions, stiffening out rigidly. If not treated, she will often die.

The bitch should be taken to the veterinarian, where she can receive an intravenous injection of calcium. Most bitches will instantly respond and rapidly become normal in their actions. Some or all of the puppies should be weaned at once. If they are allowed to continue nursing, the condition will continue to recur.

EPILEPSY

Epilepsy is quite often seen in dogs, especially in some breeds of smaller house dogs. Miniature and toy poodles and cocker spaniels are quite often affected. This is not to say many of these dogs have epilepsy, but that it is more common in them than in huskies or Great Danes.

A dog with epilepsy will have recurrent "fits" or convulsions. The dog shakes, stiffens out, falls, and jerks its legs; its head often tips backward. Excitement may trigger these seizures. They may occur only once a year, or several times daily. They don't last long each time they come.

There are oral drugs that can be given when epilepsy has been diagnosed. Primidone and Dilantin, which are used with human epilepsy victims, if given regularly will usually keep the dog from having seizures. After the drug has been given for a few months, it has been my experience that it can be cut down gradually while still maintaining a level that does not allow seizures.

FLEAS

When a dog parasite is mentioned, everyone immediately thinks of fleas. But only with a few dogs are they ever much of a problem, as long as a few preventive measures are taken. There are some dogs that develop an allergy to fleas. These poor dogs break out with a rash, scratch, and are miserable if even one flea takes up residence in their coat.

Fleas are little, quick-moving, flat insects that suck blood and annoy dogs and people. Dog fleas will bite people! Sandy, dry areas are favorite spots for fleas. Fleas do not spend their life on the dog, but hop off and on. This is why, when treating the dog with a flea spray or powder, you should also treat its bedding, rug, or sleeping place.

Powders containing rotenone are safe and effective. A dusting should be done weekly for three weeks for surest results in severe infestations. Should the home get infested with fleas, which can happen even with no animals in the house, it is best to call an exterminator. Most fly sprays on the market will kill fleas, but the exterminator will be experienced in knowing the favorite hiding places and will know how to get maximum kill.

FLIES

Biting flies are often a problem for the outdoor dog. Dogs with erect ears in particular are often attacked so badly on the ear tips that they bleed and scab over. These scabs in turn attract more flies. A daily application of a wipe-on insect repellent, such as that used for horses, will prevent this. If the dog should receive some fly bites prior to the application of the repellent, daubing scarlet oil on the raw spots will not only help heal the raw spots, but will help repel the flies.

FUNGUS INFECTIONS

Fungus infections are often mistaken by people for mange. There are many types of fungal infections that can attack dogs, but perhaps the most common is the fungus that causes "hot spots." Hot spots often appear very suddenly during the summer and fall. They are bald, angry red spots that have a moist whitish look in the center. They either itch intensely or are very tender, causing pain if touched. They spread outward, usually keeping a roundish shape. They usually occur on the neck and back.

The hair must be clipped away from the spot, being sure the entire red area is hairless. You can't treat hair. Your veterinarian, on examination of the dog, can prescribe an antifungal, which quickly clears up the trouble.

GUNSHOT WOUNDS

For some reason, dogs receive more gunshot wounds than any other animal. Perhaps it is because they do more "roaming" into other people's yards and are "chased off" at gunpoint. Also, during hunting season, hunters often shoot at anything, just for fun (?), be it sparrow or dog. Knowing where your dog is at all times will protect it from gunshot wounds.

Being shot with birdshot is often more dangerous than being struck by a rifle. The one reason for this is that the rifle wound is more often noticed. The pellets from birdshot penetrate the body, leaving very little sign.

If you suspect your dog has been shot, examine it carefully. Really pick and feel. With birdshot, you will want to know about where the majority of shot struck. With a rifle wound, you will look for an entrance wound and exit wound. The exit wound may not be in line with the entrance wound, the bullet having been deflected by bone or angle.

Keep the dog warm and calm. Stop any bleeding that is present, using a pressure pack. Then call your veterinarian.

HEMATOMAS (BRUISES)

Dogs sometimes get bruises, like people do. However, a dog's skin is looser, allowing more bleeding under the skin (a bruise *is* bleeding under the skin). These bruises fill with blood, making a lump called a hematoma. They are often found on ears, due to flopping the ears in attempts to get rid of itching ear mites or dirt accumulation. They're also commonly found on the neck from collar injuries, such as occur when a dog lunges on a chain.

With an ear hematoma, the layers of skin pull away from the ear cartilage, and this can cause severe thickening and deforming of the ear flap. The ear hematoma can sometimes be eliminated without surgery, if caught early, but often surgery is required to save the normal appearance of the ear.

No bump should be drained unless it has been checked to see if it is an abscess or hematoma. Many animals have bled to death when a person has lanced a hematoma, thinking they were lancing an abscess, because once relieved of the pressure that stopped the bleeding under the skin, the animal continues to bleed, sometimes so much that it is fatal.

HEPATITIS

Hepatitis is caused by a virus and therefore is easily spread, often by the urine of infected dogs. Its symptoms resemble those of distemper. There is usually a fever, inflamed eyes, vomiting, no appetite, and diarrhea. The dog may develop white eyes, which can cause temporary blindness. This usually follows the acute period of the disease, where the dog is the sickest. If it is not treated, it will usually disappear in a week or two. This condition is called "blue eye." The same condition sometimes arises following vaccination. It, as well, usually clears without treatment. Do not put cortisone ointments into the eye or give injections of cortisone, as this sometimes causes scar tissue to form, making the eye permanently blind.

The only safe means of prevention is to vaccinate any susceptible dogs. Treatment consists of blood transfusions, intravenous fluids, and broad-spectrum antibiotics to prevent secondary infections. Since distemper often follows or accompanies hepatitis, it is usually a good idea to give globulin to prevent it.

HIP DYSPLASIA

Hip dysplasia is a problem of the hips, not always causing noticeable signs without X-ray, except when the dog is severely affected. It is an hereditary condition, and, as with most hereditary conditions, it is found most often in registered dogs of certain breeds. German shepherds, Old English sheepdogs, and St. Bernards are a few of those breeds with a high incidence of hip dysplasia. Inbreeding or linebreeding on lines with even a scattered incidence of the condition can produce a litter with several pups affected with various grades of hip dysplasia, with the rest of the pups being carriers of the condition.

It is recommended that every bitch and male used for breeding be X-rayed at 24 months of age—*before* being bred. An earlier X-ray can be incorrect. It is not enough to say that the animal appears sound. These X-rays may be taken at your local veterinarian's office or a state veterinary school. They can then be sent into the Orthopedic Foundation for Animals, where the dog is issued an OFA number. If all breeding animals were examined in this way, hip dysplasia would gradually be weeded out. But this is a utopian dream, as it is nearly impossible to get all breeders (or all people for that matter) to cooperate.

INTERVERTEBRAL DISC LESIONS

Certain breeds are quite prone to back problems arising from protrusion of a spinal disc, which puts pressure on the spinal cord. It can arise from an injury and seems hereditary in a certain sense, as cockers, Pekingese, and most often dachshunds are affected.

Jumping on and off furniture, stairs, and uneven ground often causes an attack. First noticed is severe lameness, an unwillingness to stand, and finally paralysis. When let go a few days, the dog will often assume a froglike position, with the hind legs out behind the body.

Surgery is sometimes used, but as with humans, not all back surgery is successful. Very often, though, these back injuries can be healed to the point that the dog can walk and lead a normal life by means of drugs, good nursing, and physical therapy.

LEPTOSPIROSIS

Leptospirosis is caused by a bacteria and can be passed to humans. There are many locales where there is a high incidence of this disease, higher than most people realize. The dog may suddenly become sick. There will often be a fever, diarrhea and increased urination, bloody or discolored urine, vomiting, and weakness. There is often permanent kidney damage, even if the sick dog survives the disease. The mucous membranes in the mouth may become inflamed, sore, and later slough off.

Prevention consists of vaccination and of keeping the dog away from places rats are known or suspected to frequent, as rats are often the carriers of this disease, spreading it through contamination with their urine. Cattle and other dogs may also spread the disease. Treatment is exacting, and if you suspect this disease, your veterinarian should be called immediately.

LICE

Lice are small, slow-moving, grayish parasites that occasionally infest dogs. They are most often seen on medium-coated or long-coated breeds, as the long hair enables them to hide from the light. When lice are bothering a dog, the dog will usually begin to scratch excessively. On parting the hair, you will see the tiny lice and the little specks which are their eggs. A severe infestation of lice can kill a dog through severe anemia. I once had a dog die on the examination table from lice.

When lice are discovered on a dog, the entire dog should be clipped short. With no hair to hide in and protect them from an insecticide, the lice are usually easily taken care of. There should be a repeat treatment every week for three weeks to kill any new lice that have hatched out. The dog's bedding should be burned and its bed dusted with the same powder or spray you used on the dog. Don't mix insecticides, as switching from one to another can be dangerous for the dog.

MANGE

Mange is quite common in dogs. Perhaps this is because they have such close contact with people! You see, people can often carry the mange mites on their skin and not realize it because the mites don't bother people. In vet school, we took skin scrapings from our whole class. Over 90 percent had mange mites! And, this was *before* we had any actual contact with dogs. (We also weren't a dirty, scruffy bunch!)

These mites are so tiny they can not be seen with the naked eye. They burrow into the skin, causing intense itching. A mange session often follows a period of severe stress. Malnutrition, followed by poor skin health, often lets the mites get a head start and cause problems. Any skin eruptions, especially about the face, legs and belly, should be regarded as suspicious. Pustules, scabby areas, thickened, grayish areas, and baldness are all symptoms of mange.

Mange is very contagious to other dogs, so it is best to isolate the suspect until a proper diagnosis is made by a veterinarian. The *only* way to make a right diagnosis is by examination of a skin scraping under a microscope. Do not let a neighbor tell you that a dog has mange, as there are several other skin troubles that *look* like mange.

A dog affected by mange should be clipped entirely. This is often hard for an owner to agree to, especially if the dog has a long, beautiful coat, but it is the only way to stop the mange at once. You can't treat spots for mange if you can't find them, and you can't treat through hair and do any kind of a good job.

The use of medicated shampoos, along with ointments containing rotenone, malathion or pyrethrins, will usually effect a cure. Sometimes it is necessary to use a lindane preparation. This is very toxic, both to humans and dogs, so it must be used under veterinarian supervision.

Also see "Fungus Infections" earlier in this chapter.

METRITIS

Metritis is inflammation of the uterus. There are two types, acute and chronic. With acute metritis, the bitch is very sick. She has often retained a placenta or fetus. The foul uterine discharges are absorbed making the bitch extremely toxic. She will vomit, have diarrhea, run a high fever, and act listless. Any bitch that has recently whelped and acts dull or has abnormal uterine discharges with a foul odor should be examined by a veterinarian. It could save her life.

In chronic metritis, there is often a low-grade infection present. The bitch can go a long time with a mild infection without acting sick. Sometimes the only sign of trouble is breeding difficulties. The bitch may be bred several times and not conceive. If she does conceive, the puppies may either be stillborn or die shortly after birth. Although antibiotic therapy can be used, the best course of action in many cases is to remove the uterus. Sometimes the low-grade infection can "blow up" into an acute attack, and the bitch will be lost. It is very hard to get rid of a chronic metritis without removing the uterus.

PORCUPINE QUILLS

Nearly every farm dog sooner or later runs into a porcupine, provided, that is, it lives in an area where there are porcupines. These slow-moving animals prefer to just go about their business, but when harassed by a dog, they can quickly slap a lot of quills into a dog's nose. Porcupines do not throw their quills, but they can slap that long-quilled tail faster than you can see, leaving around a hundred quills imbedded firmly.

Many dogs know to quit after they've gotten four or five quills stuck into their nose. But once in a while, a dog really gets mad and tries to tear the porcupine up. The usual result is a dog with a mouth, nose, and throat full of quills. This is the dog that should be taken to the veterinarian for quill pulling. Any attempt to remove the quills at home will be futile.

Porcupine quills have tiny barbs that are imbedded in the flesh, making them hard to pull. If they are grasped firmly and pulled very slowly, the barbs will be released. But if yanked, which is not uncommon if the dog is struggling, the quills will snap off, leaving a large amount of each beneath the skin. These quills often become infected, causing swelling and pain. There are also tiny quills that get into the skin when the dog bites at the porcupine. These are little bigger than a hair, but if left in or broken off, they can cause as much trouble as the three-inch-long ones. This is why it is usually best to take the dog to your veterinarian where it will receive a general anesthetic, to be relaxed while the painful operation of quill pulling is done.

Once in a while, a dog gets into quills so badly that it goes into shock. Here, it must be treated at once or it will die. If the dog suddenly becomes shaky, pale, and acts strangely, get it to your veterinarian right away.

RABIES

Rabies is caused by a virus that is very highly concentrated in the saliva of infected animals. It used to be called hydrophobia because the paralysis of the throat made it hard or impossible for a rabid dog to drink.

There are two types of rabies: dumb rabies (the dog just sits, mouth often hanging open, and has a peculiar look in its eye) and furious rabies (the dog hallucinates, snaps at imaginary objects, wanders, and becomes irritable). Often, the dumb rabies is the most dangerous, as many people pry into the mouth, thinking the dog has something in its throat or mouth. Getting the dog's saliva into a small cut or scratch can give you rabies, so NEVER stick your hand into such an animal's mouth.

Not all rabid dogs attack people and have frothy mouths. A rabid dog often has a personality change. A timid, fearful dog will get brave and friendly. A normally friendly dog will get surly and timid. A rabid dog will often leave home and wander until exhausted. Skunks, foxes, and bats often have rabies, so never try to pick up or catch a "friendly" wild animal. Keep your dog away from them also.

There is no treatment for rabies, once symptoms have developed in dog or man. Vaccination will protect your dog and thus you from the disease, as dogs and cats are the contact between wildlife and humans in rabies.

STRYCHNINE POISONING

Although strychnine poison was used on rats and mice in the past and has been replaced with such products as warfarin, there are still some malicious people in the world that use strychnine to poison neighborhood dogs. The poisoned dog will usually begin to show symptoms an hour or so after having eaten the tainted food. It will begin to tremble, pant, and act nervous. As the symptoms progress it will respond to any loud noise, such as a car horn beeping, by having convulsions. As the condition worsens, even clapping the hands can produce a severe convulsion.

If the dog can be taken immediately to a veterinarian, it can be given sodium pentobarbital, a general anesthetic, to keep it from having convulsions until the poison is removed by bodily processes. If left untreated, the dog will suffer one convulsion after another, until it dies from exhaustion. It is a cruel death that not even a rat should suffer.

TICKS

Ticks are quite a problem for dogs in many areas. There are several types of ticks that infest dogs. All are basically the same. They are blood-sucking parasites that attach themselves to an animal. In small numbers, they generally cause no trouble except irritation. In large numbers, however, they can produce anemia and extreme agitation. Scratching and digging at the tick bites break off the tick heads, irritate the skin, and aggravate the situation. Secondary infections often follow. Some ticks get into the ear canal, causing ear infections and irritation.

Ticks may be removed simply by pulling slowly but firmly. If they are yanked off, the mouth may remain attached, causing infection and soreness. Where ticks are a problem, it is usually best to dip the dog with rotenone or pyrethrin once every two weeks during tick season to keep it free of the pests. The dog should be checked in between dips, though, as some ticks are resistant to various insecticides.

TONSILLITIS

Tonsillitis occurs often in dogs. Usually it is caused by a bacterial infection. I have seen many dogs having a simultaneous anal gland infection, caused by the same bacteria infecting the tonsils. I believe these dogs had their anal gland infection first, licked the anal area in an attempt to alleviate the condition, and picked up the infection in the tonsils. In chronic cases, once the anal glands were removed, the dogs never had tonsillitis again. Coincidence? I hardly think so.

A dog affected with tonsillitis will usually cough, gag, and vomit. It may paw at its throat. Often there will be lack of appetite, dullness, and lack of energy. Often one, or both tonsils, can be felt when swollen, just below the jaw.

When taken care of promptly, most cases of tonsillitis clear up in three to four days. Use of a broad-spectrum antibiotic, plus cortisone to take the swelling out of the tonsil and throat, works in most cases. Good nursing plays an important part also. The dog can often be coaxed to eat by giving it ice cream, cold milk, and cold broth. These things are soothing on the sore throat and will encourage the dog to take more nourishment.

With cases of recurrent tonsillitis, it is often advisable to remove the tonsils surgically.

WORMS

The dog should receive a regular six month fecal exam for worms by a veterinarian. There are "shotgun" prescriptions available at many stores that claim to kill all worms. Unfortunately, they either do not, or worse, kill the dog also. Each worm is affected by different wormers. Few wormers do a good job on more than three types.

Heartworm Once mainly a problem in the South, heartworm has become widespread nationwide. It is spread by the mosquito, which sucks the infected blood of one dog and transmits the microfilariae (larvae) to another dog. Here, they develop into mature heartworms. These in turn reproduce and there are more microfilariae to infect another dog. Heartworms infest the heart. When a badly infested dog is exercised, it may show shortness of breath, coughing, lack of stamina, and may be easily tired.

Every dog should have a yearly check for heartworm. If found free of them, it can be put on an oral heartworm preventive. This is given daily throughout the mosquito season. Treatment for heartworm can be tricky. The drug which kills the adult heartworm must be used with extreme care, because if too many worms are killed quickly, they leave the heart, causing blockages in the bloodstream, like a spring log jam. This can result in death.

Hookworm Hookworms cause unthriftiness, diarrhea, blood in the stool, and death in young puppies, due to anemia. They are one of the most severe intestinal parasites. Puppies can be infected before being born and become reinfected very early. Death may result. Hookworms enter the body by penetrating the skin. In this way, they can also infect people.

All puppies should receive a fecal examination for worms at weaning, but if there has been trouble with hookworm in the past, this examination should be done at two to three weeks of age. If you wait until eight weeks, there may not be any puppies left.

Strict sanitation measures are necessary when hookworm has shown up. As the larvae are in the soil, the dogs should be moved to a new, clean area after having been wormed. Regular stool checks should be done after that, to insure that the parasite is really gone, not just in hiding.

Roundworm Roundworm is the most common parasite affecting dogs. Most puppies are born with them, even when the dam has been faithfully wormed before she was bred. These worms are quite large, white, and tapered at both ends, resembling a bean sprout. They are often coughed up or seen in the stool, especially in puppies. A small puppy can harbor huge amounts of these parasites, which harm the digestive tract and cause malnutrition. After all, you can't feed a puppy what it needs if the worms beat it to the food.

The worm makes a migration through the bloodstream and thus can be difficult to treat. One worming is not enough. That only kills the worms present in the stomach and intestine, but it does not kill the larvae in other places or destroy the eggs that will hatch and soon reinfest the dog.

Tapeworm Tapeworms are carried to the dog by the flea. The flea larva ingests tapeworm eggs, becomes an adult, and is ingested by the dog; then the eggs hatch, starting the cycle. The adult tapeworm is large and flat and can grow to a length of several feet. It is made up of segments, each containing eggs. These sections are passed in the stool; they are whitish pieces which look like inchworms when first passed and quickly dry to look like grains of rice. They are often found in the hair around the dog's rectum and tail, or in its bedding. Rabbits also serve, along with fleas, as an intermediate host of the tapeworm, so rabbit entrails should never be fed to dogs.

Whipworm Whipworm is less often seen than the other worms. It can be hard to get rid of, though, because it lives in the colon and cecum (a blind pouch resembling the appendix in humans). Often the most common sign of whipworm is the liquid, foul-smelling stool. Unthriftiness and anemia follow.

CATS

General Care and Management

Although the average cat is very independent of people, it does require care to remain happy and healthy.

The house cat should have a litter box available, or have use of a pet door to be able to go outdoors when necessary. A scratching post is appreciated, both by the cat and its owners, because without a scratching post to use for cleaning the claws and for exercise, the cat will often use the furniture or carpet.

FEEDING

The old idea that a hungry cat is a better mouser is untrue. The well fed but not fat cat gives the best in its hunting. The female cat, hunting instinctively for her kittens, will hunt all day. She should have adequate nourishment to do this. Her kittens should also receive additional food, as often one kitten who is most aggressive will grab all the prey the mother brings, leaving its brothers and sisters hungry.

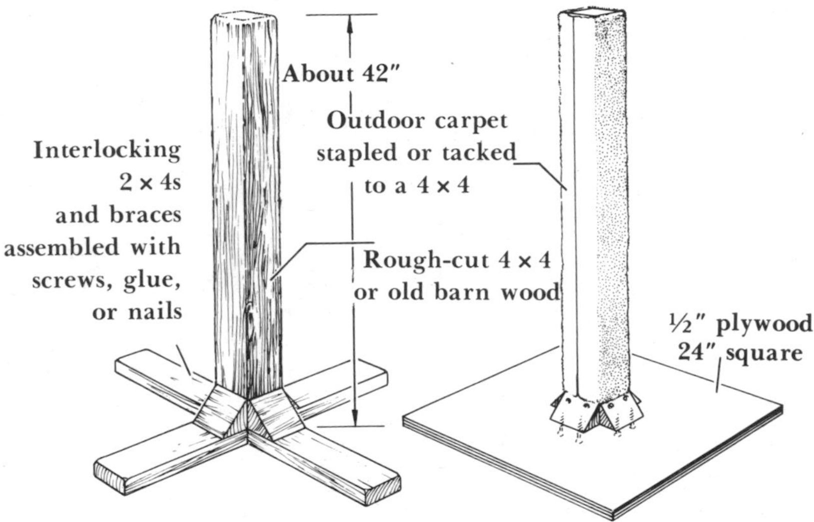

Two scratching posts—most cats like at least one of these surfaces to use for cleaning their claws.

Cats do not like sour or moldy food. Never leave moist food such as canned cat food in a bowl for longer than 12 hours. If it is too much for the cat to eat in that period, feed less food. Sour or moldy food can be filled with bacteria that will make the cat sick or even kill it.

Cats should not be fed any cooked fish or poultry containing the bones. Small, sharp bones can not only cause stomach pain, but also impaction of the intestine and death. Highly seasoned foods should not be fed to cats. Remember, nature did not intend cats to eat hot peppers, bologna, and sausage. Gastric upsets often result, which can lead to more serious troubles.

Cats should always have access to fresh, clean water. If they do not receive adequate water, they may become dehydrated and susceptible to illness. Urinary calculi can be caused by inadequate water consumption, especially when a diet high in minerals and ash is fed. Dry cat foods have also caused trouble in this way. If the cat does not drink adequate water to compensate for the lack of moisture in dry boxed foods, it is more likely that urinary calculi will form. (For more on urinary calculi see **Diseases and Other Problems** later in this chapter.)

RESTRAINT

Occasionally it becomes necessary to restrain the cat. Examinations, either at home or by a veterinarian, minor treatment, such as clipping nails, combing a snarl out, or medicating the cat, are all made easier by using tried and true methods of restraint.

Sometimes there is a certain knack to just holding onto a cat. When it has decided that it would rather be elsewhere, a cat can turn into a slippery, twisting bundle with claws. Being a naturally nervous animal, many things often upset a cat, even if it normally has a calm disposition. A loud noise, a moving car, barking of dogs, and strange surroundings can all bring on the desire to "escape" and hide. The best way to hold a cat that may wiggle away is to grasp the forefeet with one hand and the hind legs and tail with the other hand. The cat uses the tail for balance when jumping, and the hind legs for ripping and clawing when frightened or angry. Restraining both front and hind legs, plus the tail, will enable the average person to hold onto all but the most frightened or vicious cat.

This hold, however, gives no protection to you against bites. Most cats will not bite unless hurt first. When a cat is given an injection, no matter if it is just an inoculation against distemper, some will try to claw or bite. The easiest way to hold the cat for a procedure such as this is to grasp the skin firmly behind the neck and just in front of the tail, placing the cat on a slippery table or other surface.

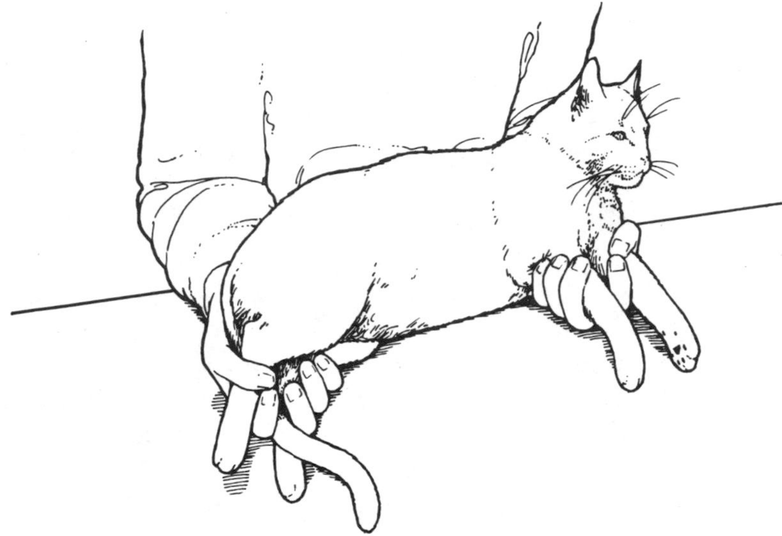

Restraint for Cats

Wrapping the cat in a towel sometimes aids in minor treatment, but will not work with a very frightened cat. Calmly slipping the cat into a canvas bag with a drawstring at the top, allowing the head to come out, then closing the bag snugly (but not too tightly), not allowing enough room for the front legs to be worked free, works well for medicating ears, cleaning teeth, giving oral medicines and examination of the head. A subcutaneous injection may also be given using this method of restraint by pulling the neck skin out just behind the ears.

Once in a while, it becomes necessary to prevent a cat from scratching at its ears, eyes, or licking medication off its body. Although tranquilizers can sometimes prevent this, many a cat will continue to bother, even though really drugged. It might not hit the right place, but it will continue to try, sometimes causing damage.

The easiest way to keep the cat from bothering medication or self-mutilation due to an itching problem such as ear mites, is to make an Elizabethan collar. This can be made of a variety of materials, but usually plastic, such as that cut from plastic pails, or heavy cardboard. The collar is made in the shape of a circle, perhaps twelve inches in diameter, with a hole in the center, which fits snugly around the cat's neck. A cut is made in

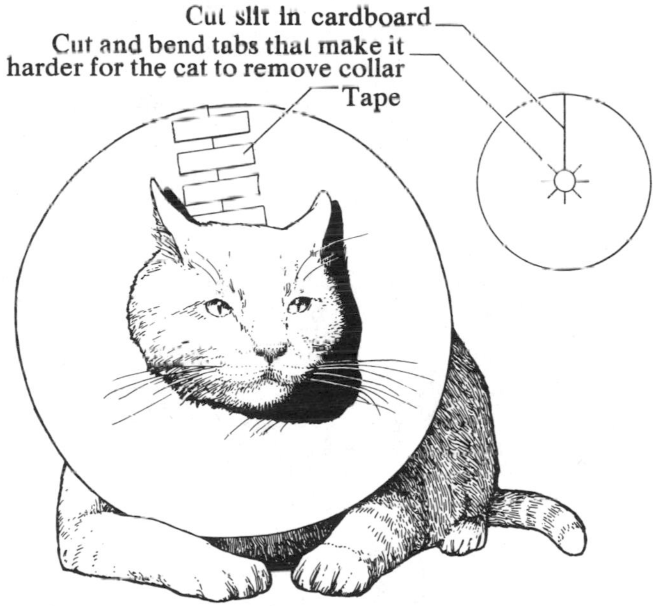

Elizabethan Collar

the collar, from neck hole to the outside rim. Then the collar is fitted on the cat, the cut edges overlapped and taped together, forming a cone-shaped arrangement. When well fit and the right size, only the most determined cat will be able to get it off or get around it with feet or mouth.

TRANSPORTING

It sometimes is necessary to take a cat some distance by car. By nature, few cats enjoy riding in a car and are made nervous and possibly even sick by the motion and noise. The first reaction of the cat is to try to escape, and if this fails, the cat will usually hide under a seat (becoming almost impossible to reach when you want to get it out).

There are many types of cat carriers on the market, and if you do much travelling with your cat you should get one. Prices range from a mere $1.50 on up. They are a great convenience and a great protection to a cat, making accidental escapes nearly impossible. A cat likes to feel hidden and secure, so, lacking a ready-made cat carrier, one can be improvised out of a heavy cardboard box, or best of all, a beer case. A beer case is a boon to many cat owners. It is easy to carry, heavy duty, and easily begged from a beer drinker. The cat is placed in the case with a towel or blanket, the top is shut down and tied with twine, then the whole thing is slowly turned upside down when put in the car. The reason for this is that the cat will try to escape upward, and if the strongest side is up there will be very little chance of escape.

BREEDING

The queen or female cat will come into heat every two to three weeks, most often in the winter, spring, and summer. She is in heat for a period of three to six days. Signs of heat are arched back, with hindquarters high in the air, calling, rolling about on the floor, holding the tail upward, and treading the hind legs.

Left to her own resources, the queen will find a mate (or he will find her) and be bred. When a breeding is desired, it should be planned for. The queen should be in the very best health possible. She should be checked for worms and other parasites, *before* she even is due to come into heat. She should carry immunity to the diseases she is able to be vaccinated against (many kittens are lost at an early age due to distemper and like diseases), and she should be in good flesh, but not too fat.

Arrangements should be made with the stud owner (unless the queen makes them, unknown to you!) in advance of the time she is due to come into heat. If she is to be bred to one certain male, she should be kept isolated in a secure room to prevent an accidental mating with another male cat.

Following a successful breeding, the queen will often seem to suddenly go out of heat. This is because copulation stimulates ovulation.

Pregnancy can often be detected by an experienced person at about three weeks. If the abdomen is gently palpated, the marble-sized lumps in the uterus can be felt. The abdomen should not be squeezed roughly or very hard, as damage to the queen or the kittens can result.

The pregnant queen should receive a balanced diet and be encouraged to eat high-protein foods such as liver. A good vitamin-mineral supplement should be given to aid the developing kittens, and the queen. Her appetite will increase with her abdomen, and she should receive plenty of quality food. It is natural for her to slow down, not playing or running about, as she may have done prior to feeling her pregnancy.

As her time draws nearer, she will seek out a quiet secluded "nest," a stump, hole in the hay, or dresser drawer, and beginning a few days before she has the kittens, she will spend more and more time there. Fifty-eight to 68 days after breeding, she will be ready to give birth to her kittens. Her temperature will drop sharply 12 to 24 hours preceeding birth. The kittens are usually born with no trouble due to their shape and size, but sometimes a physical defect in the queen or other problem will hinder birth. If she labors for longer than half an hour with a kitten, producing nothing, call your veterinarian. He may advise a little more time, an injection to help uterine contractions, or possibly a caesarean, should it be impossible for her to make a natural delivery.

DELIVERY

Because of the very small size of the vagina and the pelvic opening in the queen it is best to take the queen to the vet at once when there are birth difficulties. With other animals, it is easier to assist a difficult birth without instruments or knowledge (or experience). A queen tires quickly in a difficult birth and can be easily injured by inexperienced attempts to help her. Many a uterus has been ripped by too forceful an extraction of a fetus, and many a queen has been lost due to shock and exhaustion.

If the difficulty is just a larger kitten becoming stuck at the vaginal opening, this is generally no problem. The head or legs are grasped by a dry towel and gently, but firmly pulled on as the queen strains. The kitten usually is then quickly expelled. Do not just yank the kitten out. This will cause damage or bleeding.

In most cases, however, the kittens are born easily. It is a good idea to keep an eye on the queen while she is having them, as you can often help save a kitten. Once in a while, a queen may be busy cleaning one kitten, ignoring the fact that she just had another one. If the membrane is not removed from the kitten's head after the umbilical cord breaks, it will often drown on the amniotic fluid. If the queen does not remove the sac, you should do it for her, drying the head (especially the nose and mouth) well.

Each kitten is followed by a placenta, or afterbirth. These should be counted, as once in a great while a queen will retain one or more placentas. This can cause an inflammation and infection of the uterus. Don't, by the way, be alarmed at the color of these placentas. They are often a horrible greenish black. Also, don't be alarmed when the queen eats them; this is normal. Eating the placentas stimulates her milk letdown.

The kittens will be born with their eyes shut tightly. These will open in about two weeks, and the kittens will begin to move about.

At this time it is easiest to sex your litter of new kittens, if it is desired. Right after birth, the testicles of the male are readily apparent. Hold the kitten up, upside down. In the males, you will see the testicles as tiny bulges just below the anus, on either side of the penis. To the inexperienced, sexing kittens is more difficult than other animals are, other than rabbits, because of the close external similarity between the male and female genital areas. With the male cat, the penis is not exposed as in other male animals, but hidden in a fold of skin which resembles the vulva of the female. This is the reason it is easiest to look for the testicles.

As soon as they will eat semisolid food, they should be given several small feedings daily to relieve the queen of the strain of producing milk.

Kittens can be weaned at eight weeks of age, when adequate care is given them. Small kittens should be fed four or five times daily. When they are about three months old, cut down to three meals a day, and at six months, feed them twice daily. They need a 30 percent protein diet, so feeding a dry food with 14 percent protein will not maintain a kitten nor allow it to grow. Inadequate protein intake will usually result in death. Feeding such foods as liver, kidney, raw beef (ground for kittens), and small amounts of milk will boost the protein intake. Too much milk, cereals, or vegetables will cause indigestion and diarrhea.

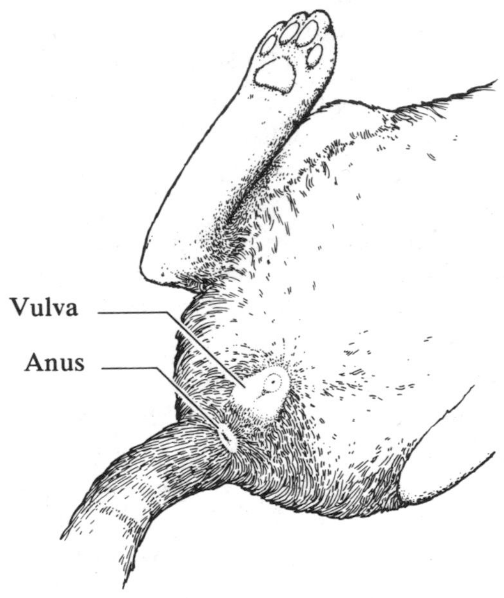

Orphan Kittens Once in a while, whether due to lack of milk on the queen's part or due to her death, it becomes necessary to raise the litter by hand. This is quite a job, so be prepared!

The kittens should get about 1 to 2 cc. of preferably goats' milk every two hours, day and night, for the first week. This can be given easily, either by tube feeding (see puppies), or by using a doll bottle with a small rubber nipple. An eye dropper is no good, as it gives the milk too fast, causing inhalation pneumonia, as the milk droplets enter the lungs.

After the first week, the milk should be increased to three to four cc., depending on the size and health of the kittens.

Kittens being fed the right amount of milk will feel full and round, with tight skin. They will squirm and mew angrily when hungry. Too much milk will cause diarrhea, which is often fatal.

The amount of milk should be gradually increased, and the number of feedings decreased as they get their eyes open. At three to four weeks, semisolid foods can be added to their dict in the form of mashed liver.

One word here: If the queen can not be around to take care of cleaning the kittens, you are elected. Not just for pretty kittens, but for their very life. Kittens need to be stimulated to urinate and defecate for a week or more after birth. The mother does this by licking the genital areas. You will have to use a slightly damp wash cloth after each feeding. If this is not done there will be serious gastric troubles and often death.

NEUTERING: SPAYING AND CASTRATION

Any pet cats, especially those kept in the house, should be neutered. Otherwise, the male will begin to spray urine (which doesn't smell like cologne!) about the house, marking his "territory," at about nine to 12 months of age. It is the rare male that does not do this. It is an odor that is lingering and hard to remove from fabric, such as rugs and drapes. The male that is not neutered will also begin roaming, seeking romance. Unfortunately, other toms have the same idea about the same female, and fighting results. The pet male often returns from these brawls scratched, bitten, and torn.

A quite inexpensive and safe operation done on the male at about eight months of age will end these problems before they begin. Castrating an older male who is set in his ways may slow him down, but may not completely alter his habits.

With the female, there are other problems. Once every two to three weeks she will be in heat, rolling about yowling constantly. Trying to find a place to put her out of hearing, but still away from the visiting males, is a problem. If the door is left open she will be out like a flash, presenting you with a litter of two to six kittens in two months.

The spaying procedure is briefly outlined under neutering in the dog chapter. The same procedure is generally used on a cat. The operation is usually safer with a cat, due to the smaller size of the uterus and blood vessels. Spaying should be done between five and ten months of age if possible. It is not necessary for her to have been in heat or to have had a litter.

TRIMMING CLAWS AND DECLAWING

Due to the extreme sharpness of a cat's claws and the tendency for some cats to use those claws, on people (even if in play) or on the furniture and drapes, people often want them dulled or removed. There are two choices here: declawing, which is the surgical removal of the claw and first joint of each toe, or trimming the nails.

I would recommend trying to trim the claws before deciding to declaw the cat. Declawing *is* permanent and does remove the cat's prime defense. A declawed cat can hunt and climb trees, but is a bit hampered, compared to its clawed brother.

A cat is usually easy to work on when trimming the claws. The cat's claws are retractile, so you have to press upward between the toes to unsheath the claws. Most cats have light colored claws, making it easy to see the pink blood vessel that runs part way down inside the claw. Clip off the hook on the end of the claw, staying away from the blood vessel. Should the vessel be nicked, touching a styptic pencil to the end will stop the bleeding. One claw is clipped at a time until all four feet are finished. The hind claws are not as long or as sharp as those on the front claws.

Should it be necessary, the cat can later be declawed by a veterinarian.

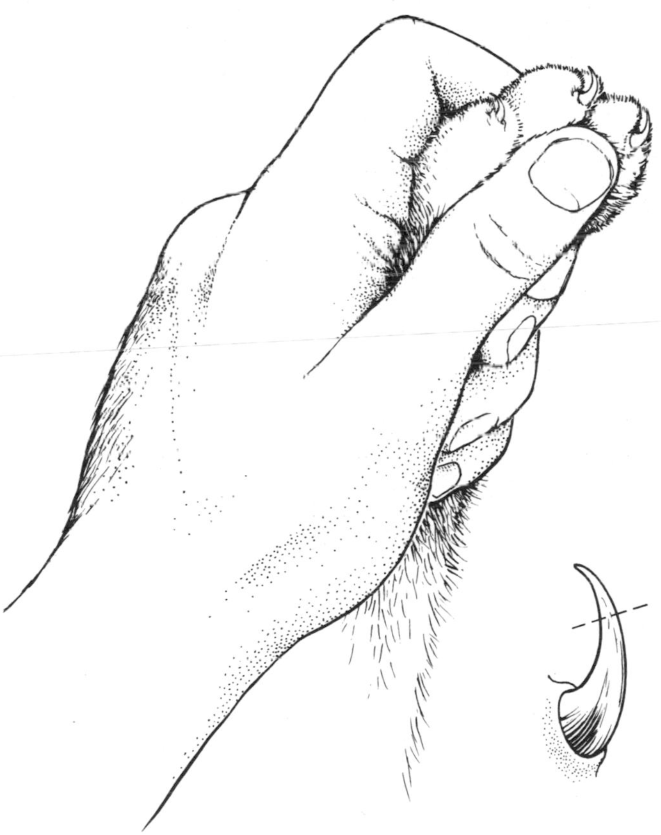

Trim a cat's claws by pressing the paw with your thumb to expose the claws. With a nail clipper, take off the end only, staying well away from the visible blood vessel.

DENTAL PROBLEMS AND CARE OF THE TEETH

Today's cat is often prone to dental problems. A soft diet, such as canned cat food, does not massage the gums or clean tartar deposits from them. These tartar deposits build up and irritate the gums. Swelling, bacterial infections, and abscesses are often a result.

A cat that drools either when eating or just resting should be examined for tooth and gum problems. Foul breath is also a sign of dental trouble. Often a cat with bad teeth will eat hard food such as dry cat food with its head cocked sideways as it tries to avoid chewing on the sore tooth.

A cat's mouth should be checked periodically, and the cat should be taken to the veterinarian if any redness of the gums, foul breath, or decayed teeth are noticed. If the teeth appear brownish or yellow they should be cleaned. This is easiest and best done by your veterinarian using a general anesthetic. Spots of tartar can be removed at home by scraping the tooth with the edge of a dime. But this is only to be used if there are only a few spots of tartar on one or two teeth. To do a good job the cat must not wiggle and squirm.

Giving the cat dry food from time to time will aid in preventing tartar buildups and gum troubles because it keeps the teeth scraped clean.

Diseases and Other Problems

ABSCESSES

Cats are often seen with abscesses, particularly males. Fight wounds, such as bites and scratches that puncture the skin but do not tear, often get dirty and close up, sealing bacteria under

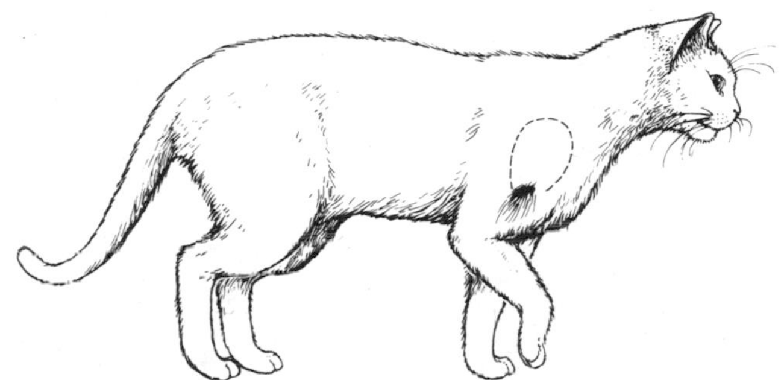

This cat has developed an abscess on the shoulder. The abscess causes pain so the cat has licked it open and drainage has started. Without thorough antibiotic treatment and flushing, however, the opening won't heal properly, and the abscess will recur.

the skin. Such punctures will later abscess. With the normal loose skin of the cat, the abscess can spread under the skin and fur, until all of a sudden a large bulge becomes noticeable. The abscess may break and drain, but often it will ooze through perforations in the skin and not drain adequately.

The abscess should be lanced near the bottom with a sterile instrument. This is best done under an anesthetic, so that the area can be thoroughly flushed and cleaned. The abscess should be kept clean and open until healed from the inside. Antibiotic therapy is a good idea to prevent a septicemia.

Never lance a bump, unless you are positive it *is* an abscess. Hematomas, or blood-filled bruises, look like abscesses, but if they are lanced the cat may bleed to death. Therefore, it is not wise to attempt home treatment.

BROKEN LEGS

Legs are the most often broken bones in the cat. Maybe this is because they are long and thin, and the other bones are not positioned in such a way that they get caught and wrenched as do the legs. The tail is one exception, and it does frequently suffer breaks, usually due to having been slammed in a door.

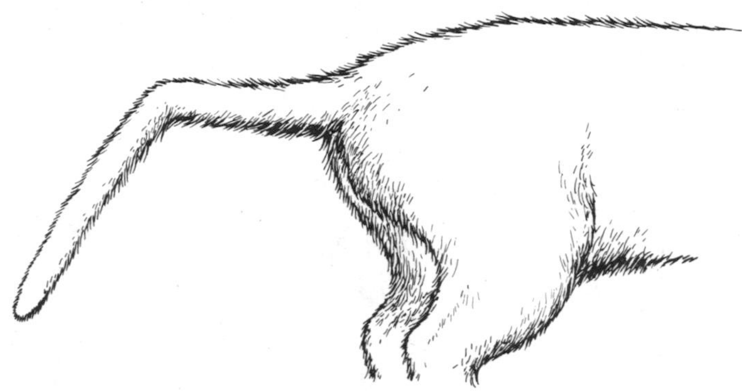

An unfortunate cat that has a new understanding of slamming doors; its tail has been broken.

The cat with a broken leg will usually limp very badly, holding the leg off the ground. The leg will usually dangle unnaturally. When finding such a cat, quietly get hold of it and carefully place it in a closed room or secure box or carrier. Many injured cats desire to go away and hide when the initial shock wears off. Cats that are seriously injured and left untreated can develop complications and possibly die.

The veterinarian should be called immediately. *Do not attempt to put a splint, temporary or not, on the cat.* Many serious complications have arisen following improper placing of a home splint. It is better just to allow the cat to remain quietly in a box with a towel than to place a splint on the leg that may upset the cat, causing damage to the leg.

Most broken legs can be quite easily set on a cat, by means of an intramedullary pin, light aluminum or plastic splint, or light plaster cast.

CAR ACCIDENTS

More cats are injured by cars than any other way. Because cats are hunters, it is natural for them to seek out the grassy roadsides to hunt on. And unfortunately, many times they are frightened by cars, then panic, run on the road, and are hit.

Any outside cat that suddenly acts in pain, is lame or listless should at least be suspected of having had an encounter with a car. The body should be inspected closely for abrasions, bald spots, bruises or swellings. The gums should be checked, as pale gums indicate either shock or internal bleeding. The eyes should be checked to see if one pupil is more dilated than the other, indicating a concussion. Where both are dilated, there may only be shock, or possibly there is a head injury.

After a quick, but fairly thorough examination, such a cat should be taken to the veterinarian for a thorough examination and possibly observation for a day or so. Sometimes, seemingly minor injuries can worsen with time with bad results.

Cats seem to have a problem with fans in cars. They like to get up under the hood, especially in cold weather, and when the motor is started they get caught in the fanbelt. Should this happen, do not panic. A seemingly horribly torn-up cat may live and make a complete recovery in a few weeks. Don't listen to well-meant advice to "put the cat away," unless it comes from a veterinarian (unless, of course, the cat is really torn up, intestines torn, abdomen opened, head split or something of the like).

Place the cat in a quiet, dark box with some light bedding and drive to your veterinarian. I've had some really cut-up cats recover in a short time—no scars even! Cats have a good healing ability when given a chance—and good nursing.

CAR SICKNESS

Cats, on the whole, are not good travelers in the family car. They often get extremely nervous at the sight and feeling of the movement of the car. They can get so frightened they go berserk, clawing and yowling.

A more common reaction is for the cat to hide under the seat, yowl and drool. The cat is often nauseated, and sometimes vomits.

The cat can be given a tranquilizer a while before the trip is taken, but it sometimes has the opposite effect than you had hoped for. If the cat is to be tranquilized, it is best to try out the tranquilizer on your cat before the day the cat rides in the car.

Often car sickness can be avoided by placing the cat in a dark, closed-in box or cat carrier. Feeling hidden and more secure, the cat will not be as nervous and get car sick.

If the cat is going to have to ride periodically, it may be a good idea to get it slowly used to riding in the car. Short trips, like going to the corner store, school, or park are easier on the cat's nervous system and soon it will nearly relax in the car. Slowly lengthen the trips as the cat remains calm and appears relaxed.

CONJUNCTIVITIS

Conjunctivitis is the inflammation and often reddening of the conjunctiva (the light pink lining around the eyeball). Simple conjunctivitis is often caused by dust, weeds, pollen or other foreign bodies irritating the area, causing inflammation. Tearing and squinting are commonly found with this problem. Bacterial infections often follow the initial irritation, causing even further irritation and swelling. The cat may rub its eye with a paw, or rub its head on the floor. This only serves to irritate the area further.

Most cases of simple conjunctivitis or conjunctivitis complicated with a bacterial infection will clear up when an antibiotic ointment is used for a day or two. There are some excellent ointments on the market now that are inexpensive and contain not only an antibiotic, but a local anesthetic to deaden the pain and itching.

You should be aware, however, that conjunctivitis is often just a symptom of a disease, such as rhinotracheitis. So, if it does not clear up with minimum treatment, the cat should be taken to your veterinarian. If the cat acts sick at the same time the conjunctivitis is noticed, it is a sign that the conjunctivitis is coming along with some other disease, so take your cat to your veterinarian *before* attempting treatment.

CONSTIPATION

Constipation is another problem that is often associated with improper diet. Feeding too much dry food with not enough water intake, or small bones will often cause constipation. Never feed fish, chicken or chop bones to your cat. Not only do they cause constipation, but they can puncture the intestines and kill the animal. When feeding a dry cat food, alternate it at least twice a week with a canned food. If the cat is often bothered by constipation, it may be wise to put about a teaspoonful of vegetable oil in its food daily or feed more canned food. Milk added to a dry diet will also help prevent constipation.

CUTS

Cuts do happen in cats; they are often caused by hay mowers, fights, and the like. Should your cat get a cut, first stop any bleeding that may be present. This is usually quite easily done by means of a pressure bandage, which is simply a piece of gauze held firmly against the cut with your hand. Severe bleeding can be controlled by methods used on humans for first aid: tourniquet and the use of pressure points, between cut and heart or behind cut, depending on the vessel cut.

If the cut is a fairly fresh one—not more than a day old—it may heal best if stitched up. Many cuts do not. Included in these are cuts that are dirty, cuts over joints, and cuts over heavily muscled areas. Often a bad-looking cut will heal completely in a month, without suturing and without a scar. When the same wound is sewn up, healing takes about six weeks and leaves a scar. One reason for this is that the outside of the cut heals before the inside, sealing in a few bacteria. These bacteria soon multiply and cause an infection. A very mild infection can retard healing for a lengthy period. So, let your veterinarian make the decision whether to suture that cut or not. Many times I've been nearly ordered to sew up a cut that I knew would not heal properly and would become infected, or that I knew the cat would remove the stitches from. People think the wound looks better if it is not gaping open, I guess. What they don't realize is that it would be around a shorter period of time if left open and treated with an antibiotic.

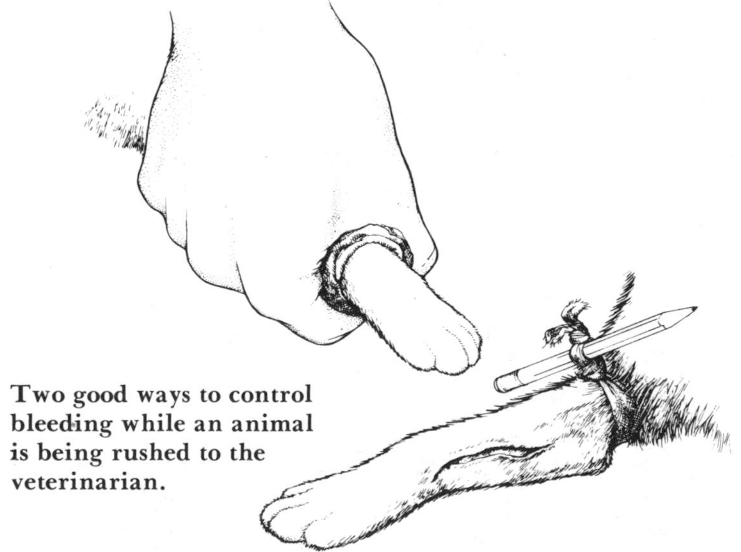

Two good ways to control bleeding while an animal is being rushed to the veterinarian.

Of course, some wounds are better sewn up. The point is: go to your veterinarian with an open mind, and just ask his opinion.

Bandages are another no-no. In few instances is a wound better off covered. A bandage retards healing by not allowing air to circulate freely around the wound. A bandage *is* useful to hold a pressure pack in place or to protect the animal from self-mutilation.

DIARRHEA

Diarrhea can be a problem or it can be a *symptom* of a problem. Like humans, cats occasionally are bothered by diarrhea. Pampered housecats are most susceptible to this problem. Improper feeding is the most common cause of simple diarrhea. Feeding such things as bologna, hotdogs, fried fish, spiced foods, and so on to a cat is just asking for gastric upsets.

When a cat is bothered by diarrhea, take *all* food away from it. Be sure to leave a full water dish out. Insufficient water intake, along with diarrhea, can cause dehydration. Give one teaspoonful of kaolin-pectin every three hours. If this does not stop the diarrhea in 12 hours, contact your veterinarian.

Diarrhea can be a symptom of many illnesses, some serious. Feline distemper and severe parasitic infections often have an accompanying diarrhea.

EAR INFECTIONS

Ear infections in cats are often brought about by ear mites. They burrow into the ear and provide places for bacteria and fungus to enter. Cats do not have the ear problems so often as dogs, because their ears stand erect and do not hang down like those of many breeds of dogs. The hanging ear makes a warm, moist incubator for bacteria and fungi.

When the cat shakes its head, scratches at the ears with its hind legs, and yowls, it pays to check the ears. Sometimes there is just an accumulation of wax and dirt in the ear canal. Swabbing the ear, first with a dampened ball of cotton (use alcohol or peroxide), then with a dry ball, will usually take care of a wax and dirt build-up. Go down into the ear as far as you can reach. If you aren't too forceful and don't use anything smaller than a cotton ball and your finger, there's little chance you'll do any damage to the ear while cleaning it. This cleaning may need to be repeated daily for two or three days.

If just cleaning the ear does not bring relief promptly, the cat should be taken to the veterinarian for closer examination and proper diagnosis. Treating the ear for ear mites will not help the cat infected with a fungus infection or bacterial infection which can only be correctly diagnosed by a vet. Ear infections left untreated, or treated improperly, can result in deafness or central nervous conditions.

FELINE DISTEMPER OR PANLEUKOPENIA

Panleukopenia or feline distemper is a very contagious disease that can strike unexpectedly, killing cats before any sign of illness is noticed. Symptoms include diarrhea, vomiting, weakness, depression, and quick death. This disease is often confused with poisoning, as it strikes so quickly and has such a high mortality rate.

Antibiotics to prevent secondary bacterial infections, fluids, and blood transfusions help a cat over the crisis. Good nursing and treating the symptoms, such as giving an antidiarrheal to combat fluid loss and drugs to quiet the stomach, are often essential. If the cat survives the first 48 hours after treatment has begun, its chances for recovery are usually quite good.

It is safer and far less expensive, though, to have your cat protected by a vaccination. The weanling kitten is usually vaccinated, then given a booster vaccination from two to 12 weeks later, depending on the product used. An annual booster following this is recommended for optimum protection.

FISHHOOK IN THE MOUTH

Cats, being curious and also hunters, often get tangled up in fishing tackle such as treble-hooked lures. Sharp, barbed hooks become imbedded very easily in the lips, but are very hard to remove, particularly from the mouth of a frightened cat. If only one hook is into the skin, it is sometimes possible to wrap the cat in a sturdy towel and clip the barbed point off with a pair of side cutters.

If the cat is too frantic or there is more than one hook in the skin, it is best to take the cat to a veterinarian for the hook removal. He can give the cat a slight injection of a quick-acting anesthetic that will immobilize it temporarily while the hooks are taken out.

FLEAS (AND OTHER EXTERNAL PARASITES)

Fleas are the main external parasites that bother cats. Ticks are rarely a problem, nor are lice under most circumstances. If watched for and not allowed to infest the cat in large numbers, fleas are quite easily controlled in cats. Dusting or spraying with a rotenone compound is safe and quite effective, should the cat pick up fleas. Remember, fleas do not stay on the cat exclusively and can be in the rug or in the cat's bedding. Be sure to spray these places at the same time the cat is de-flead.

Bathing the cat in a flea dip can be used, but many cats resent a bath, and for an inexperienced person, this method of flea control is not desirable.

There are, of course, flea collars on the market, but I hesitate to recommend their use, as some cats are adversely affected by them. Some cats are allergic to the chemicals contained in the collars, either developing rash or skin lesion around the neck where the collar fits, or developing respiratory problems. The collars especially cause problems in some cats after they have become wet. It seems to intensify the chemical residue left on the cat's neck. If a collar is used, be sure to remove it if the cat has been in the rain.

Some anesthetics are not safely given if the cat has been recently wearing a flea collar, so be sure to inform your veterinarian of this, should the cat require surgery.

I really would not recommend the usage of a flea collar, unless there is a severe flea allergy problem with a cat that other methods of flea control do not seem to help.

FLY LARVA

There is a fly larva that is sometimes seen in cats, quite often in kittens. It is the cuterebra. There is often only a tiny hole, in the neck area or under the chin. There may be a slight wetness in the area. The larva is large, sometimes nearly an inch long. On close examination, the larva can be seen moving around in the opening in the skin.

The larva should never be squeezed, as this can cause anaphylactic shock and kill the cat. The opening should be enlarged, and the larva removed slowly with a forceps. The wound should then be flushed out and treated with an antibiotic ointment or powder. Once the larva is removed, there are seldom any complications.

HAIRBALLS

Hairballs are a common problem in cats, especially long-haired cats. As the cat cleans itself, any hairs that are shed are often swallowed. In the stomach they mass together, forming a wad which in some instances may be as large as six or eight inches long and two or three inches in diameter. The cat may vomit these or show gastric distress from their presence. When passed further down the digestive tract, they can cause constipation or even complete intestinal blockage.

There are special preparations with a palatable base that are useful in expelling hairballs before they become a serious problem. Mineral oil, milk of magnesia, and castor oil will generally bring relief from the hairball, but are hard to give many cats.

HYPOCALCEMIA

Hypocalcemia is rarely seen in cats, but when it is, it must be treated soon after symptoms appear or the cat will die. It is seen just following the birth of kittens, from a week to three weeks following birth. It is most frequently seen where there is a very large litter of healthy, hungry kittens. The queen is called on to produce immense quantities of milk to supply these kittens, and she depletes the normal calcium in her bone, and begins drawing it from her blood.

She becomes incoordinated, stiff, shaky, and nervous. She may have fits or go into a coma.

Treatment by a veterinarian is needed at once to save her. Calcium is given by intravenous injection. Recovery is fast. On no account should the kittens be allowed to continue nursing, as the queen will have the same problem again, and this time it may kill her.

MANGE

Mange is not often seen in cats, but it does occur. Mange is caused by several different types of mites, but the results are about the same. The first signs of mange are usually scabby spots, often around the face, where the hair suddenly has fallen off. There may be a foul discharge, intense itching, thickened skin, large crusty areas, and large areas of hair loss.

The mites burrow into the skin, making them difficult to treat with common insecticides, such as those used for fleas. And the cat, being especially sensitive to toxic compounds, is sometimes difficult to treat effectively.

A malathion solution or rotenone solution is often used with good results, but should be used by your veterinarian so the cat can remain under his supervision following treatment, should a sensitivity to these compounds show up in the animal. The hair should be clipped completely and the scabs removed before treatment is begun, as it is hard enough to treat mange without trying to treat through matted hair.

The only way for a positive diagnosis to be made is by a skin scraping. Other problems can arise that *look* like mange, but they are not related, other than the fact that they cause skin lesions. Such things as fungal and bacterial infections, and flea allergies resemble mange, but will not be cured by the use of a mange remedy. A word of caution: *Do not use a dog mange remedy on a cat unless directed to by a veterinarian.* The wrong compound can kill the cat.

MASTITIS

Mastitis is inflammation of one or more mammary gland. It is often caused by a bacterial infection which invades the gland due to stress. Some common types of stress are injury such as bruising, falls, being stepped on, cat bites, getting banged in a door, copious milk supply not taken by kittens, and wounds to the teats.

When first noticed the affected gland is often swollen and hard. There is usually heat in the area of infection. The cat may act sick or in pain. The kittens may also be affected and act listless. They should be removed to a warm nest right away and kept off the mother until she is better. They can be fed by bottle.

Treatment often consists of giving a broad-spectrum antibiotic, hot packs and massage, plus squeezing as much milk from the affected gland as possible several times during the day.

PHENOL POISONING

Cats are highly susceptible to phenol and phenol compounds, as well as to iodine. Many household cleaners contain phenol, and many cats are poisoned unintentionally when drinking out of a toilet bowl containing Lysol or another cleaner. Never use a phenol shampoo, such as is often used on dogs, on a cat. Floors mopped with a phenol cleaner should be well rinsed and dried before allowing the cat into the room. Licking wet paws containing a heavy phenol concentration can cause serious gastric upsets.

A cat that has ingested large amounts of phenol will often sustain such extensive damage before the illness is discovered that it is very difficult to treat it successfully. When smaller amounts are taken, induction of vomiting, fluids given parenterally, preparations to soothe the stomach and intestines, and good nursing will often bring relief.

PNEUMONITIS

Pneumonitis is caused by a virus. It is very contagious and is spread by direct contact. The first signs noticed are usually sneezing and coughing. There is often a discharge from the eyes and nose. Kittens often have weight loss as they lose their appetite. There is also a temperature of from .5 to two degrees above normal, which is short lasting. Adult cats are not hit as hard as kittens, as they generally stay in good condition.

Treatment with a broad-spectrum antibiotic to prevent secondary invasions such as pneumonia, plus good nursing, are important. Most cats treated fairly early in the course of the disease recover with little trouble.

It is important to remember that there are other feline diseases that have symptoms like pneumonitis, and not every disease causing sneezing, coughing, and runny eyes and nose is definitely pneumonitis. Be sure to consult your veterinarian.

RABIES

Rabies is not as often seen in cats as it is in bats, skunks, fox and dogs. But, unfortunately, it can and does occur. It is always fatal, once signs of the disease appear. And, of course, it can be spread to man with fatal results unless treatment is given immediately, before symptoms occur.

There are two types of rabies: dumb rabies and furious rabies. With furious rabies, really fewer people are endangered, because they naturally avoid a biting, yowling, scratching cat. But with dumb rabies, the cat sits around with its lower jaw hanging down and saliva running out of its mouth. Often such a cat is thought only to have a bone stuck in its throat, and a person becomes infected by being scratched slightly and having the disease-spreading saliva rubbed into the abrasion.

Rabies is spread most often by a bite, contaminated by saliva which carries the virus. Exposure is possible from other routes, but it is uncommon. Many rabid animals develop a complete personality change. A quiet, loving cat will become shy or vicious. A nasty cat will suddenly become loving and want attention. There is often a change in the voice, due to paralysis of the throat. The rabid animal will often either quit eating or develop a depraved appetite. There may be stiffness in the hind limbs.

Any animal with the above symptoms should be treated with caution and either isolated in an escape-proof cage or taken to a veterinarian for a check-up. Don't, however, think your female in heat has rabies, because of her "change in voice" and strange behavior!

If bitten by a suspected rabid cat, try to capture the cat and contact your veterinarian and physician immediately.

There is no treatment for rabies in the cat, but there is a very effective vaccination available. And with cats being the natural hunters they are, it is a very good idea to have one vaccinated, not only to protect the cat, but to protect your family as well.

RHINOTRACHEITIS

Rhinotracheitis resembles pneumonitis, as the cat has mattered eyes, a copious discharge from both nose and eyes, and coughs and sneezes. It is also caused by a virus. There is no vaccination to prevent it as there is for pneumonitis. Treatment is more difficult, and it is often good nursing rather than drugs that brings a cat through the disease. Cats that recover from it can be carriers and transmit the virus to others.

RINGWORM

Ringworm is caused by a fungus, often *Microsporum canis.* It is *not* a "worm" nor is it caused by a worm. It is a circular lesion appearing often quite suddenly. The skin is often rough, the hair gone from the spot. If left untreated, the spot gets larger and larger, usually retaining the circular pattern.

Ringworm, or rather, some types of ringworm, are contagious to humans. All can be passed back and forth among animals of a like species. So, if ringworm is suspected, isolate the affected cat immediately, and then check all the other cats and kittens right away.

Iodine preparations are often used in ringworm in cattle and dogs. But, many cats are highly sensitive to iodine, and have severe trouble resulting from its use.

Diagnosis is made by either a skin scraping and examination under a microscope or ultraviolet light. Treatments vary, from soaking the animal in a medicated shampoo to treating the spots alone with a good, low toxicity fungicide. If the spots are treated at home, be sure to use rubber gloves and apply the medication from the outside of the spot toward the inside of the spot. If the opposite is done, the fungus can be spread.

URINARY CALCULI

Urinary calculi most often causes trouble in male cats rather than female cats. There is a divided opinion as to whether or not castration affects the incidence of the problem. Some studies have been done, and they reveal no significant difference in the size of the urethra, but many veterinarians do believe there is a definite connection between castration of young males and urinary calculi. I personally have found that 90 percent of the cats affected by urinary calculi have been altered males.

Castration is generally recommended for cats between seven and nine months of age, and not younger. Feeding a diet of only dry food will often contribute to the problem. When fed a moist diet, such as canned food or meat, the cat gets additional moisture through the food. When eating dry food, the cat often does not drink enough additional water.

A change in the pH of the bladder, whether due to an infection or other causes, can contribute to urinary calculi. As the pH in the bladder becomes more alkaline, salts, crystals, and calcium precipitate out, forming the calculi.

Many times the cat has passed several smaller calculi before one lodges and blocks the urethra. The usual symptoms first noticed are straining at the litter tray, dullness, and loss of appetite. The distended bladder can be felt as a hard, roundish bulge in the abdomen. The cat must be taken immediately to the veterinarian for treatment. When the problem progresses, the cat becomes toxic by absorbing the waste material. When it becomes very ill from uremia, treatment is difficult, and the cat often dies.

Treatment consists of emptying the bladder, by use of a catheter, direct tap, or by flushing the urethra to dislodge the plug. An attempt is made to acidify the bladder by use of oral medication. Antibiotics are often given to take care of any infection present or possibly following the trauma of the blockage.

The cat, once again in the home, should be placed on a strict diet of meat, boiled eggs, or a prescription diet. Feeding cat food with fish, dry foods, and high ash diets can contribute to a recurrence of the problem. Some cats must receive a daily medication to keep the urine acid enough to prevent calculi.

WARFARIN POISONING

Even though supposedly safe for children and pets, warfarin can sometimes poison cats. There are two popular rodenticides which usually cause trouble. Most often the cat either eats the rodent bait or eats a rodent which is already sick from the poison. Continuous feeding on poisoned rodents can kill cats. Warfarin and other rodenticides contain a drug, dicoumarin, which causes hemorrhage throughout the body. Affected cats appear weak, anemic, and depressed. They do not appear in pain or to be severely distressed.

When you suspect that the cat may have had access to a rodenticide or to poisoned rodents, warfarin poisoning should be kept in mind and the cat taken immediately to the veterinarian. Blood transfusions, vitamin K, fluids, and confinement will all aid in helping the blood to clot. No rodenticides should be left where it is at all possible for pets or children to reach them.

WORMS

Although cats are less often severely bothered with worms than dogs, there are several types that do infest them on occasion.

Hookworm Hookworm can be found in cats. Anemia, bloody stools, diarrhea, and unthriftiness are symptoms.

Young kittens are the hardest hit and often die suddenly. These worms are not seen in the stool nor are they normally visible with the naked eye.

Roundworm Roundworm is the most common. This worm is visible to the naked eye and looks like a bean sprout. It is most often seen after being vomited up, often along with a hairball. A severely infested cat will have a potbelly, bad haircoat, and act listless.

Tapeworm Tapeworm, which quite often infests cats, is carried into the cat via the flea. While cleaning itself, the cat can swallow a flea containing tapeworm larvae. Soon the cat is infested with an adult tapeworm up to two feet in length. Tapeworm can also be passed to the cat through infested rabbits or other rodents eaten by the cat. Tapeworm segments are eliminated with fecal material and often cling to the rectal area. When just passed, they look like an inchworm. When dry, they look like small grains of rice. The cat with tapeworm may just appear unthrifty, or it may have digestive or nervous disorders. Some cats do not show signs of trouble, but still are infested with a tapeworm.

There are many other worms and intestinal parasites that can and have infested cats. A few of them are threadworms, lung flukes, liver flukes, *Giardia,* coccidia, lungworms, heartworms, and *Babesia felis.* Many come from eating infested rodents. Others are picked up when the cat licks the eggs off its feet while washing.

When suspecting intestinal parasites, be sure to take a fecal sample to your veterinarian for examination. Each worm or group of worms has one or two worm medicines that work best.

Some worms have rather complicated treatments. Just buying a "shotgun" wormer at the drugstore will do your cat no good and may even be dangerous, should the cat be severely debilitated or sick with, say, a bacterial infection rather than worms.

The cat should have a fecal examination for worms and other intestinal parasites at least yearly. Many parasites do not cause visible damage until there is not much that can be done to improve the cat's health after removing the worms. Lungworms cause scarring and infections in the respiratory tract. Many protozoa cause ulceration in the intestinal tract, which can become infected. Many worms cause digestive upsets as they burrow into the mucous lining of the stomach and intestines, sometimes severe enough to kill the cat. Hookworm can cause anemia severe enough to bring on sudden death. Migrating large and dead adult worms can cause plugs in blood vessels or heart attacks. And so on.

The point is, the few minutes it takes to collect a small fecal sample and take it to your veterinarian could easily save the cat's health, if not its life.

SOME BASICS FOR THE LAYPERSON

DRUG ADMINISTRATION

Oral Liquid Oral medications are used primarily either to give treatment for gastrointestinal troubles such as diarrhea or worms, or to institute systemic therapy for bacterial infections.

If it is not done properly, giving farm animals liquid orally can be a problem because of their size and strength. Restraint is essential. You just can't chase an animal around with a drenching bottle or syringe stuck in its mouth. When giving a liquid orally, the head should be tilted upward, but the mouth should not be higher than the eyes. If the head is tipped upward too far, large amounts of liquid can choke the animal, or worse, get into the lungs and cause inhalation pneumonia.

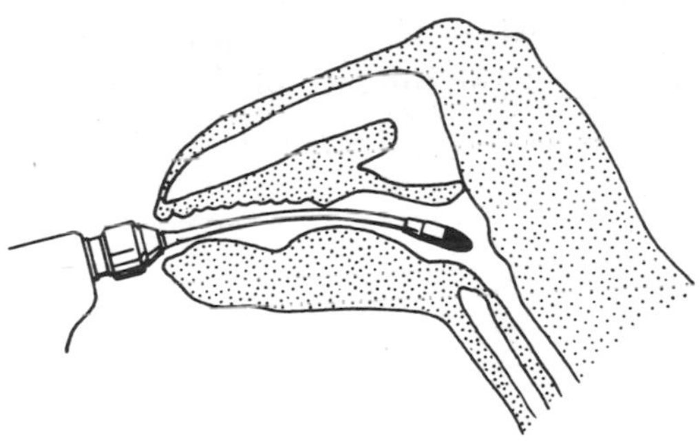

Drenching with Head in Normal Position

The medicine is usually more readily acceptable if mixed with diluted honey or molasses. Small amounts should be given at a time, allowing the patient to swallow before more is given. The animal should be kept calm and unexcited to prevent gasping, which would otherwise allow droplets to get into the lungs. A glass bottle should not be used, especially by the novice, as it can break if it's knocked against the teeth or bitten by the patient.

A dog will take liquid easier if you can form a pouch with the lower lip to receive the liquid. Administer a small amount then tilt the head slightly back and stroke the throat. When swallowing occurs, give it the rest of the medicine in the same way.

Cats are a little harder to dose with an oral medicine. An eye dropper or syringe is often easier to give medicine with than a spoon, due to the size of the mouth. An unruly cat can be wrapped up in a heavy towel to avoid scratches with the hind feet.

Small amounts of oral medicine can be mixed with a sticky substance such as honey and smeared on the nose or front paws. The cat, when cleaning itself, will lick off the medicine. Do not use this method on a very ill cat, as the cat will not feel like cleaning itself when very sick, and the medicine will do no good and will only make a mess.

Oral Pill Pills are often used to get oral medicine into small animals. Under the term "pill" we also include tablets and capsules. Dogs are quite easy to give pills to, with the exception of the very neurotic dog or the mean dog. The average family pet, if eating, can often be given a pill wrapped up in some hamburger, or better yet, a chunk of hot dog. (This has a strong odor which masks any odor the pill may have.) When capsules and pills come with instructions that they should not be chewed, they obviously should not be given in food. Some dogs are very clever about taking medicated food. They may take the meat, then spit out the pill. Most pills can be crushed, which eliminates the feel of a lump in the meat. With the wise dog, give a small ball of unmedicated food, quickly followed by a medicated ball, then quickly give another unmedicated ball. In its haste to get all the meat, the dog will usually gobble up the medicated ball with no hesitation.

The cat can be treated in this way also. Cats are especially careful of what they eat, so try to be particularly careful when you conceal the medication.

Sometimes it is necessary to give the pill by hand, as with the very sick animal that refuses to eat. With a dog, the best method is to simply push the pill down its throat as far as you can. Just putting it into the dog's mouth is not enough, as it will chew it, spit it out, and may put up a fight when you further try to give it more medication. If the dog is not excited and the pill is quickly slipped down its throat, most dogs will instinctively swallow without a struggle. If the dog must receive more than one pill, give only one at a time. An exception can be made for very tiny pills. But even with these, no more than two should be given together, or the dog may have some trouble swallowing. If swallowing is uncomfortable to the dog, it will not be easy to dose the second time.

Cats don't often take pills easily. If the top lip is curled around the top canine teeth and the paws are restrained by an assistant, the mouth can be quickly opened and the pill inserted down the throat with the thrust of one finger. The mouth is quickly shut, and the throat stroked to encourage swallowing. This method may also be used on a dog that struggles or tries to bite when being dosed.

Oral Bolus Because of their large size, farm animals receive a bolus rather than a pill. The bolus (say bowl-us) is usually a large oblong pill. Again, restraint is very important in proper administration.

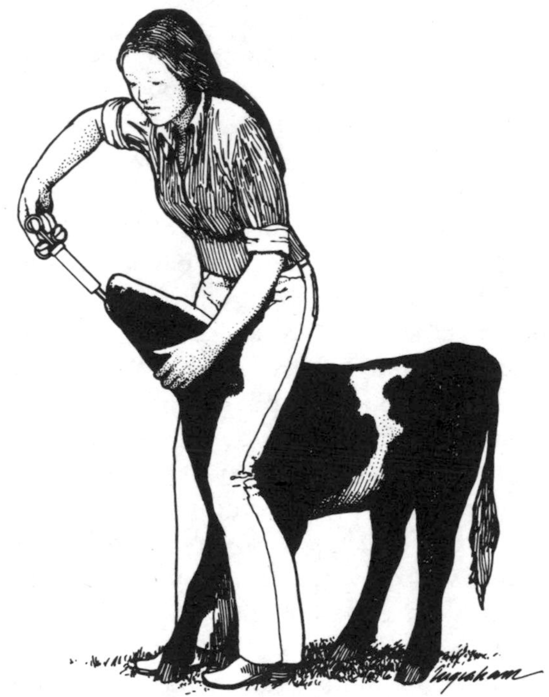

The bolus is most easily given with the aid of a balling gun. The bolus fits into the gun, which is inserted into the mouth and thrust behind the tongue. The bolus is then popped down the throat. There is usually little objection from the animal when a balling gun is used. It is a lot easier than trying to avoid the sharp teeth while dosing.

It is usually easiest to lubricate the bolus with shortening or lard before placing it in the balling gun. The bolus will slip down the throat easier, and when the animal comfortably swallows the bolus, it will be easier to dose the second time.

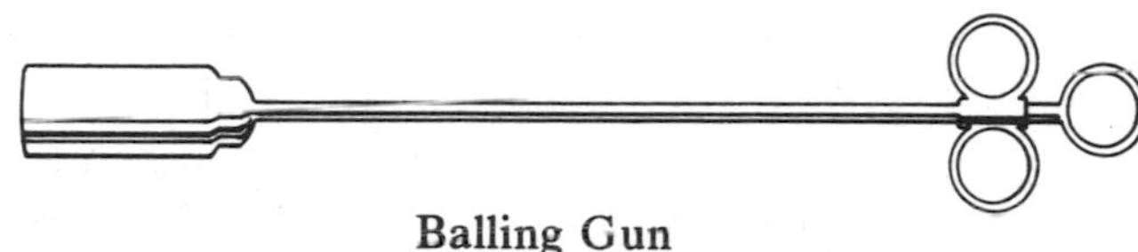

Balling Gun

Medicated Feed or Water There are many medications, either liquids or powders, that are meant to be mixed with the feed or water. Objectionable tasting medications are often hard to give in this way. Sometimes the addition of Kool-Aid to the drinking water one or two days before medication is to be given and then on the day of medication will mask the odor and taste of the drug in the water. When medication is given in dry feed, you can often mask its taste and smell by either adding molasses to the feed, or by smearing a strong smelling ointment such as Vicks or camphorated oil on the animal's nose. In any case, there should be no other source of feed or water available until the medication has been taken.

Medication via the Stomach Tube A stomach tube is often used by veterinarians to administer large quantities of

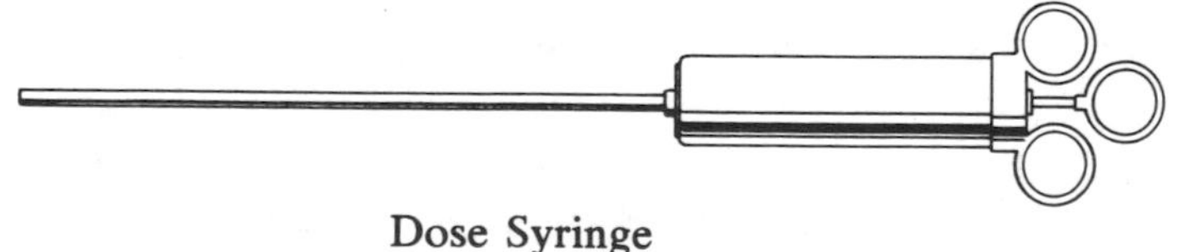

Dose Syringe

liquids, particularly to large animals. When a ruminant such as a goat or cow is treated by use of the stomach tube, a mouth speculum is frequently used. This is a short, pipelike instrument used to keep the animal from biting the flexible tube, thereby making it easier to slip the tube down the throat. Horses usually receive the stomach tube through the nostril. In such cases no speculum is used. Once in the stomach, the medication is pumped down. Care must be used that the tube does not go into the lung. If that were to happen, death would be the result after the medication had been administered. Never use a milk hose or garden hose when attempting to administer drugs. These have sharp edges and may cut or scrape the esophagus, resulting in death.

Intramuscular Injection The intramuscular (IM) injection is often used with many drugs, due to the ease of administration and the rapid absorption of the medicine. Any large muscle mass can be used for the intramuscular injection, but those most often used are in the side of the neck and in the hindquarters.

The hair is cleaned of any dirt or debris. I do not use the term sterilized, because it is impossible to sterilize skin, especially skin that is covered by hair. What is done is not sterilization but mechanical removal of bacteria, along with the dirt.

With large animals it is usually easiest to take the needle off of the syringe, give the animal a couple of slaps with the back of your hand, then quickly plunge the needle into the muscle. The nerves in the skin will still be tingling from the slaps, and the animal will not feel the needle enter the body. Then the needle is reattached to the syringe. To be certain you have not hit a blood vessel, draw back on the syringe. If blood enters the syringe, you are into a blood vessel and should retract or advance the needle.

The drug is then injected. On pulling the needle out of the skin, it is often a good idea to massage the area to aid absorption and to reduce leakage through the puncture in the skin.

Intravenous Injection The intravenous (IV) injection often is used to administer large amounts of a drug or to get a drug into the bloodstream more quickly. It is harder to learn to do properly, and it takes more caution in administering than other parenteral treatment. Only those solutions recommended for intravenous use should be given in that way, as many drugs will kill when given improperly. An intravenous injection is usually given to horses, cows, sheep, and goats in the jugular vein. Dogs and cats most often receive an intravenous injection in the large vein in the front leg. Other veins are used occasionally; ear, hind leg, tongue, and milk veins are sometimes chosen. The vein is often popped up, by use of a tourniquet or by manual pressure, behind the injection site. The needle, with syringe attached, is pushed into the vein. (In cattle, it is not necessary to use the syringe, as a larger needle is used from which the blood flows when the needle enters the vein.) When the needle enters the vein, blood will enter the

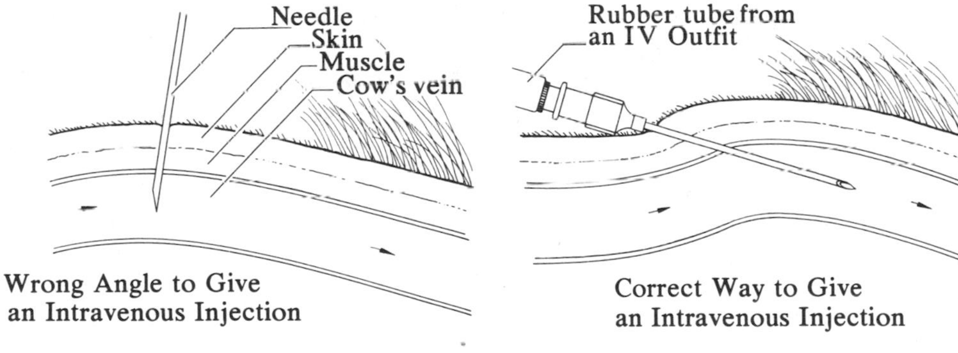

Wrong Angle to Give an Intravenous Injection

Correct Way to Give an Intravenous Injection

syringe immediately, especially if a little suction is applied by drawing back on the plunger of the syringe.

The needle is threaded up through the vein, with the needle parallel to the vein. This holds it in place, should the animal make a sudden move. The drug is then administered. When large volumes of medication are needed, the needle should be taped to the skin. Ether—such as that used to start cars—is sprayed on the tape to increase the tape's sticking ability.

No intravenous solution should be administered rapidly. Some drugs can cause serious discomfort, or even kill the animal, if they hit the heart too rapidly. Do not let the needle slip from the vein or be stuck all the way through to the other side. Some intravenous drugs are irritating to the muscle and there can be serious irritation, should the drug leak out of the vein.

Intraperitoneal Injection When it is not possible to give an intravenous injection, the intraperitoneal route (injection into the abdominal cavity itself) is often chosen. There is rapid absorption, and large amounts of fluid can be given in this way. Fluids such as electrolytes are often given by this method.

A long needle is usually needed in order to penetrate the skin, muscle, and peritoneum sufficiently to administer the drug or fluid easily. The needle is slowly but firmly inserted through the abdominal wall. Do not jab, or you may hit an intestine or other body organ. When the needle is in place, administration of the drug is started.

An intraperitoneal injection will sometimes cause temporary abdominal cramps. These will pass as the fluid is absorbed. Slow administration of the drug will often prevent this.

Subcutaneous Injection Subcutaneous injection is recommended for many drugs. Because the drug is administered just under the skin, the injection is usually quite painless and easily given. Care should be taken to read labels. Drugs not meant for subcutaneous injection can cause irritation and abscesses. The subcutaneous injection should be given in an area where there is loose skin. The neck, flank, and withers are all routinely used. If large volumes of fluids are to be given, it is best to use several injection sites rather than one, as excessive irritation may result.

After the injection is complete, rub the site vigorously, as this aids absorption and prevents leaking. Leaking is often a problem in subcutaneous injections, due to the back pressure of the drug as it lays under the skin. Again, vigorous massage will help prevent this.

Intradermal Injection Intradermal injection is made *into* the skin, as compared to *under* the skin, as in a subcutaneous injection. Intradermal injection is most often used in certain vaccinations and in the TB test. Very few drugs are administered in this way.

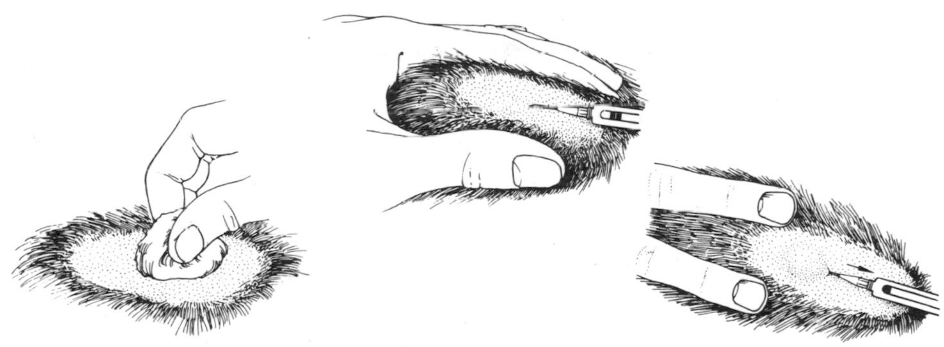

Making an Intradermal Injection

Epidural Injection This is the "spinal" often given to large animals during some obstetrical work and when the uterus has been thrown out and must be replaced. The anesthetic is administered in between the vertebrae and numbs the entire rear quarters, eliminating straining.

ANTIBIOTIC COMPATIBILITY

There are certain antibiotics that enhance each other's action. These drugs are often commercially mixed or given simultaneously. Such drugs are penicillin-streptomycin, penicillin-neomycin, and neomycin-polymixin B.

There are also some drugs that are antagonistic toward each other, interfering with each other's action. An example of this is penicillin with tetracycline. When used together or at the same time, or even closely following one another, each may negate the effects of the other. A typical example of this is when scouring calves are treated. Often Terramycin is given as a bolus, and Combiotic (penicillin-streptomycin) is given parenterally. Studies have been done which indicate the futility of such treatment; the one cancels out the other. Be sure, when using more than one antibiotic or when changing antibiotic therapy, that you consult your veterinarian. There is no need to waste money and time by using any other than the most compatible of drugs.

ACTION OF A VACCINE

A vaccine is made up of the agent that causes the disease. It is either live, attenuated (weakened), or dead. When administered, it initiates the production of antibodies by the host's body against that specific agent. Antibodies are produced by a natural body defense mechanism to combat a disease or foreign protein. Sometimes it is necessary to give a "booster" vaccination. This is a repeat of the first vaccination. After the first vaccination, the body builds up a level of protective antibodies, which, depending on the vaccine, may or may not drop after a period of time. If it drops, a "booster" is given to raise the level, keeping the animal safe.

VIRUS OR BACTERIA?

Virus The virus reproduces itself and thus is considered living. Viruses have no energy of their own, so they obtain energy from body cells which they enter. Different viruses have preferences for different parts of the body. For example, rabies affects the central nervous system, and red nose in cattle affects the respiratory system and reproductive tract. The virus disease has to run its course while the patient is supported by good nursing and given antibiotics to prevent it from picking up secondary bacterial infections, while its resistance is low.

Viruses cause damage to body cells from inside the cell, so anything that will effectively kill the virus will, 99 percent of the time, damage or kill the body cells as well. At the present time there is no specific treatment of any viral diseases, other than vaccinating against them before sickness strikes.

Bacteria Bacteria, in contrast, are known to be one-celled organisms and are members of the plant family. Many bacteria found in or on animals are harmless and even necessary, that is, as long as they stay in their normal place in the body. But if for some reason they show up where they don't belong, they can cause trouble. For example, *E. coli* is a normal gut bacteria and has essential functions in the alimentary canal. If *E. coli* should suddenly be transferred to the urinary tract and then the bladder, the results may be cystitis, or inflammation of the bladder.

Bacteria cause trouble in different ways than viruses do. While viruses work from within a body cell, bacteria work by overwhelming the body by sheer numbers (as weeds do a garden), or by producing a toxin which is detrimental to the health of the host. An example is the clostridia organisms, of which certain species produce toxin which in turn can cause tetanus, botulism poisoning, gas gangrene, blackleg, and so forth.

Bacteria are classified in various ways. The classification is based on the way the organisms stain with the Gram stain, which is a routine stain used in all diagnostic laboratories. All bacteria are either Gram-positive or Gram-negative and remain thus. This staining characteristic is also closely connected to the susceptibility of the organism to a particular drug or antibiotic. Some antibiotics are primarily effective only against Gram-positive organisms—for example, penicillin. Other drugs are mainly effective against Gram-negative organisms. Then there are broad-spectrum antibiotics which are effective against both types of organisms.

However, all antibiotics effective primarily against Gram-positive organisms are not effective against *all* Gram-positive organisms, and not all antibiotics effective against Gram-negative organisms are effective against *all* Gram-negative organisms. Nor are the broad-spectrum antibiotics effective against *all* organisms. Sensitivity tests can be run in a laboratory to determine which antibiotic is more effective against a certain organism. For example, *Staphylococcus aureus* is a common skin contaminant and is a Gram-positive organism. It should, by reason, be sensitive to penicillin, and it quite often is. But you can run into a staph aureus that might be sensitive only to an antibiotic that is very rarely used because its effectiveness is not as consistent as that of another antibiotic, say, penicillin.

This is why, when at all possible, it is best to first have a culture taken to identify the organism, then a sensitivity test run on it so that the infection can be treated effectively and without loss of time.

HANDLING THE ANIMAL WHEN IN SHOCK AND WITH POSSIBLE INTERNAL INJURIES

Shock is a condition often brought about by trauma, which shows itself in reduced circulation, rapid breathing, rapid pulse, often subnormal temperature, weakness, vomiting, and prostration. It can be difficult, without running tests, to determine the difference between shock and internal bleeding, which may happen after an accident involving a car and an animal. Drugs given to increase blood pressure, which are needed in shock, will only serve to increase hemorrhage if there already is internal bleeding. Therefore, it is important to differentiate between the two. Remember also that shock can be brought about by hemorrhage.

The cause of the shock should be determined, if at all possible. If the cause of the shock can be removed, such as severe chilling (due to falling through ice or being stuck in a snow bank) or heat exhaustion, for instance, the recovery will be much aided. The patient should not be excited or moved unnecessarily. With small animals, a blanket slipped under it like a stretcher will make moving safer. Large animals should be left where they are and covered with a blanket to prevent chilling, unless, of course, it is very hot outdoors in which case any additional heat can add to the shock.

In either case, the animal should receive prompt veterinary attention. There are many drugs used to combat shock and internal hemorrhage, but they are of no use when the animal has been in severe shock for so long a period that it is past the point of no return.

Any injured animal should be checked for paleness of the gums and mucous membranes before being moved. Paleness may indicate internal bleeding, and if there is internal bleeding, moving the animal might be very dangerous.

ELECTROLYTES IN THE BODY

Electrolytes are normal bases, acids, and salts found in the blood. The loss of fluid due to scours, fever, etc., is the loss of water and electrolytes. Seldom is there a loss of water alone. And in electrolyte therapy, not only does the water have to be replaced, but also sodium, magnesium, potassium, and calcium, combined with sulfates, chlorides, bicarbonate, phosphate, along with amino acids and proteins. When the animal is dehydrated to a critical point, cellular death occurs. Replacement of water and electrolytes, to compensate for their loss until the condition causing the loss is corrected, is necessary to prevent irreversible damage. Electrolytes are often given intravenously over a period of several hours as a continuous drip. They are also used subcutaneously and intraperitoneally in many cases for ease of administration by the layman.

The use of oral electrolytes in the place of milk for scouring calves is becoming popular. The electrolytes replace the irritating milk which is only making the scours worse, and at the same time they aid in restoring the electrolyte balance in the body.

THE IMPORTANCE OF BODY TEMPERATURE

Although it will vary from individual animal to individual animal, there is an average normal temperature for each kind of animal. It is a good idea to have on record each of your animal's normal temperature. Of course if you own many animals this may not be possible.

When an infection or septicemia is present in the body, very often there will be a rise in temperature. This temperature rise is a body defense mechanism which tries to kill the bacteria by heat. It does not, however, work in all cases. When an animal appears sick, take its temperature before any treatment is begun. If the temperature is up one or two degrees and treatment is started, the temperature should be on the decline in 24 hours. If it is not, or if it continues to rise, there may be a need to change antibiotics. If the temperature is down, you will have a good idea that the antibiotic you are using is doing its job. A very high temperature can destroy brain cells, so it may be necessary to use alcohol baths or aspirin to reduce the fever until the antibiotic begins to work.

A slight subnormal temperature is often a sign of shock. One or two (or more) degrees subnormal usually is a sign that the animal is dying. An effort should be made to raise the temperature to near normal by means of heat lamps or heating pads. Just using blankets will not work, as the animal has lost the ability to produce its own heat, and unless an electric

NORMAL TEMPERATURE RANGE

Cows	101°-102°F.	*Chickens	105°-109°F.
Goats	102°-103°F.	Dogs	100°-103°F.
Horses	99°-101°F.	Cats	100.5°-102.5°F.
Sheep	101°-102°F.	Rabbits	101°-103°F.
Pigs	101°-102.5°F.		

*This temperature range holds true for all poultry. Although, generally speaking, the smaller the bird, the higher its normal temperature. For example, a starling's normal temperature is 110°F. and a swan's is 106°F.

blanket is used, the blanket cannot produce heat of its own. When an animal's temperature has remained subnormal for quite some time, irreversible damage is usually done, and nothing can save it.

Taking an Animal's Temperature Any animal that acts abnormal should have its temperature taken as the first step. No medication should be given prior to this, for if it is given it will never be known if the animal had a temperature before the medication was given and the medication knocked down the temperature, or if the animal never had one in the first place. An above-normal temperature indicates a bloodstream infection or sickness in the animal. A below-normal temperature indicates shock and often a dying animal.

Any thermometer can be used—it matters not if it is a human oral thermometer, which is most often handy. But the animal must have its temperature taken rectally. The thermometer is

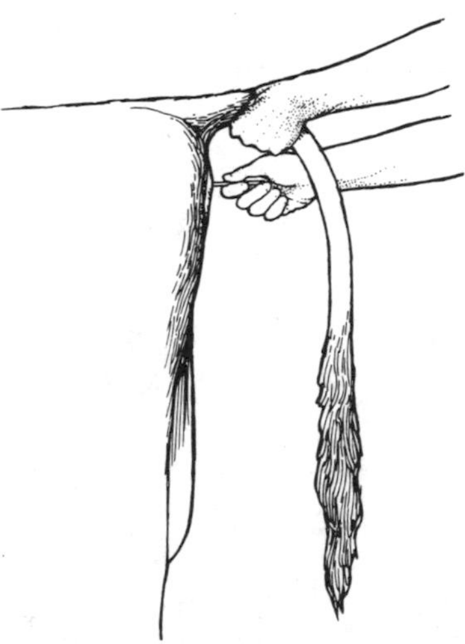

When taking rectal temperature, shake thermometer down and insert it halfway into the rectum, while holding the tail to steady the animal.

shaken down to below normal for that animal. The tail is grasped, and the thermometer is inserted an inch or two into the rectum. It is left in place for three minutes, while the animal is held quietly. Most animals are quite easy to handle during this process.

ARTIFICIAL RESPIRATION

There are some instances where it becomes necessary to give an animal artificial respiration. Quite often it is necessary in newborn animals that have not begun to breathe, animals that have received an electrical shock, or those that have drowned. With small animals, there are two methods that are used.

One is the mouth-to-mouth method, where you cup your hands around the mouth and blow directly in. The amount of

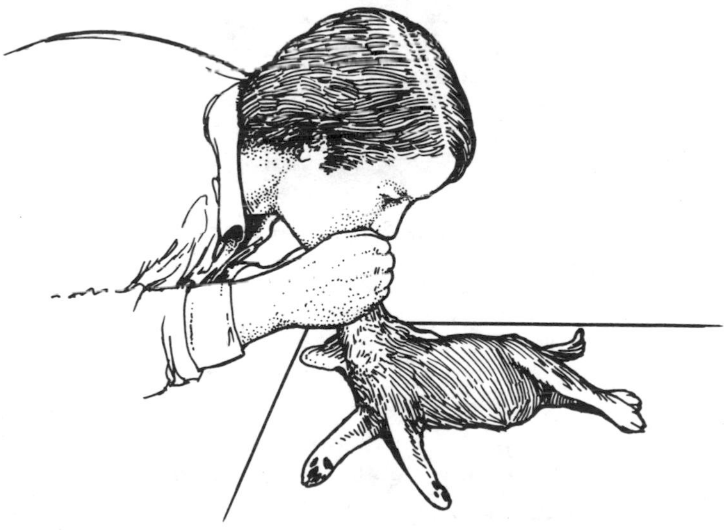

When giving artificial respiration to a small animal, cup your hands to prevent air from escaping when you blow.

air needed varies with the size of the animal. The chest should expand to natural size with each breath. Be sure the mouth and throat are clear of fluids and mucus. Should the animal have drowned, be sure to drain the lungs and air passages of water by holding the animal upside down by the hind legs. Quickly wipe the mouth clear, then begin artificial respiration.

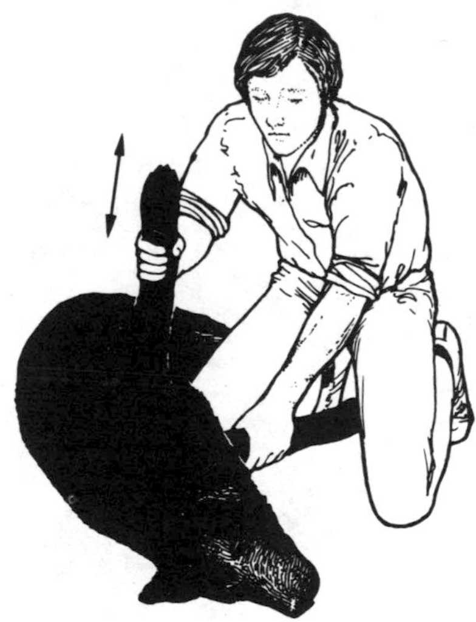

Artificial Respiration on Larger Animals

The second method used on small animals is also the one used on larger animals. The animal is laid on its side, and the top foreleg is raised, while the bottom one is held down. The animal is "played" like an accordian, pressing down and pulling up on the top leg every four seconds. This allows the lungs to fill and compress.

Sometimes pain will work to get the animal breathing again when nothing else will. This is especially true of newborns.

(Remember, the human doctor smacks baby's bottom at birth if breathing has not started well.) Poking a finger up the nose or down the throat, biting or pinching an ear, or slapping the chest may cause the animal to gasp, and breathing will start. As long as there is a heartbeat, there is life and a chance to save the animal.

As soon as the animal begins to breathe, keep it warm and visit your veterinarian to guard against pneumonia that sometimes follows.

ACCIDENTS TO WHICH ALL ANIMALS ARE SUSCEPTIBLE

Beesting When an animal is stung by a bee or wasp the area should be inspected for the stinger. When located, it should be scraped out, using a fingernail. Don't pick it out with the fingers because extra poison may be squeezed into the wound if the poison sac is still attached to the stinger. The hair then should be clipped allowing access to the sting. Often a cold pack, along with a paste made from a little baking soda mixed with water applied to the sting, will quickly relieve the pain.

In cases of severe sting it may become necessary to give the animal an injection of antihistamine to combat the allergic reaction, which could kill the animal.

Burns Animals most often receive burns by having some hot liquid spilled on them or by stepping on a hot stove, fire, etc. With good nursing, most burns heal rapidly and well. Soon after the burn is received the hair in the area should be clipped off. The area should then be flushed with cool, soapy water, then rinsed. With small areas, an ointment containing antibiotics and a local anesthetic, such as tetracaine, should be used.

When a larger area is to be treated it is best to consult with your veterinarian. Many animals suffer shock when a large area is burned. Often using cloths soaked in a mild saline solution on the burn area and giving systemic antibiotics and fluids will save an animal that might have otherwise died. Good nursing is very important in severe burn cases. A high protein diet with a good vitamin-mineral supplement will aid healing.

Poisoning In cases of poisoning (be sure the animal was poisoned and is just not ill) encourage the animal to vomit (unless otherwise indicated on the poison product's label) by giving it a couple of tablespoonsful of salt on the back of the tongue, mustard and water, or warm salt water. This will get the toxic material out of the stomach, preventing more from being absorbed into the system. Then rush the animal to the veterinarian. *Do not give emetics if the animal is having convulsions or is stiff.* Such symptoms indicate strychnine poisoning. With this poison, the animal's nerves are supersensitive, and even slight stimuli, such as light or a small noise, can throw it into a convulsion. Giving an emetic can cause so violent a convulsion that the animal may die.

There are many hundreds of toxic materials, many specific to a certain area; among these are poisonous plants. It is a good idea to see your local veterinarian or county agent concerning them. Some are only poisonous at a certain time of the year; in others, only one part of the plant (roots or leaves, etc.) is toxic. A few plants that are toxic to livestock are chokecherries, lupines, cocklebur, bracken fern, lechuguilla, rubberweed, milkweed, water hemlock, lambkill, castor bean, sorghum, Sudan grass, jimsonweed, and buttercup.

Lead poisoning used to be very common, especially when young cattle licked and chewed at barn walls and fences that had been painted with a lead-based paint. Lead poisoning should still be considered if the buildings have old paint on them and the animals exhibit illness in the form of weakness, staggering, and diarrhea.

Clay pigeons used in trapshooting will poison hogs, as will molds growing in corners of feeders. Moldy sweet clover hay, stunted sorghum, and wilted chokecherry leaves often poison cattle. Rat poisons and fly bait sometimes kill more poultry than vermin. Doubling up on organophosphates have killed horses and small animals. Insecticides, such as fly sprays and flea collars, can kill an animal that has been given a general anesthetic. Chemical fertilizers and herbicides should be stored carefully because cattle can die from eating the bags in which these toxic substances are packed. Salt can poison, especially if too much has been accidently mixed with the feed. Few animals will poison themselves on salt if they are fed it free choice. Alkali poisoning is a problem in some areas. Rhubarb leaves can poison an animal eating even just a few of them.

The above are listed just to give you an idea of a few of the many toxic materials quite readily available to animals. Most have different symptoms. If you are aware of what actions are normal for your animals and check them daily, you should be able to spot any unusual signs before the animal is past help. When in doubt, call your veterinarian and ask his opinion.

Prolapsed Eyeball Certain traumas can cause the eyeball to prolapse, or in other words, pop out of the socket. Bumping the eye just so or severe strain, especially with such breeds of dogs as Pekingese, can cause a prolapsed eye.

The two most important things here are to keep the animal calm and restrained, and to try to get the eyeball back into the socket as soon as possible. The wild animal can tear the eyeball off on a fence or furniture, and the longer the eyeball is out of the socket, the less chance there is of getting it back in.

Often the eyeball can be replaced by simply holding a warm, damp cloth over the eyeball, and firmly, but gently pressing inward. With a large animal such as a cow or horse, adequate restraint measures should be taken first. The veterinarian should be called immediately. If you cannot replace the eyeball with one or two tries, the vet must be ready to do so. Aftercare consists of bandaging the head to keep out dirt and light and keeping the eyeball in place. Antibiotics are often given to prevent infection, and cortisone is given to prevent swelling and pain. (Note: The prolapsed third eyelid mentioned elsewhere in this book is not a problem in itself, but a symptom of tetanus. This third eyelid is the thin "skin" or membrane in the corner of the eye which falls over the eye when an animal develops tetanus.)

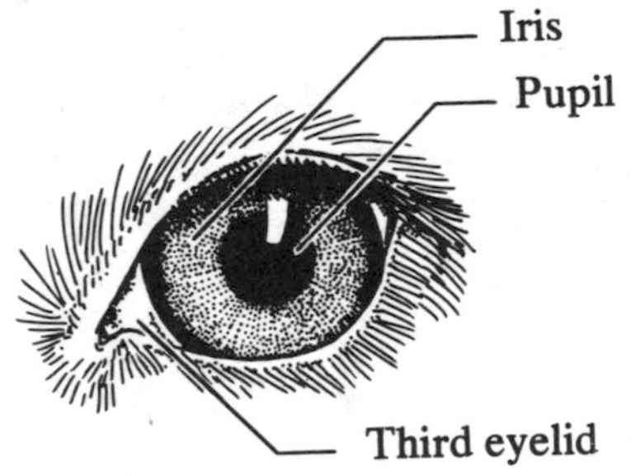

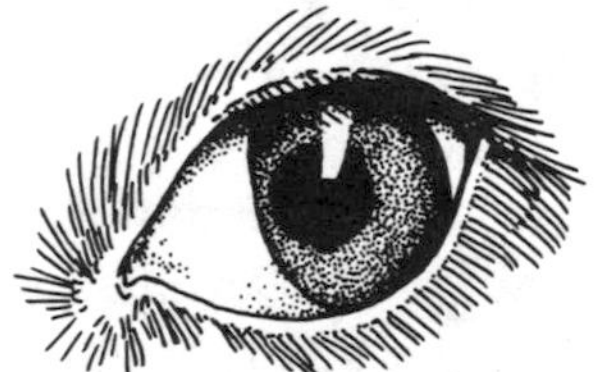

The third eyelid falls over the eye when an animal develops tetanus

Snakebite Animals are bitten by poisonous snakes as often as are humans. They are most often struck on the legs, udder (cattle and goats), nose, and belly. It is important to be able to recognize a poisonous snake and the bite marks, as even the harmless garter snake will fight and strike if threatened. In the United States, there are four families of poisonous snakes:

copperheads, rattlesnakes, water moccasins, and coral snakes. The first three have large fangs which leave a double puncture wound. The coral snake does not have these large fangs and must hang on longer to make its poison effective. It cannot bite through heavy hair and has a relatively small head which doesn't allow for a good hold on a quick moving animal. Coral snakes are, however, the most poisonous of all North American snakes, being related to the cobra.

If an animal is seen being struck by a snake use the same first aid that is used on a human. Keep the animal calm, use a tourniquet if possible (depending on location of the bite), incise the wound, and encourage bleeding. Rush the animal to a veterinarian or call him out, depending on the size of the animal. Antivenin should be administered as soon as possible.

A large animal such as a cow or horse will often live through the bite itself, but get into severe trouble later as the bite area becomes necrotic and develops a bacterial infection. Lameness or swellings on the lower extremities or face merit quick inspection, keeping snakebite in mind. Bites on the lips or into blood vessels are often fatal if not treated immediately.

Dogs, being smaller, often die soon after being bitten. The amount of poison injected at the time of the bite is the determining factor here, as well as the location of the bite and how quickly first aid is given.

GLOSSARY OF COMMONLY USED VETERINARY TERMS

Abdominal cavity that part of the body that contains such organs as stomach, liver, kidneys, spleen, uterus in female, intestines.

Abomasum the fourth or true digestive stomach of a ruminant.

Abortion the termination of a pregnancy before due date because of injury, the mother rejecting an abnormal fetus, fatigue, viruses, etc.

Abscess a localized collection of pus surrounded by inflamed tissue.

Acetonemia another name for ketosis in cattle; see *ketosis.*

Acute sudden onset, short duration, severe.

Aerobic organism one which grows in the presence of oxygen.

Afterbirth the placenta which is expelled after the birth of a mammal.

AI abbreviation for artificial insemination; see *artificial insemination.*

Alimentary canal the tubular passage from the mouth to the anus which functions in digestion and absorption of food and elimination of residual waste.

Amniotic fluid the liquid surrounding the fetus in the uterus.

Anaerobic organism one which grows in the absence of oxygen.

Anal glands two scent glands, one on either side of the rectum, in dogs; these empty into the rectum during a bowel movement or at times of fright.

Anaphylactic shock extreme sensitivity of an animal to a drug or foreign protein causing severe shock or death.

Anemia a condition in which the blood is deficient in red blood cells, in hemoglobin, or in total volume causing lack of vitality.

Aneurysm a localized, saclike dilation of the blood vessel.

Antibiotic a substance produced by a microorganism and able in dilute solution to inhibit or kill another microorganism.

Antibody any of the body globulins that combine with antigens (a protein or carbohydrate substance) and neutralize toxins or bacteria, and precipitate soluble antigens.

Antiserum a serum containing antibodies against a particular disease which is used to treat that disease.

Antivenin an antitoxin to a venom (poison); an antiserum containing this antitoxin.

Artery a vessel carrying blood away from the heart through the body.

Arthritis a crippling of the joints caused by various organisms; characterized by puffiness at the joints and pain; treated in the early stages with antibiotics; in the later stages with daily exercise, light casts, or surgery; prevention is the best treatment; also called joint ill.

Artificial insemination (AI) or breeding the introduction of semen into the uterus by other than natural means.

Ascarids large, round worms in the intestinal tract of almost all species of animals, including humans; characterized by loss of appetite, unthriftiness, and inactivity; treated with a wormer.

Ascites the accumulation of serous fluid in the abdominal cavity.

Aspiration pneumonia pneumonia caused by breathing foreign matter into the lungs, such as amniotic fluid at birth, dust, or liquid from an improperly given drench; also called inhalation pneumonia; see *pneumonia.*

Atrophic rhinitis a condition in pigs similar to necrotic rhinitis, but without the swollen snout or face; see *necrotic rhinitis.*

Atrophy a decrease in size or wasting away of a body part or tissue; as happens to testicles after castration by clamping.

Avian relating to birds.

Avian leukosis complex a disease in poultry affecting the nerves, eyes, and/or internal organs; characteristics differ according to body parts affected; no treatment available.

Azoturia lameness in a horse characterized by profuse sweating, trembling, incoordination, and darkening of the urine; treated with rest, oral electrolytes, sodium bicarbonate, and injectable thiamine.

Bacteria one-celled organisms belonging to the plant kingdom.

Bacterin suspension of killed bacteria used to immunize against a specific disease.

Balling gun an inexpensive instrument used to insert medicine through an animal's mouth down into its throat.

Bedsore an ulceration of tissue deprived of nutrition caused by prolonged pressure; prevented and treated by changing positions.

Benign mild, nonspreading, and nonrecurring.

Blackhead a destructive disease of turkeys and chickens caused by a protozoa, which is carried by the cecal worm, that invades the intestines and liver; characterized by droopiness, sulfur-colored diarrhea, and weight loss; treated with drugs and a wormer.

Blackleg a sudden-appearing disease in cattle caused by a clostridia organism which enters the body through the digestive tract or a small puncture wound; characterized by a purple-looking leg; prevented by vaccination; no sure treatment.

Blister, external an ointment or salve applied to the skin surface to produce heat in the area, and in turn increase circulation to promote healing; often used in treating lameness in horses; also called external blister.

Bloat an accumulation of gas in the rumen of cattle, goats, and sheep which have overeaten, eaten grain followed by drinking water, or have indigestion; characterized by staggering, panting, and finally collapse; treated with a defoaming agent, a stomach tube, or a trochar and cannula; also called gastritis.

Blood poisoning another name for septicemia; see *septicemia.*

Blue comb a disease in chickens and turkeys caused by a virus or by stress; characterized by watery or pasty diarrhea, weight loss, blue comb, and depression; treated with molasses and antibiotics.

Boar an uncastrated male pig.

Bolus large pill often oval in shape.

Bots fairly large, grublike fly larvae which attach themselves to the stomach lining of horses causing pitting and scarring; treated with a wormer.

Bovine relating to cattle or oxen.

Bovine virus diarrhea (BVD) a viral disease in cattle; characterized by fever, loss of appetite, diarrhea, and sometimes sores around the mouth, nose, and eyes and drooling or foaming at the mouth; treatment is difficult; protected by vaccine; also called infectious bovine diarrhea (IBD).

Bowed tendon lameness in a horse caused by severe strain or overwork; characterized by the tendon below the knee bowing outward and soreness; treated with cold and rest.

Breech presentation an abnormal birth position; the buttocks appear first.

Brisket the breast or lower chest of livestock animals.

Brucellosis a disease in pigs, cattle, and man caused by the organisms brucellae; characterized and treated according to type and animal infected.

Bull-nose another name for necrotic rhinitis; see *necrotic rhinitis.*

"Bump" the calf during the fifth or sixth month of a cow's pregnancy if you make a fist and gently but firmly bump into her right flank side, you will feel a hard, abnormal lump bump you back. This is the calf.

BVD abbreviation for bovine virus diarrhea; see *bovine virus diarrhea.*

Caesarean section the removal of a fetus through an incision in the mother's abdomen and uterus.

Caked bag another name for udder edema when the bag becomes swollen just before or after freshening due to fluid retention.

Calcification the process of depositing calcium salts to make inflexible; as in the healing of a bone.

California Mastitis Test (CMT) a test used to determine if a cow has mastitis; see *mastitis.*

Cannibalism when an animal devours its own kind; occurs in young chicks that are overcrowded and bored; prevented by providing less crowded quarters, a well-balanced ration, and a chunk of soil or grass to pick on; debeaking will also help; see *debeaking.*

Cannula a small tube which is attached to and inserted by a trochar into an animal and then left in place to allow drainage from an affected area, such as the stomach.

Capped elbow or hock lameness in a horse caused by bruising; characterized by swelling on either the elbow or hock; treated with ice, cortisone, mild exercise, and rest from work.

Caprine of, relating to, or being a goat.

Caruncles cup-shaped, spongy-textured lobes or "buttons" on the uterus which attach to the placenta; commonly, but mistakenly, called cotyledons.

Caseous lymphadenitis a serious abscess infection in the lymph glands of sheep and goats caused by various bacteria; characterized by a thinning animal; treated by isolation and by opening, draining, and packing with antibiotics the external abscesses in the intestines, liver, kidneys, or lungs; also called wasting disease.

Cast stuck in a down position, such as when a horse gets stuck in a stall or fence, or in deep snow or mud.

Castration removal or destruction of the testicles; neutering a male animal.

Catheterize insertion of a tube into a body passageway or cavity to permit injection or withdrawal of fluids, as into the urethra to drain the bladder.

Caustic ointment a paste applied in a ring around the base and on the button of a young animal's horn buds to prevent them from growing; a method of dehorning.

Cautery a hot iron, caustic, or other agent used to burn, sear, or destroy tissue.

Cecal worm a worm that infests the ceca of chickens and turkeys causing inflammation of the cecum and unthriftiness; treated by good sanitation, and a wormer; a carrier of the protozoa that causes blackhead disease.

Cecum the blind pouch that begins the large intestine; resembles the appendix in humans.

Cervix the narrow outer opening of the uterus.

Chorea a nervous disorder marked by spasmodic movements of the limbs or facial muscles and by incoordination.

Chorioptic the most common type mange found in cattle; see *mange.*

Chromosome microscopic body containing genes which determine hereditary factors.

Chronic slow onset, long duration, somewhat resistant to treatment.

CMT abbreviation for California Mastitis Test; see *California Mastitis Test.*

Coagulant powder a powder used to slow down and stop bleeding by causing it to clot.

Coccidia protozoa; one-celled parasites in the digestive membrane of birds and animals.

Coccidiosis infestation with coccidia; characterized by stunted growth, diarrhea, and unthriftiness; treated with sulfas.

Coggins test a blood test for swamp fever or EIA.

Colic a bellyache caused by overeating, eating grain then drinking large quantities of water, drinking water while overheated, constipation, or impaction; characterized by pacing, sweating, kicking, hard breathing, and rolling; treated with injections to calm the stomach and relieve the pain.

Colostrum the first milk secreted by a mother after giving birth; characterized by high protein and necessary antibodies for the newborn.

Comminuted fracture a smashed bone containing many fragments.

Compound fracture a break in both bone and skin.

Congenital a condition existing at birth, but not hereditary.

Conjunctiva the mucous membrane covering the eyeball and the inner side of the eyelid.

Conjunctivitis inflammation of the conjunctiva caused by irritation of foreign matter, such as dust; characterized by mattery or runny, itchy eyes; treated with an anesthetic ointment.

Constipation abnormally delayed or infrequent passage of dry hardened feces.

Corns a painful foot condition in cattle characterized by an extra chunk of tissue extending from between the toes; usually removed surgically.

Coronet the lower part of a horse's pastern where the horn terminates in skin.

Cotyledons knobs on the placenta or afterbirth; also the name mistakenly used to refer to caruncles.

Creep-fed method of feeding growing young animals which allows access to feed by young while excluding adults by size and placement of feeder.

Creep-fed ration a ration for growing animals meant to be fed free choice.

Cross ties a restraining device made of two ropes from each side of an aisle that snap on the side halter rings.

Cuterebra a large fly larva that appears in a hole in the neck or chin area of cats; treated by forceps removal, flushing the area, and applying an antibiotic solution.

Cyanosis a bluish or purplish discoloration due to deficient oxygenation of the blood; used to describe blue comb in chickens or turkeys; see *blue comb.*

Cystic ovaries ovaries containing cysts; characterized by a female that is continually in heat; treated with hormones.

Cystitis inflammation of the bladder.

Debeaking trimming back the top beak of a chick to prevent cannibalism.

Dehorning iron an electric instrument used to burn (kill) the horn cells of a young animal; also called disbudding iron.

Demodectic a type of mange found in animals; see *mange.*

Dermatitis inflammation of the skin caused by an irritation.

Dermatosis any disease of the skin not necessarily with inflammation.

Descenting the removal of the major scent gland located on the head of a goat by burning or surgery.

Dewclaw on the leg above the hoof of a mammal, a toelike projection that doesn't reach the ground.

Diabetes a disease in dogs and humans characterized by increased thirst, frequent urination, weight loss, and weakness; treated by diet control, medication, and/or insulin injections.

Diarrhea abnormally frequent bowel movements with more or less fluid stools.

Distemper a contagious disease in dogs of the central nervous system caused by a virus; characterized by running, mattery eyes, plugged crusty nose, diarrhea, vomiting, and twitching; treated with antiserum or globulin, antibiotics to prevent secondary infections, and good nursing.

Distemper another name for strangles in horses; see *strangles.*

Diuretic a substance taken to increase the flow of urine by drawing fluid from the body.

Dock to cut off the end of a body part, such as the tails of sheep.

"Downer" cows cows unable to stand after calving because of injuries to ligaments, muscle, and bone.

Drake a male duck.

Drench to give a liquid medicine to an animal.

Eastern equine encephalomyelitis (EEE) a virus-produced disease spread from mosquitoes to birds, back to mosquitoes, then horses, and sometimes to man; characterized by depression, incoordination, drooping lip, high fever, pushing against a wall, or being down and unable to rise; treatment involves good nursing and isolation.

Eclampsia a condition in a newly whelped bitch; characterized by panting, walking with a stiff gait, stumbling, falling, being unable to rise, and convulsing; treated by weaning the puppies and giving an intravenous injection of calcium; similar to milk fever; see also *milk fever.*

Edema the accumulation of fluid in tissues caused by poor circulation in an area due to sprain, injury, tight leg wraps, or pregnancy; characterized by swelling; treated with diuretics; called stocking in horses.

EEE abbreviation for eastern equine encephalomyelitis; see *eastern equine encephalomyelitis.*

EIA abbreviation for equine infectious anemia; see *equine infectious anemia.*

Elastrator an instrument which places a rubber band between the body and body part, such as horns or testicles, to be removed from a young animal. The band shuts off circulation and eventually the body part falls off.

Electrolytes normal bases, acids, and salts found in the blood.

Emasculatome a clamp used to crush the cords to the testicles causing them to atrophy and shrink up; used in the clamping or "pinching" method of castration.

Emasculator an instrument that crushes and cuts both the cord and blood vessels in the testicles; used in surgical castration.

Embryotomy knife a special curved knife with a small blade used to cut the skin of a dead fetus without damaging the uterine wall.

Emetic an agent that induces vomiting.

Emphysema a condition of the lung characterized by distension and frequently by impairment of heart action.

Enterotoxemia a disease of some animals, most often young goats, calves, and lambs, caused by an organism; characterized by diarrhea, circling, convulsions, incoordination, and weakness; prevented by vaccination and exercise; treatment is inadequate; also called overeating disease.

Epidural injection an injection between the vertebrae; also known as a spinal.

Epilepsy seizures that occur in dogs that may be triggered by excitement; characterized by shaking, stiffening, falling, and jerking; treated regularly with the oral drugs Primidone or Dilantin.

Equine infectious anemia (EIA) another name for swamp fever; see *swamp fever.*

Erysipelas an acute infection in young pigs caused by organisms living in the joints or heart; characterized by high temperature, pain, and diamond-shaped purple blotches on the sides, belly, and back; treated with penicillin and serum.

Estrogen a female hormone.

Eversion turning inside out; as the eversion of the uterus in cattle.

Expectorant a substance which clears the air passages of secretions.

External blister another name for blister, external; see *blister, external.*

Farrow to give birth to pigs.

Fecal pertaining to the bowel movement or excreta.

Feline distemper another name for panleukopenia; see *panleukopenia.*

Fetlock a projection bearing a tuft of hair on the baek of the leg just above the hoof of a horse or similar animal.

Fetus an unborn, developing animal.

Firing the method of applying a firing pin to the skin surface to produce heat which in turn increases circulation to promote healing; used to treat lameness in horses.

Firing pin a hot electric point used in firing horses; see *firing.*

Flatulence a digestive upset characterized by gas in the stomach or intestincs.

Float a special file about four inches long on the end of a long handle which is used to file down sharp edges on horses' teeth.

Flush to prepare an animal for breeding by putting them on full feed and usually lush pasture so they are gaining weight when bred.

Foot rot a fungus infection that attacks the feet of cattle, goats, and sheep causing a sudden lameness; usually treated with an antibiotic.

Founder lameness in a horse caused by overeating lush pastures or grains, drinking water when overheated, or by a retained placenta; characterized by a reluctance to move and above-normal temperature; treated with antihistamines, rest, and cold; also called laminitis.

Fowl cholera a fast-hitting, bacterial disease with a high mortality rate in poultry; characterized by bluish combs and wattles, fever, increased water intake, difficult breathing, drowsiness, and emaciation; treated by controlling with vaccination, cleanliness, good feeding practices, and isolation of infected birds.

Fowl typhoid a disease in poultry caused by *Salmonella gallinarum*; characterized by depression, ruffled feathers, and a yellowish or greenish diarrhea; treated by controlling sanitation and bedding, and by isolation.

Freshen when an animal gives birth and comes into milk.

Frog the triangular, elastic, horny pad in the middle of the sole of a horse's foot which absorbs shock while the animal is moving.

Front presentation the normal, front end delivery of a calf or kid; front legs followed by the head and the shoulders, and finally the hips and back legs.

Frostbite the freezing of some part of the body, such as the ears and feet of newborn goats; characterized by stiffness, swelling, tenderness, and heat; treated by soaking in warm water, rubbing with towels, placing in warm surroundings, and by injecting cortisone intramuscularly; prevention is best.

Fungus a simple plant, lacking chlorophyll.

Gall a skin sore caused by chronic irritation.

Gander the adult male goose.

Gangrene the decay of soft body tissue due to disease or shut-off of blood supply.

Gapeworm a parasite that migrates to the lungs and then imbeds in the trachea of poultry causing blockage which inhibits breathing and sometimes eating; characterized by sneezing, coughing, neck stretching, loss of appetite, and dullness; treated with thiabendazole and by controlling snails and slugs with insecticide.

Gastritis inflammation of the mucous membrane of the stomach; another name for bloat; see *bloat.*

Gelding a castrated male horse.

Genes the parts of chromosomes carrying hereditary factors.

Gilt a young female pig that has not farrowed or has just farrowed the first time.

Globulin any of a class of simple proteins that are insoluble in water but soluble in dilute salt solutions, and that occur widely in plant and animal tissues.

Glucocorticoid another name for glucocorticosteroids; see *glucocorticosteroids.*

Glucocorticosteroids the cortisone that has an effect on glucose metabolism in the body; also called glucocorticoid.

Gouger a simple instrument with two round wooden handles with a sharp blade which fits down over a horn button. When the handles are pulled apart quickly, the horn button is gouged out; used to dehorn young animals; also called scoops.

Gram-negative bacteria which does not hold the purple dye when stained by Gram's method.

Gram-positive bacteria which holds the purple dye when stained by Gram's method.

Gram's method used in diagnostic laboratories as a means for the differential staining of bacteria by which some species remain colored and some are decolorized by treatment with Gram's solution (iodine and the iodide of potassium) after staining with gentian violet.

Granulation the process of the minute red granules of new capillaries forming on the surface of a wound in healing.

Grease heel another name for scratches; see *scratches.*

Grubs parasitic fly larvae that live under the skin on the back of cattle causing few problems; treated with sprays, pour-ons, or powders.

Gruel any softened, moistened, easily mouthed feed.

Hairballs a wad made of hair swallowed by a cat which collects in the digestive tract; characterized by vomiting and gastric distress or constipation and intestinal blockage; treated with mineral oil, milk of magnesia, or castor oil.

Hardware disease a condition in cattle caused by swallowing metal objects, such as nails, wire, bottle caps, etc.; symptoms and treatment vary depending on the location of the metal.

Heartworm a parasite, spread by the mosquito to dogs, which infests the heart; characterized by shortness of breath, coughing, lack of stamina, and tiring easily; treated with extreme care with a drug and with an oral preventative during mosquito season.

Heaves a chronic pulmonary emphysema of a horse characterized by difficult breathing, heaving of the flanks, and a persistent cough.

Heifer a young cow; one that has not had a calf.

Hematoma a swelling due to the collection of blood under the skin; a large bruise.

Hemorrhage heavy or uncontrollable bleeding.

Hemorrhagic septicemia another name for shipping fever in cattle; see *shipping fever* and *pneumonia.*

Hepatitis inflammation of the liver caused by a virus; characterized by fever, inflamed eyes, vomiting, no appetite, and diarrhea; treated with blood transfusions, intravenous fluids, and antibiotics to prevent secondary infections; prevented with vaccination.

Hermaphrodite an animal with both male and female reproductive organs.

Hernia a protrusion of the bowel or other organ through a weak spot in the muscle or wall of the body cavity.

Hip dysplasia a hereditary condition of the hips, most often found in registered dogs of certain breeds.

Hobbles a restraining device, usually made of leather, fastened around a horse's pasterns to keep the legs together to prevent straying or kicking or to throw a horse to permit working on it.

Hock the tarsal joint in the hind limb of animals, such as a horse, corresponding to the heel and ankle of man, except that it is elevated and bends backward; a joint of a fowl's leg that corresponds to the hock.

Hog cholera a highly infectious often fatal virus disease of pigs; characterized by high fever, diarrhea, and weakness in the hind legs; treated with hog cholera serum.

Hookworms severe intestinal parasites that penetrate the skin of animals, including humans; characterized by unthriftiness, diarrhea, blood in the stool, and death due to anemia; treated with a wormer and strict sanitation measures.

Hot spots a common fungal infection in dogs often mistaken for mange; characterized by sudden-appearing red spots with a moist, whitish center that occur on the neck and back resulting in itching or tenderness; treated with an antifungal agent after clipping away the hair.

Hutch burn a condition in rabbits kept in wooden hutches caused by exposure to urine; characterized by the genital-anal area being red, chapped-looking, and having brownish crusts; treated with a bland ointment and proper sanitation; called scab nose when the infection spreads to the nose.

Hydrophobia another name for rabies; see *rabies.*

Hypocalcemia a deficiency of calcium in the blood seen in heavy milking sows with large litters, around weaning time; characterized by thinness and weakness in the hindquarters; treated by weaning the pigs and providing good nursing, and with injections of calcium; also named posterior paralysis.

IBD abbreviation for infectious bovine diarrhea; see *infectious bovine diarrhea.*

IM abbreviation for intramuscular; see *intramuscular.*

Impaction the lodgment of something in a body passage or cavity, such as feces in the bowel, often caused by improper feeding; characterized by small, scant, hard droppings, followed by pain; treated with mineral oil or occasionally an enema.

Infectious bovine diarrhea (IBD) another name for bovine virus diarrhea; see *bovine virus diarrhea (BVD).*

Infectious keratitis another name for pinkeye; see *pinkeye.*

Infertility the inability to reproduce.

Inguinal pertaining to the groin area, such as the inguinal canal.

Inhalation pneumonia another name for aspiration pneumonia; see *aspiration pneumonia.*

Intervertebral disc lesions a back problem in dogs arising from protrusion of a spinal disc which puts pressure on the spinal cord; caused by injury or may be hereditary; characterized by lameness, unwillingness to stand, and finally paralysis; treated with drugs, good nursing, physical therapy, and occasionally surgery.

Intradermal injection an injection into the skin, not under it; as in a TB test.

Intramedullar pins stainless steel pins which are run through the marrow of the bone to repair fractures.

Intramuscular (IM) situated in or entering through a muscle, as in an intramuscular injection.

Intraperitoneal situated in or entering through the cavity of the abdomen, such as an intraperitoneal injection.

Intraperitoneal injection injection into the abdominal cavity; the organs are not injected, just the cavity.

Intravenous (IV) situated in or entering through a vein, as in an intravenous injection.

IV abbreviation for intravenous; see *intravenous.*

Jenny burro a female donkey.

Johne's disease a chronic, often fatal, inflammation of the intestines (esp. in cattle) caused by bacteria; characterized by persistent diarrhea and gradual emaciation; no treatment available.

Joint ill another name for arthritis; see *arthritis.*

Jugular vein the large veins on each side of the neck that return blood from the head.

Ketosis a metabolic disturbance with an abnormal increase of ketone (acetone) bodies in the blood, urine, and milk; causes, symptoms, and treatments vary according to the animal.

Laminitis another name for founder; see *founder.*

Laparotomy a surgical incision into the abdominal cavity.

Leptospirosis a bacterial disease in animals (including humans) characterized by fever, diarrhea, increased urination, bloody or discolored urine, vomiting, weakness, and inflamed mouth membranes; prevented by vaccination.

Lesion an abnormal change in tissue due to injury or disease.

Lice various small, flattened, oval-shaped, bloodsucking, gray insects that are parasitic on warm-blooded animals; characterized by rubbing, itching, and patchy, bald spots; treated with louse powders.

Ligate tie off, as in surgery.

Liver fluke a parasitic flatworm that invades the liver in mammals, destroying liver tissue; treated with intramuscular injections.

Lockjaw another name for tetanus; see *tetanus.*

Luxation of the patella another name for stifling; see *stifling.*

Malignant spreading deterioration.

Mange a persistent, contagious skin disease caused by mites that burrow into the skin; characterized by itching, scales, crusty spots, pustules, or thickened skin; treatment varies according to the animal.

Mastitis the inflammation of the mammary gland caused by bacteria which results in changes in the milk; symptoms and treatment vary according to the type mastitis, i.e., acute, chronic, or gangrene.

Mastitis tube a syringe with a flexible tube, containing antibiotics to inject directly into the teat canal.

Metritis an inflamed uterus, preventing conception and often normal heat cycles; characterized by pus and exudate in the uterus; treated with hormones or antibiotics.

Microfilariae the minute larvae of various nematodes (that develop in biting insects) that as adults are parasites in the blood and tissues of mammals.

Milk fever a disease of recently calved cows (occas. sheep or goats) caused by low blood calcium during the establishment of the milk flow; characterized by an ascending paralysis, beginning with the hind legs, and *no* fever; treated with a calcium solution given intravenously.

Milk vein a very large blood vessel on each side of a cow's underside.

Mites small parasites that feed on blood and live in the roosts and litter of poultry; cause birds to be anemic and appear unthrifty; treated by fumigating the poultry house and dusting the birds.

Molt to periodically shed hair, feathers, shell, horns, or an outer layer.

Mucoid enteritis a disease in rabbits with no known cause; characterized by humped-up-sitting, acting as if in pain, teeth-grinding, ear-drooping, and eye-closing; there may be diarrhea or constipation; treated with antibiotics, good sanitation and husbandry, and isolation of affected animals; no known cure.

Navicular disease lameness in a horse caused by trauma, hard work on unyielding surfaces, or faulty conformation; characterized by unnatural stance, short strides, and narrow, long hooves; no permanent treatment.

Neck rope used with a halter to tie a horse; a strong rope with a loop with a ring tied in it about two feet up from the snap.

Necro another name for necrotic enteritis; see *necrotic enteritis.*

Necrotic pertaining to dead tissue.

Necrotic enteritis the inflammation and decaying of intestinal tissue in pigs caused by dietary deficiency or bacterial infection; characterized by lack of appetite and energy, high temperature, and diarrhea; treated by improving the diet and giving antibiotics or sulfa drugs; also called necro.

Necrotic rhinitis a condition in pigs caused by an organism introduced through an injury; characterized by a swollen snout or face, a nasal discharge, sneezing, or occasional bleeding; treated with antibiotics or sulfas.

Neural pertaining to the nerves.

Neuter a spayed or castrated animal.

Newcastle a sudden-appearing, quick-spreading viral disease in poultry; characterized by respiratory distress followed by nervous disorders and then death in chicks; no treatment available.

Nictitating membrane a thin membrane at the inner angle or beneath the lower lid of the eye of many animals; also called third eyelid.

Ocular pertaining to the eye.

Oocyst an encysted fertilized egg of certain one-celled animal parasites.

Ophthalmic relating to the eye; for use on or in the eye, such as an ointment.

Osteomyelitis inflammation of the bone.

Ovariohysterectomy the removal of the ovaries and uterus; spaying.

Overeating disease another name for enterotoxemia; see *enterotoxemia.*

Oxytocin a hormone used to aid new mothers having difficulty letting down their milk or to cause uterine contractions in a difficult birth.

Panleukopenia a very contagious, quick-striking, high mortality disease in cats; characterized by diarrhea, vomiting, weakness, depression, and quick death; treated with good nursing, and antibiotics to prevent secondary infections; prevented by vaccination; also called feline distemper.

Parasite an organism, living in or on another organism, which depends on its host for support and/or existence without making a useful return and usually causing injury; such as ticks, lice, and worms.

Parenteral situated or occurring outside the intestines; introduced otherwise than by way of the intestines, such as intravenously or intramuscularly.

Pastern the part of a horse's foot extending from the fetlock to the bone within the hoof.

Pasteurellosis another name for snuffles; see *snuffles.*

Patella the kneecap.

Pediculosis infestation with lice.

Pen-strep shortened form for penicillin streptomycin, a common broad-spectrum antibiotic.

Pericardium the membrane that encloses the heart and its surrounding blood vessels.

Peritoneal cavity the membrane lining of the abdomen of mammals.

Peritonitis inflammation of the abdominal membrane caused by various means, such as uterine tears or strings of afterbirth remaining in the uterus after delivery, by the piercing of the membrane by wire in hardware disease (see *hardware disease*) or by bots in horses (see *bots*); treated with antibiotics.

Phenol poisoning cats are highly susceptible to this form of poisoning; characterized by gastric upsets; treated by inducing vomiting, giving fluids parenterally, and good nursing.

Pinkeye an infection in cattle spread by flies; characterized by watery eyes which may become bloodshot; treated with eye powders; also called infectious keratitis.

Pinworms intestinal parasites that cause intense itching around the anus (of a horse); treated with a wormer.

Placenta the milky membrane that contains the fetus in the uterus.

Pneumonia a disease of the lungs caused by a bacteria, a virus, or stress; characterized by fever, quick breathing, puffing, a drop in milk production, and coughing; treated with antibiotics or sulfas.

Pneumonitis a contagious viral disease in cats; characterized by sneezing, coughing, a discharge from the eyes and nose, a fever, and weight loss; treated with good nursing, and antibiotics to prevent secondary infections; prevented with vaccination.

Polled having no horns as a result of dehorning or being born without them.

Posterior paralysis another name for hypocalcemia; see *hypocalcemia.*

Posterior presentation another name for rear presentation; see *rear presentation.*

Poult a young turkey.

Pregnancy disease another name for ketosis in sheep; see *ketosis.*

Prolapse the dropping down or slipping of a body part from its usual position; sometimes used to describe an organ that is in fact everted, as with a uterus.

Prolapsed eyeball a condition caused by trauma in which the eyeball pops out of its socket; treated by keeping the animal calm and restrained, calling the vet, and replacing the eyeball; aftercare consists of bandaging the head and giving antibiotics to prevent infection and cortisone to prevent swelling and pain.

Proud flesh an excessive tumorlike growth of granulation tissue produced in the healing of a wound; characterized by oozing, bleeding easily, enlarging, and being easily injured; treated surgically.

Pullet a hen less than a year old.

Pullorum a destructive poultry disease caused by a bacteria; characterized by diarrhea, huddling together, and droopiness; treated with sulfas.

Pyometra an infection of the uterus preventing conception and often normal heat cycles; characterized by pus in the uterus; treated with hormones or antibiotics.

Quarter crack another name for sand crack; see *sand crack.*

Queen a female cat.

Rabies a disease caused by a virus that is highly concentrated in the saliva of infected animals; characterized by personality change and various symptoms depending on type of rabies; no treatment available; prevented by vaccination; also called hydrophobia.

Rear presentation a less frequent normal delivery position of a calf or kid; backward, with the underside of the hooves coming first, followed by the tail instead of the head; also called posterior presentation.

Reportable disease a serious, usually highly contagious, disease that must be reported to the state veterinarian; an affected flock is quarantined.

Retained corpus luteum a reddish yellow mass of tissue forming a ruptured cyst in the ovary preventing a female from having heat cycles; treated with estrogen injections.

Retained placenta when the placenta has not been expelled a short time after birth; indicated by it hanging out of the vulva or being retained internally; treated by manual removal, a hormone injection, and boluses or powder to prevent infection.

Reticulum the second stomach of a ruminant.

Rhinotracheitis a viral disease in cats; characterized by a discharge from the eyes and nose, coughing, and sneezing; treated by good nursing.

Rickets a disease caused by failure to assimilate and use calcium and phosphorus due to inadequate sunlight or vitamin D; characterized by soft, deformed bones.

Ring-bone lameness in a horse caused by infection after injury, rickets, hard work, kicks, or arthritis; characterized by swelling or ridges in the pastern area; treated with pasture rest and cortisone.

Ringworm a contagious skin disease caused by a fungus; characterized by circular crusty spots; treated by cleansing and applying an antifungal drug.

Rooter the hard ridge of cartilage near the snout that a pig roots with.

Rotenone solution a plant-derived insecticide of low toxicity.

Roundworm the most common parasite in dogs and cats; quite large, white and tapered at both ends; seen when coughed up or in the stool; harms the digestive tract and causes malnutrition; treated with a wormer.

Rumen the large first stomach of a ruminant.

Rumenotomy a surgical incision into the rumen.

Ruminants animals that chew a cud, such as cattle, goats and sheep.

Ruptured pig an inherited defect characterized by an enlargement and softness in the testicle(s) due to the presence of intestines in the scrotum along with the testicle(s); treated surgically.

Saddle sores an irritation developing on the back of a horse at the points of pressure from an ill-fitting saddle; treatment is rest from the saddle.

Sand crack lameness in a horse; characterized by cracks running up the hoof from the toe to near the coronet; treated with moisture and a hoof dressing; also called quarter crack.

Sarcoptic a type mange found in goats; see *mange.*

Scab or scabies another name for mange; see *mange.*

Scab nose hutch burn infection of the nose; see *hutch burn.*

Scirrhous cord a buildup in the scrotum of fibrous scar tissue from the incomplete healing of the testicle cord and tunic after castration; treated by dissecting it away from the skin and body tissue with the fingers to prevent hemorrhage.

Scoops another name for gouger; see *gouger.*

Scours severe diarrhea in farm animals; also called winter scours or winter dysentery.

Scratches a condition on the back of a horse's pastern characterized by sores or roughness, swelling, tenderness, lameness, and crusts of dried serum; treated with daily washings, hair clipping, and alternate use of astringent and antibiotic ointment; also called grease heel.

Screwworms the larvae of blowflies which live in a wound causing it to ooze; treated with a fly repellent.

Scrotum the external sac or pouch containing the testicles.

Scurs misshapen horns, often small, knotted and twisted, often caused by injury to the horn bud by improper dehorning.

Septicemia an invasion of the bloodstream by microorganisms from an infection; characterized by chills, fever, and prostration; also called blood poisoning.

Septum a dividing wall or membrane between body spaces or masses of soft tissue, as between the nostrils.

Serum the watery portion of the blood left after the cells clot.

Sheath the tubular fold of skin into which the penis of many mammals is retracted.

Shipping fever another name for a pneumonia in cattle and goats; accompanied by diarrhea; caused by a stress, but not always the stress of moving or shipping; also known as hemorrhagic septicemia; see *pneumonia.*

Shipping fever another name for strangles in horses; see *strangles.*

Shock a condition brought about by trauma which results in reduced circulation, rapid breathing, rapid pulse, subnormal temperature, weakness, vomiting, and prostration; must be treated immediately.

Simple fracture a break in a bone without a break in the skin; a break without secondary complications.

Slicker a flat brush with bent metal pins used for removing dead hairs and stimulating the skin of medium-coated dogs.

Snuffles a common contagious rabbit disease caused by the organism *Pasteurella* following stress; characterized by sneezing, wheezing, coughing, and running eyes; treated with antibiotics, proper nutrition, and protection from stress; also called pasteurellosis.

Sore hocks injured, chaffed, or bruised hocks in rabbits that may become infected; characterized by bald, red, scabby or swollen hocks; treated with a sulfa or antibiotic plus an ointment or powder.

Soremouth a contagious, viral disease in sheep; characterized by swollen lips with scabs which may extend into the mouth and may be on the feet, between the toes, and on the nose; treated by keeping the animal's strength up with moist foods until virus runs its course; vaccination available.

Sow a female pig that has farrowed at least once.

Spay the removal of the ovaries and uterus neutering a female animal.

Speculum an instrument inserted into a body passage for inspection or medication, as a mouth speculum used for dental work.

Splints lameness in a horse caused by hard work on hard or rough surfaces, blows or injuries; characterized by small inflamed spots; treated with pasture rest and liniment.

Sprain a sudden or violent twist or wrench of a joint with stretching or tearing of ligaments; characterized by lameness, heat, and tenderness; a fresh sprain is treated with cold, alcohol, cooling liniment, and cortisone injections; after swelling occurs, treat with heat, heating liniment, hot udder ointment, and massage.

Stanchion a device that fits loosely around an animal's neck and limits forward and backward motion (as in a stall).

Stifle the joint above the hock in the hind leg of animals; corresponds to the knee in man.

Stifling lameness in horses and cows caused by a conformation weakness, often hereditary; characterized by a hind leg being "stuck" straight; treated by replacing the dislocation with a rope and a neck loop; also called luxation of the patella.

Stocking (stock up) another name for edema in horses; see *edema.*

Stool a bowel movement.

Strangles a contagious disease of horses caused by bacteria; characterized by heavy mucous secretions from the nose, cough, fever, and enlargement or abscesses of the lymph glands; treated by isolating and good nursing; also known as shipping fever.

Stress a mental or physical disruption upsetting the well-being of an animal, such as moving, changes in the weather, a switch in feed, etc.

Strongyles a group of roundworms which migrate through the bloodstream of horses causing scarring of the vessel walls; treated with a wormer.

Strychnine poisoning characterized by trembling, panting, acting nervously, followed by convulsions; treated with a general anesthetic.

Subcutaneous injection an injection given just under the skin.

Subcutaneous tissue tissue between the skin and muscle.

Suture to sew (verb); the material used for closing wounds (noun).

Swamp fever a viral disease in horses spread by biting insects; symptoms vary according to the form of the disease; no treatment or vaccination available; also called equine infectious anemia (EIA).

Syringe an instrument used to inject into or remove fluid from the body.

Tapeworm a large, flat, long, segmented parasite that enters the digestive tract of dogs and cats by being ingested with a flea containing tapeworm larvae; seen as white ricelike pieces in the stool; treated with a wormer.

TB abbreviation for tuberculosis; see *tuberculosis.*

Tendotomy surgery on the tendons.

Tetanus an acute infectious disease caused by an organism usually introduced through a wound; characterized by stiffness, poor coordination, and inability to eat; treated with antitoxin; also called lockjaw.

TGE abbreviation for transmissible gastroenteritis; see *transmissible gastroenteritis.*

Thoracic cavity in mammals the area between the neck and abdomen where the heart and lungs lie.

Thrombosis the formation or presence of a blood clot within a blood vessel.

Thrush a diseased condition of the feet in various animals characterized by pus.

Ticks any of numerous bloodsucking, disease-carrying, flat, parasitic insects that attach themselves to warm-blooded vertebrates; treated with a dip, spray, or powder insecticide.

Tonsillitis inflammation of the tonsils caused by bacteria; characterized by coughing, gagging, vomiting, lack of appetite and energy, and dullness; treated with an antibiotic, cortisone, and good nursing.

Torsion twisting, as when the uterus twists on itself preventing the birth of an animal.

Transmissible gastroenteritis (TGE) a rapidly spread, contagious disease in pigs caused by a virus; characterized by diarrhea, vomiting, severe dehydration, and weight loss; prevention with vaccination is the best treatment.

Trauma a wound or stress.

Trochar an oval-shaped, pointed instrument used to insert a tube (cannula) into an animal to allow drainage from an affected area, such as the stomach.

Tuberculosis (TB) a contagious disease in animals and man caused by the tubercle bacillus; characteristics and treatment vary according to the animal affected.

Tumor an abnormal mass of tissue that is not inflamed, arises with no known cause from the cells of preexisting tissue, and has no physiologic function.

Tunic the white tough membrane surrounding the testicle.

Twitch a restraining device made of a hardwood handle with a chain loop on one end which is slipped over a horse's upper lip and twisted until quite tight.

Udder the organ of milk production; a mammary gland.

Udder edema another name for caked bag; see *caked bag.*

Umbilical pertaining to the depressed area in the center of the abdomen; the "belly button" or navel.

Unthriftiness unhealthy appearing; exhibiting a coarse coat, a potbelly, a lack of luster, dullness of spirit, etc.

Urea a soluble weakly basic nitrogenous compound that is the chief solid component of mammalian urine; used as an animal protein supplement.

Uremic poisoning in kidney disease the accumulation in the blood of constituents normally eliminated in the urine, causing a severe toxic condition; also called uremia.

Urinary calculi deposits of calcium carbonate, calcium, sodium, calcium phosphate, or cystine in the urinary tract that can make urination difficult and sometimes impossible.

Urinary incontinence the inability to completely control urination; characterized in older dogs by dribbling urine; treated with diethystilbestrol and geriatric tablets.

Uterus a muscular, fleshy pouch in the female where the fetus grows.

Vaccine a suspension of live, killed, or attenuated (weakened) virus or bacteria administered to the body to build up immunity to diseases caused by those organisms.

Vagina the canal in a female animal that leads from the uterus to the external opening of the genitals.

Vaginitis inflammation of the vaginal walls caused by a bacterial or a viral infection; characterized by failure to conceive; treated by not breeding for several weeks and with douches.

VEE abbreviation for Venezuelan equine encephalomyelitis; see *Venezuelan equine encephalomyelitis.*

Venezuelan equine encephalomyelitis (VEE) similar to EEE, but found mainly in the Southwest; see *eastern equine encephalomyelitis.*

Virus a microorganism that reproduces itself and obtains its energy from the body cells it enters, causing damage to the body cells from within; no specific treatment for any viral infection.

Visceral pertaining to the liver, kidneys or other body organs.

Vulva the external parts of the female genital organs; also, the opening between the projecting parts of the external organs.

Warfarin a crystalline anticoagulant compound used as a rodent poison.

Warfarin poisoning seen in cats which eat the rodent poison or ingest rodents sick from the poison; causes internal hemorrhages; characterized by weakness, anemia, and depression; treated by a veterinarian with blood transfusions, vitamin K, fluids, and confinement.

Warts a horny projection on the skin caused by a virus; treated with a wart vaccine.

Wasting disease another name for caseous lymphadenitis; see *caseous lymphadenitis.*

WEE abbreviation for western equine encephalomyelitis; see *western equine encephalomyelitis.*

Western equine encephalomyelitis (WEE) similar to EEE but found mainly in the West and Midwest; see *eastern equine encephalomyelitis.*

Wether a male goat or sheep castrated before sexual maturity.

Whelp to give birth to puppies; used when speaking of dogs.

Whipworm a parasitic worm in the liver and cecum of dogs; characterized by a liquid, foul-smelling stool, unthriftiness, and anemia; treated with a wormer.

Wind puffs lameness in a horse caused by strain; characterized by puffy swellings on the lower leg; treated with cold, rest, and astringents.

Withers the high point just behind the neck formed by the shoulder blades.

INDEX